PHARMACOLOGY – RESEARCH, SAFETY TESTING AND REGULATION

TOPICS IN MEDIATOR PHARMACOLOGY

PHARMACOLOGY – RESEARCH, SAFETY TESTING AND REGULATION

Additional books in this series can be found on Nova's website under the Series tab.

Additional E-books in this series can be found on Nova's website under the E-books tab.

Pharmacology – Research, Safety Testing and Regulation

Topics in Mediator Pharmacology

Jagdish N. Sharma

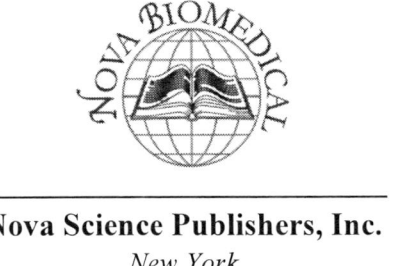

Nova Science Publishers, Inc.
New York

Copyright © 2011 by Nova Science Publishers, Inc.

All rights reserved. No part of this book may be reproduced, stored in a retrieval system or transmitted in any form or by any means: electronic, electrostatic, magnetic, tape, mechanical photocopying, recording or otherwise without the written permission of the Publisher.

For permission to use material from this book please contact us:
Telephone 631-231-7269; Fax 631-231-8175
Web Site: http://www.novapublishers.com

NOTICE TO THE READER

The Publisher has taken reasonable care in the preparation of this book, but makes no expressed or implied warranty of any kind and assumes no responsibility for any errors or omissions. No liability is assumed for incidental or consequential damages in connection with or arising out of information contained in this book. The Publisher shall not be liable for any special, consequential, or exemplary damages resulting, in whole or in part, from the readers' use of, or reliance upon, this material. Any parts of this book based on government reports are so indicated and copyright is claimed for those parts to the extent applicable to compilations of such works.

Independent verification should be sought for any data, advice or recommendations contained in this book. In addition, no responsibility is assumed by the publisher for any injury and/or damage to persons or property arising from any methods, products, instructions, ideas or otherwise contained in this publication.

This publication is designed to provide accurate and authoritative information with regard to the subject matter covered herein. It is sold with the clear understanding that the Publisher is not engaged in rendering legal or any other professional services. If legal or any other expert assistance is required, the services of a competent person should be sought. FROM A DECLARATION OF PARTICIPANTS JOINTLY ADOPTED BY A COMMITTEE OF THE AMERICAN BAR ASSOCIATION AND A COMMITTEE OF PUBLISHERS.

Additional color graphics may be available in the e-book version of this book.

LIBRARY OF CONGRESS CATALOGING-IN-PUBLICATION DATA

Sharma, Jagdish N.
 Topics in mediator pharmacology / Jagdish N. Sharma.
     p. ; cm.
 Includes bibliographical references and index.
 ISBN 978-1-61668-961-2 (hardcover)
 1. Inflammation--Mediators. 2. Bradykinin. I. Title.
 [DNLM: 1. Inflammation--physiopathology. 2. Inflammation Mediators--metabolism. 3. Inflammation Mediators--pharmacology. QZ 150 S539t 2010]
 RB131.S53 2010
 616'.0473--dc22
                                                            2010025962

Published by Nova Science Publishers, Inc. † New York

"This book is dedicated to my beloved father late Shri Hrydaya Narayan Sharma and my beloved mother late Shrimati ShahodraDevi Sharma for their excellent guidance, care, support and dedication"

Contents

Preface		ix
Acknowledgments		xi
Chapter 1	Pathogenic Responses of Bradykinin System in Chronic Inflammatory Rheumatoid Disease	1
Chapter 2	Interrelationship Between the Kallikrein-Kinin System and Hypertension	23
Chapter 3	The Role of Chemical Mediators in the Pathogenesis of Inflammation with Emphasis on the Kinin System	43
Chapter 4	Mediation of Kallikrein-Kinin System in the Mechanism of Action of Angiotensin Converting Enzyme Inhibitors	77
Chapter 5	The Kinin System and Prostaglandins in the Intestine	91
Chapter 6	Pro-inflammatory Actions of the Platelet Activating Factor: Relevance to Rheumatoid Arthritis	105
Chapter 7	Role of Tissue Kallikrein-Kininogen-Kinin Pathways in the Cardiovascular System	111
Chapter 8	Role of Nitric Oxide in Inflammatory Diseases	125
Chapter 9	The Role of Leukotrienes in the Pathophysiology of InflammatoryDisorders: The prospects of Leukotrienes as Therapeutic Targets	141
Chapter 10	Therapeutic Prospects of Bradykinin Receptor Agonists in the Treatment of Cardiovascular Diseases	153
Chapter 11	Therapeutic Prospects OfBradykinin Receptor Antagonists	169
Index		181

Preface

This book has been written with the aim of giving an overview of the scientific developments which have occurred in mediators pharmacology. Pharmacology can be defined as a discipline of paramedical sciences that teaches how the use of drugs can bring about changes from pathological to physiological states. Mediators pharmacology is a subdivision of pharmacology which teaches the functions of molecules released in the body and produce profound pharmacological effects. The sustained release or deficiency of these mediators may result in pathological conditions. Agonists or antagonists of these mediators are novel therapeutic agents with potential clinical benefits. This book has not been intended to be a textbook of pharmacology or therapeutics and does not therefore describe the use of drugs in the treatment of diseases. Furthermore, this book is intended for postgraduates, higher level students in medicine, pharmacy, veterinary medicine, physiology, pharmacology, and research institutions.

Acknowledgments

The author highly appreciates and thanks Elsevier publishers and Birkhauser Verlag AG for granting permission to produce his published materials in this book. Furthermore, Dr. Parvathy Narayanan provided excellent assistance in making the book in the final form.

Chapter 1

Pathogenic Responses of Bradykinin System in Chronic Inflammatory Rheumatoid Disease

Abstract

Excessive release of bradykinin (BK) in the synovial fluid can produce oedema, pain and loss of functions due to activation of B_1 and B_2 kinin receptors. Activation of the kinin forming system could be mediated via injury, trauma, coagulation pathways (Hageman factor and thrombin) and immune complexes. The activated B_1 and B_2 receptors might cause release of other powerful non-cytokine and cytokine mediators of inflammation, e.g., PGE_2, PGI_2, LTs, histamine, PAF, IL-1 and TNF, derived mainly from polymorphonuclear leukocytes, macrophages, endothelial cells and synovial tissue. These mediators are capable of inducing bone and cartilage damage, hypertrophic synovitis, vessel proliferation, inflammatory cell migration and, possibly, angiogenesis and pannus formation. These pathological changes, however, are not yet defined in the human model of chronic inflammation. The role of kinins and their interacting inflammatory mediators would soon start to clarify the detailed questions they revealed in clinical and experimental models of chronic inflammatory diseases. Several B_1 and B_2 receptor antagonists are being synthesized in an attempt to study the molecular functions of kinins in inflammatory processes, such as rheumatoid arthritis, periodontitis, inflammatory diseases of the gut and osteomyelitis. Future development of specific potent and stable B_1 and B_2 receptor antagonists or combined B_1 and B_2 antagonists with y-IFN might serve as a pharmacological basis for more effective treatment of joint inflammatory and related diseases.

Introduction

Chronic inflammation in rheumatoid arthritis (RA) is a complex sequence of events which can be recognized by the formation of chronic synovitis and loss of functions of the affected joints due to bone and cartilage damage. The peripheral synovial joints are more commonly affected, being involved in episodes of painful synovitis. The overall pattern in classical RA is one of progression regardless of relieving symptoms with the help of analgesic and anti-inflammatory drugs. Although its aetiology remains a mystery, numerous immunological abnormalities have been suggested in the initiation and the self-perpetuation of the synovitis (Ziff 1982).

The pathogenic involvement of the kallikrein-kinin family in causing RA has been strongly advocated by six lines of findings: (I) kinins are potent pro-inflammatory polypeptides (Sharma and Buchanan 1979); (2) kallikrein and kininogen levels are markedly increased in the synovial tissue and in the plasma of patients with RA (Sharma et al. 1983; Al-Haboubi et al. 1986; Sharma et al. 1976, 1980; Zeitlin et al. 1976, 1977; Brooks et al. 1974); (3) presence of free kinin in the rheumatoid synovial fluid (Melmon et al. 1967; Keele and Eisen 1970); (4) bone resorption and lysosomal enzyme release in cultured mouse calvaria by kinins (Gustafson and Lerner 1984; Lerner et al. 1987); (5) kinin-induced release of cytokine and non-cytokine inflammatory mediators (see Sharma 1991a, b, c, 1992; Sharma and Mohsin 1990); (6) kinin receptor antagonist can inhibit the various inflammatory reactions in rat experimental arthritis (Burch and Dehaas 1990; Sharma 1993).

The present article is by no means intended to provide full coverage of the kallikrein-kinin system (KKS). It is rather a commentary, based on the recent investigations, suggesting the significant role of KKS in the genesis of rheumatoid inflammatory disease. Our speculations place emphasis on the interactions between cytokine and non-cytokine inflammatory mediators with the kinins in the aetiology of inflamed joints. Furthermore, we attempt to demonstrate the clinical relevance of kinin receptor antagonists as novel antirheumatic drugs.

HISTORICAL APPRAISAL OF THE KALLIKREIN-KININ FAMILY

The discovery of the KKS started when Abelous and Bardier (1909) detected the presence of a hypotensive substance in normal human urine which they called urohypotensin. However, investigation of the kinin-forming system may properly be said to date from 1926, when Frey and his colleagues extensively studied that intravenous injection of pancreatic extract. Pancreatic secretion and urine in anaesthetized normotensive dogs produced a fall in arterial blood pressure (Frey 1926; Frey et al. 1930: Frey and Werle 1933). On the assumption that the active principle in urine was identical with that in the pancreas they named it "kallikrein". Later it was demonstrated that kallikrein itself did not cause contractions of isolated guinea-pig ileum (Werle et al. 1937). These investigators also observed that, when kallikrein was incubated with plasma, a potent smooth muscle-stimulating substance was released. This active agent was of low molecular weight and thermostable. It was not a split product of kallikrein but a split product of a plasma protein. The agent which Werle and coworkers (1937) thought to be a polypeptide was initially called Darmkontrahierende Substanz ("gut-contracting substance" or "Substanz DK"). Werle and Berek (1948) renamed the smooth muscle stimulant as kallidin and suggested the name kallidinogen for the inactive precursor protein present in the plasma. They concluded that the pharmacologically active substance kallidin was released from its precursor(s) by the proteolytic action of the enzyme, kallikrein.

Independent of the work of Werle in Germany. Rocha E Silva and his colleagues (1949), in Brazil, found that incubating dog plasma with venoms of certain snakes as well as with the enzyme trypsin, produce an agent, probably a polypeptide, that also lowered BP and caused a slowly developing contraction of the guinea pig ileum, in vitro. Because of the slow contraction of the guinea pig ileum. they named it bradykinin (BK). Since BK and kallidin were formed under similar conditions and had the same pharmacological actions, it was suspected that they were closely related and they were derived from the same substrate (Werle et al. 1953). The purification of these substances seven years later confirmed this suspicion. Elliott et al., (1960) isolated BK formed by reacting trypsin with globulin, and it was synthesized by Boissonnas et al. (1960).

$$\begin{array}{ccccccccc} 1 & 2 & 3 & 4 & 5 & 6 & 7 & 8 & 9 \end{array}$$

Arg - Pro - Pro - Gly - Phe - Ser - Pro - Phe - Arg
Bradykinin

Lys - Arg - Pro - Pro - Gly - Phe - Ser - Pro - Phe - Arg
Kallidin (Lysyl-bradykinin)

Met - Lys - Arg - Pro - Pro - Gly - Phe - Ser - Pro - Phe - Arg
Methionyl-lysyl-bradykinin

Figure 1.1. Structures of endogenous kinin family.

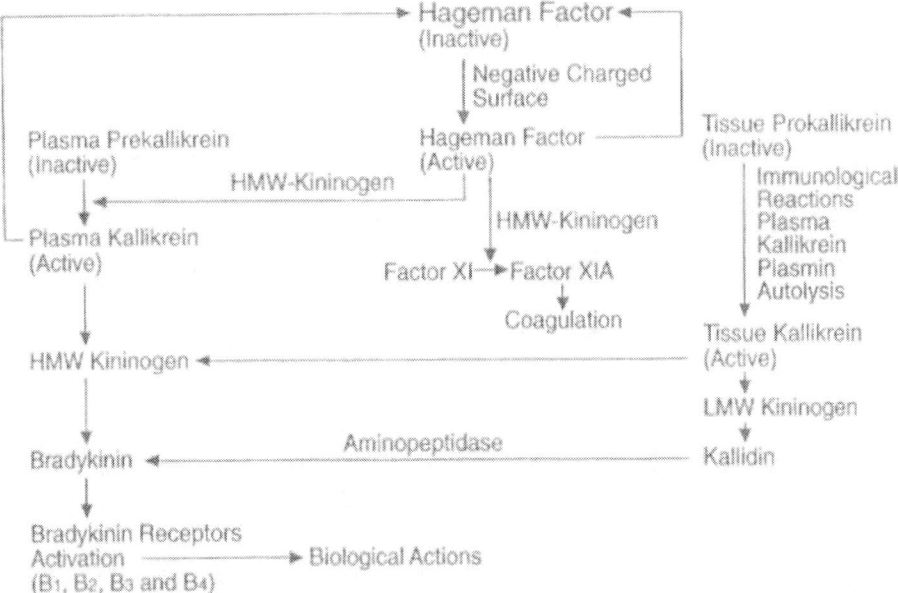

Figure 1.2. The mechanism of bradykinin formation.

THE KININ

The kinin family mainly includes BK, kallidin and methionyllysyl-BK (Figure 1.1). These are biologically active peptides derived from circulating precursors (kininogens) by the action of serine proteases, termed kallikreins (see Sharma 1988a, b). Once released in the circulation, kinins are rapidly (< 15 sec.) inactivated by a group of enzymes (Erdos 1990) called kininases.BK and related kinins can act on four types of receptors designated as B_1, B_2, B_3 and B_4, (Sharma 1992b) in inducing numerous physiopathological processes. The kinin receptor stimulation can cause activation of several second messenger systems, such as arachidonic acid products, calcium, cyclic AMP and cyclic GMP (Freay et al. 1989; Burch 1990; Schini et al. 1990). These systems have vital importance to the pharmacological activities of kinins. The mode of kinin formation is presented in Figure 1.2.

KININ-FORMING ENZYMES

Kinin-forming enzymes are known as kallikreins that are divided into two types: plasma and tissue (organ). These two kallikreins differ in their molecular weights, origins, biochemical properties, and biological actions on plasma kininogens (Schachter 1980). Plasma prekallikrein circulates in an inactive state, also known as the Fletcher factor because the deficiency of prekallikrein was first noticed by Wuepper (1973) in a patient named Fletcher. The prekallikrein is a single chain glycoprotein and synthesised in the liver. It is present in plasma as a complex bound with the high molecular weight kininogen (HMWK) (Mandle et al. 1976; Mandle and Kaplan 1977). Inactive prekallikrein can be activated to form kallikrein by activated Hageman factor (HFa or factor XIIa), and HMWK is digested to release BK (Mendle et al. 1976; Kaplan et al. 1992). Also, inactive HF becomes active by kallikrein through a positive feedback reaction (Cochrane et al. 1973). Activated HF and plasma thromboplastin antecedent (factor XI) circulate bound to HMWK (Thompson et al. 1977). Inactive factor XI is, therefore, converted to active factor XIa through HMWK to participate in the intrinsic coagulation pathway (Ratnoff et al. 1961).

Plasma kallikrein acts on HMWK to produce BK, whereas tissue kallikrein releases kallidin by the action on both high molecular weight kininogen (HMWK) and low molecular weight kininogen (LMWK) (Jacobsen 1966; Pierce and Guimaraes 1977). Plasma kallikrein is a member of single gene code (Seidah et al. 1989).

Tissue kallikrein is a single chain acidic glycoprotein that differs physicochemically and immunologically from plasma kallikrein. This kallikrein is found to be more widely distributed in the tissues (organs), such as the kidneys (urine), pancreas, salivary glands, intestine, prostate gland, and the synovial tissue (Nustad et al. 1975; Zeitlin 1971;Amundsen and Nustad 1965; Sharma et al. 1983; Al-Haboubi et al. 1986). Various organs releasing tissue kallikreins are immunologically identical within a given species (Schachter et al. 1980). The pancreatic and kidney (urinary) kallikreins are detected in the inactive form as prokallikrein (Fiedler and Werle 1967; Matsas et al. 1981; Corthorn et al. 1979), although the submandibular tissue kallikrein exists in an active form (Brandtzaeg et al. 1976). The occurrence and distribution of the tissue kallikrein genes have been extensively evaluated (see Drinkwater et al. 1988). Investigations on the complementary DNA cloning and sequence analysis have revealed that human pancreatic and renal kallikreins possess identical amino acid sequences and no more than three closely related genes (Baker and Shine 1985; Schedlich et al. 1987). In contrast with the situation in the mouse in which the kallikrein group of serine proteases consists of twenty-four highly homologous genes (Evans et al. 1987) in humans the tissue kallikrein gene family comprises the hRKALL. h GK- and PAS. These are clustered on the long arm of chromosome 19 q 13.3-13.4 (Evans et al. 1988; Morris 1989; Digby et al. 1989). However, in both mouse and rat kallikrein activity is associated with the highly conserved members of a large multi-gene family located on chromosome seven (Richards et al. 1982; Mason et al. 1983; Schedlich et al. 1988). Furthermore, research directed to investigate the structure of the kallikrein gene family may provide greater understanding of the role of various kinin-forming enzymes in specific processing of biologically active peptides in health and disease. Figure 1.3 represents the localization of plasma and tissue (glandular) kallikreins in the body.

KININ PRECURSORS OR KININOGENS

Kininogens are typical secretory multifunctional proteins containing the sequence of BK in their molecular structures. They are synthesized in the liver and circulate in the plasma and other body fluids. Immunological studies have indicated the localization of kininogens in the liver parenchymal cells (Chao et al. 1988).

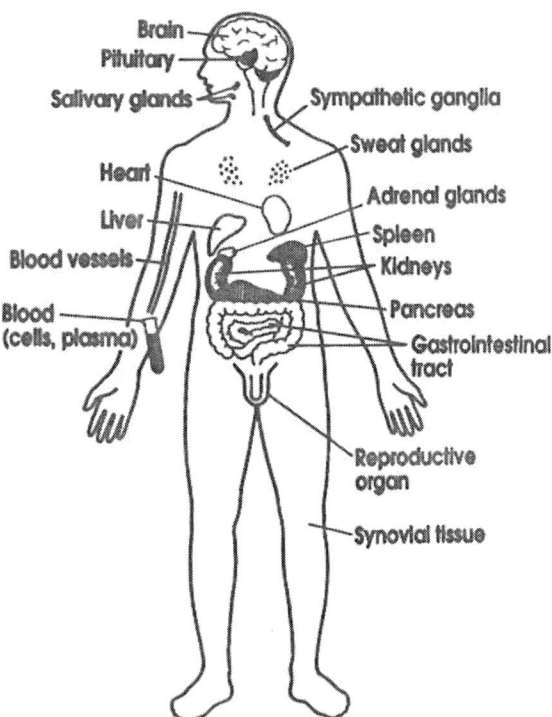

Figure 1.3. The localization and distribution of plasma and issue (organ) kallikreins in the body.

The two forms of kininogens are present in human circulation. They are designated as HMWK and LMWK (high and low molecular weight kiniogen), and differ from one another in molecular size, sensitivity to kallikreins and physiological functions (Muller-Esterl 1990). The HMWK and LMWK are single chain glycoproteins consisting of three functional domains: an amino acid domain, called heavy chain (the BK moiety released during proteolytic action by kallikreins), and a carboxyl-terminal domain, known as light chain. The third domain is of a reduced size in LMWK, but in HMWK it represents a large polypeptide chain responsible for the coagulation promoting activity of this molecule (Kellermann et al. 1987; Muller-Esterl et al. 1986). The first and third domains are bound by a disulfide bridge. The analysis of the complementary DNA data suggested a single K gene for H-and L-prekininogen in the human genomes (Kitamura et al. 1985). The HMWK and LMWK molecules are produced by alternate splicing of the gene transcript which is coded by the single K gene. In the rat, in addition to HMWK and LMWK, there are two lower molecular mass kininogen species, e.g., T-kininogen I and II which are not precursors for kallikreins. The T-I and T-11 kininogen messenger RNA are highly homologous to LMWK (0kamoto and Greenbaum 1986). The T-I and T-II kininogen genes are closely related but they have distinct genes (Enjyoji et al. 1988; Howard et al. 1990). The novel functions of these kininogens, seemingly unrelated to kinin release, are associated with the blood coagulation, cysteine proteinases inhibition, and acute phase reactions in the rat (Muller-Esterl 1990).

KININ METABOLIZING ENZYMES

Those enzymes responsible for inactivation of kinins are called kininases which are present in the plasma, urine, tissues, endothelial cells and the body fluids. Their prime function is to monitor the required BK concentrations in the body to perform the necessary physiological activities. The main enzyme which metabolizes BK in vascular beds is a dipeptidyl carboxypeptidase termed kininase II or angiotensin converting enzyme (ACE) (Erdos 1990). A slow-reacting enzyme is known to be kininase I carboxypeptidase N. The kininase I removes the C-terminal arginine of BK to leave the residual octapeptide (Erdos 1990). This enzyme may be physiologically more important in metabolizing BK, since kininase I concentration is higher the plasma (Erdos 1979). DesArg^9 BK formed by the action of kininase I on BK is inactive in vivo. However, it displays activity on various isolated vascular and non-vascular smooth muscle preparations (Regoli and Barabe 1980). Based on these pharmacological activities, Regoli and Barabe (1980) supposed BK1 receptor-mediated effects of des-Arg^9-BK, and BK2 receptor-mediated actions of BK on several isolated tissues. Kininase II and enkephalinase-A cause inactivation of kinins in removing the C-terminal Phe-Arg in the plasma and in the urine of humans and rats (Erdos 1979; Kokubu et al. 1978; Skidgel et al. 1987; URA et al. 1987). In addition, kininase II induces further degradation of des-Arg^9 to release the pentapeptide (Ser-Pro-Pro-Gly-Phe) and the tripeptide (Ser-Pro-Phe) (Sheikh and Kaplan 1986). The C-terminal phenylalanine is then cleft from each peptide leaving Arg-Pro-Pro-Gly and Ser-Pro. The Ser-Pro is also digested to Ser and Pro while the C-terminal Gly is removed from the tetrapeptide. The final plasma and urinary metabolites of BK are one mole each of Arg-Pro-Pro, Gly, Ser, Pro, and Arg and two moles of phenylalanine (Figure 1.4).

KALLIKREIN-KININ SYSTEM IN RHEUMATOID ARTHRITIS

Kinin-forming components have been known to play a major role in the pathophysiology of chronic inflammatory diseases, particularly in RA. Pro-inflammatory actions of kinins include increased vascular permeability, vasodilation, pain, oedema, loss of functions and release of numerous potent rheumatoid inflammatory mediators (Sharma 1988, 1991a, b, c, 1992, 1993; Sharma and Buchanan 1979; Sharma et al 1988; Sharma and Mohsin 1990).

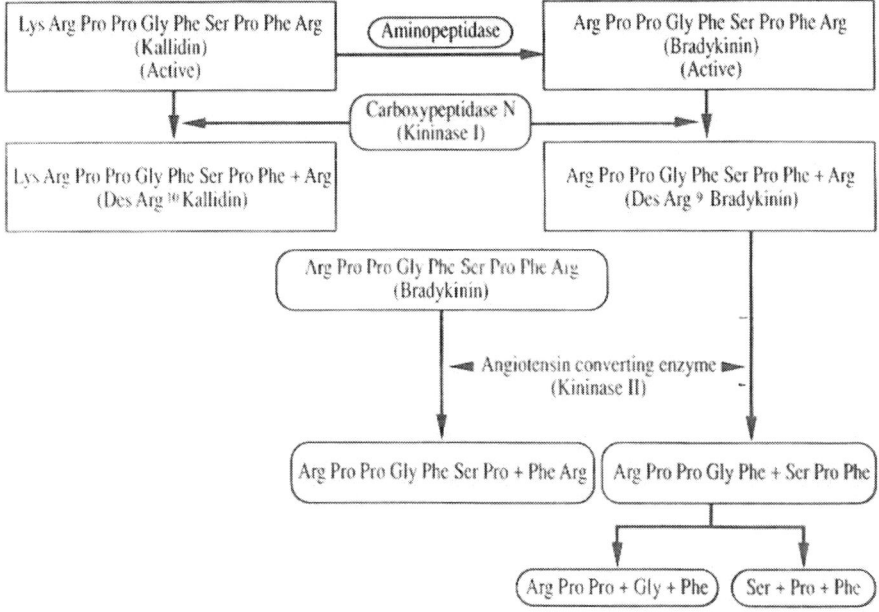

Figure 1.4. Metabolic products of kallidin and bradykinin.

Excessive release of KKS in the peripheral circulation (Sharma et al. 1976; Sharma et al. 1980; Zeitlin et al. 1976, 1977; Brooks et al. 1974) as well as within the inflamed synovial joints (Melmon et al. 1967; Keele and Eisen 1970; Sharma et al. 1983; Al-Haboubi et al. 1986) has been implicated in the genesis of RA. Suzuki et al. (1987) found higher concentrations of plasma prekallikrein levels in the synovial fluid of patients with RA, when the values were compared with the synovial fluid obtained from osteoarthritic patients. Thus, the kinin could be generated in the rheumatoid joints by active plasma kallikrein, since prekallikrein can be activated by HFa (Meier et al. 1977) because connective tissue proteoglycans and mast cell heparin can act as initiating surface for the activation of HF during immunological reactions (Hojima et al. 1984; Silverberg and Diehl 1987). In addition, plasma kallikrein may cause activation of latent collagenase into active form in vitro which could be an important action of plasma kallikrein in the destruction of the synovial tissue (Nagase et al. 1982). In rats, kininase II inhibition with the help of ACE inhibitor (captopril) treatment is accompanied by potentiation of carrageenin-induced inflammation (Boura and

Svolmanis 1984). However, the role of kininases in rheumatoid inflammation remains unclear.

Free kinin levels are raised in the synovial fluids obtained from RA and gout patients. In addition, high concentrations of kallikrein-like activity have been demonstrated in the inflamed rheumatoid joints (Sharma et al. 1983; Al-Haboubi et al. 1986). These kinin-generating components in an inflamed joint may be derived also from plasma (Jasani et al. 1969), since high concentrations of total plasma kininogen are found in the peripheral circulation (Sharma et al. 1976, 1980; Zeitlin et al. 1976; Brooks et al. 1974). Kinin release can be activated in response to tissue injury to cause stimulation of sensory pain fibre and the release of other potent mediators of inflammation (Sharma 1991a, 1), C; Sharma and Mohsin 1990). As a result, vascular permeability and blood flow to the damaged parts are increased and a full inflammatory response is obtained. The activation and release of kinin in the effusions from rheumatoid joints might be linked with the stimuli, such as interleukines and immune complexes to cause degranulation in the process of leukocyte tissue kallikrein release within the inflamed sites (Figueroa et al. 1989; Figueroa and Bhoola 1989; Epstein et al. 1968).

The released tissue kallikrein could then generate kinin from kininogens thereby providing inflammatory reactions. Interrelationship between the interleukin-1 (IL-1) and kinins is further substantiated by the fact that IL-1 is produced by the inflamed synovial tissue (Wood et al. 1985; Danis et al. 1987) and it can be detected in significant amounts in synovial fluids (Wood et al. 1983; Nouri et al. 1984). However, formation of prostaglandin E_2 (PGE_2), leukotriene B_4 (LTB_4) and prostacyclin (PGI_2) in rheumatoid synovitis may appear to be linked with the appearance of leucocytes in the synovial fluid (Higgs et al. 1974; Davidson et al. 1982). Thus, the kinin activation might be mediated by hyperimmune activity and or intrinsic coagulation pathway action.

Recently, it has been discovered that kinins mediate osteoblast formation and subsequent enhancement of bone resorption in vitro from cultured mouse calvarian bones (Liunggren and Lerner 1990). The bone resorption property of kinins has been attributed to high endogenous PGE formation in bone tissue (Ljunggren and Lerner 1990). Bradykinin is capable of stimulating bone resorption in vitro, which can be abolished by administration of several PG synthesis inhibitors (Ljunggren and Lerner 1990). Hence, the kinin action on bone resorption is mediated through high concentrations of PG formation in bone tissue. This view is compatible with the findings that PGE_2 and PGI_2 are potent mediators for bone resorption in vitro (Harvey and Bennet 1988). Kinins stimulate also PG formation in isolated osteoblast-like cells from mouse calvarial bone of neonatal mouse and in the cloned murine osteoblastic cell lineage MC3T3-EI (Lerner et al. 1989) as well as in isolated human osteoblast-like cells (Ljunggren et al. 1990; Lerner et al. 1987). Kinins are known also to cause release of cytokine and non-cytokine inflammatory mediators.

CYTOKINE INFLAMMATORY MEDIATORS RELEASE BY KININ

Kinins have significant stimulant effects on tumor necrosis factor (TNF) and IL-I release from macrophages (Tiffany and Burch 1989), and most probably from endothelial cells.

Bradykinin-stimulated release of both (TNF and IL-I) cytokines from P388-D1 and RAW264.7 murine macrophages may be mediated by the activation of B_1 kinin receptors (Tiffany and Burch 1989). Tumor necrosis factor and IL-1 can stimulate bone resorption, cartilage damage, hypertrophic synovitis, inflammatory cell migration, vessel proliferation and pannus formation (Figure1.5). Both TNF and IL-I could induce the release of at least three metaloproteinases, such as degrade gelatin, collagen and proteoglycan (Larrick and Kunkel 1988). These mediators might be released from mononuclear cells isolated from synovial tissue obtained from patients with RA and may contribute to the pathology of the inflamed joints by formation of the pannus (Larrick and Kunkel 1988). Recently, inhibitory effects of y-interferon (y-INF) on BK-induced bone resorption and PGE_2 formation in cultured mouse calvarial bone have been demonstrated (Lerner et al. 1991), although it has been shown that y-IFN can inhibit bone resorption by an unknown mechanism unrelated to PGE_2 formation (Lerner et al. 1991). Based on these findings, it is possible that the kinins might induce bone resorption by a non-cyclooxygenase pathway. The role of 5-lypooxygenase products release by kinins in causing bone resorption has yet to be investigated, since LTB_4 levels are raised in synovial fluid from patients with RA (Davidson et al. 1982). TNF receptors have been localized in the synovial tissue and cartilage-pannus junction in patients with RA that may play a major role in the genesis of RA (Delcuran et al. 1992).

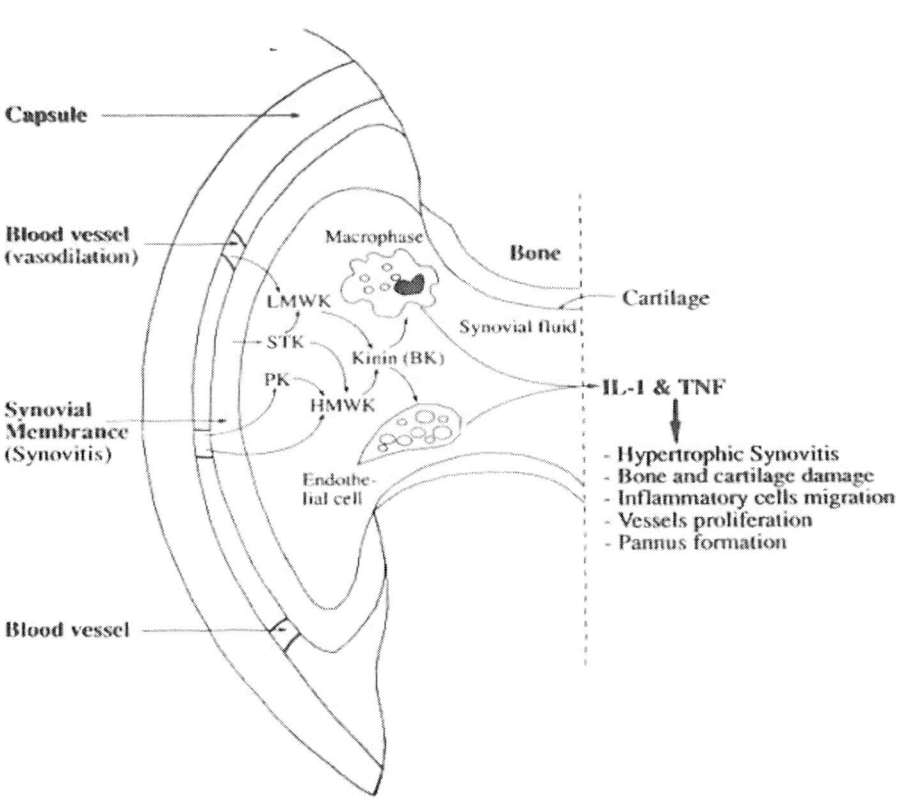

Figure 1.5. Cytokines release by kinin in the pathogenesis of rheumatoid joint disease. HMWK (high molecular weight kinninogen), LMWK (low molecular weight kininogen), STK (synovial tissue kallikrein) and PK (plasma kallikrein).

NON-CYTOKINE INFLAMMATORY MEDIATORS RELEASE BY KININ

Non-cytokine inflammatory mediators, e.g., PGE_2, PGI_2, LTs, histamine, platelet activating factor (PAF), and endothelium derived relaxing factor (EDRF) are released by kinins (Sharma 1988; Sharma 1991a, b, C; Sharma and Mohsin 1990). High levels of extracellular phospholipase A_2 have been detected from human synovial fluid (Hara et al. 1989). This might originate from macrophages. granulocytes and or lymphocytes. Phospholipase A_2 is activated by kinins to release the arachidonic acid metabolites (PGs and LTs) as well as PAF in the process of rheumatoid inflammation (Sharma 1991a, b, c). The endothelial cells and fibrobasts are capable of stimulating PG-synthesis mediated by kinins (Conklin et al. 1988).

The role of endothelium in chronic inflammatory synovitis has been discussed in detail by Ziff (1991). Increased concentrations of PGE_2, LTB_4, and PAF are present in the synovial fluid obtained from arthritic patients and adjuvant-induced arthritis in rabbits (Higgs et al. 1974; Davidson et al. 1982; Archer et al. 1985). It is possible that PAF may be involved in attracting inflammatory cells into the arthritic joint to cause oedema, vascular lesions and bone erosion (Pettipher and Higgs 1987; Sharma 1991c; Archer et al. 1985). Figure1.6 shows the kinin-induced release of PGE_2, PGI_2, LTs and PAF, and their relevance to inflamed rheumatoid joints.

BRADYKININ RECEPTORS AND THEIR ROLE IN RHEUMATOID ARTHRITIS

The BK receptore have been classified as B_1 and B_2 on the basis of the relative potencies of agonists (kinins) and antagonists (kinin analogues) on various pharmacological preparations (Regoli and Barabe 1980; Vavrek and Stewart 1985). B_1 receptors are generated de novo during incubation and antigen-induced arthritis in the vascular smooth muscle (Bouthillier et al. 1987; Farmer et al. 1991a), although it is known that B_1 receptors induction develop in nonvascular tissues and de novo formation of B_1 receptors may result from tissue injury andinflammatory reactions (Marceau et al. 1980; Couture et al., 1982). Kinin metabolites without the C-terminal arginine residue, such as des-Arg^9-BK and des-Arg^{10}-kallidin, are generated during the action of plasma kininase I (Erdos et al. 1965; Proud et al. 1987). Under physiological conditions, these kinin metabolites are devoid of biological actions. However, des-Arg^9-BK and des Arg^{10}-kallidin show significant biologcial activities (des-Arg^{10} kallidin > des-Arg^9-BK > kallidin > BK) via activating B_1 receptors in various vascular and nonvascular smooth muscles (Marceau et al. 1980; Regoli et al. 1981). The pharmacological classification of the B_1 receptor was further strengthened by the substitution of the Phe8 with leucine (des-Arg^9-[Leu8]-BK) gives rise to a potent B_1 antagonist (Regoli and Barabe 1980). B_1 receptor activation may produce stimulation of smooth muscle cells, increased cell proliferation, and high collagen synthesis (Regoli 1984). Stimulation of B_1 receptor causes release of EDRF and PGI_2 from bovine aortic endothelial cells grown in culture (D' Orleans-Juste et al. 1989). Kinins stimulate TNF and IL-1 formation from macrophages via B_1 receptors (Tiffany and Burch 1989).

Numerous studies have shown that the predominant pathological responses, such as pain (Whalley et al. 1987a), inflammation (Burch and De Haas 1990), bronchoconstriction JIN et al. 1989), and hypotension (Sharma et al. 1992) caused by BK involves B_2 receptor participation. However, it is becoming increasingly clear that B_2 receptor subtypes do exist (Llona et al. 1987; Plevin and Owen 1988; Farmer et al. 1989). The B_2 receptor is thought to mediate contraction of the rat uterus, cat and guinea-pig ileum (Barabe et al., 1977; Farmer et al. 1991b) and guinea-pig tracheal strips (Farmer et al. 1991b). Subsequently, it has been demonstrated that B_2 receptors can cause increased vascular permeability after application of kinins in rabbit skin (Schachter et al. 1987; Whalley et al. 1987). Kinins act on B_2 receptors to release conjointly EDRF and PGI_2 from bovine aortic endothelial cells in vitro (D'orelans-Juste et al. 1989). B_2 receptors exhibit much higher affinity for kallidin or BK than for des-Arg^{10}-kallidin or des-Arg^9-BK [(Tyr (Me)^8]-BK = kallidin > BK > des-Arg^{10}-kallidin > des-Arg^9-BK) in rabbit jugular vein preparation (Regoli et al. 1989).

Recent findings by Farmer et al. (1989) suggest that pulmonary tissues, particularly in the large airways, contain a novel B_3 receptor which might be involved in BK induced bronchoconstriction. These investigators noted that several B_2 antagonists (D-Arg[Hyp3, D-Phe7]-BK and D-Arg [Hyp3 Thi^{5,8} D-Phe7l-BK) as well as the B_1 antagonist (des-Arg^9[Leu^8]-BK) did not inhibit BK-induced guinea-pig tracheal contraction. The presence of B_3 receptor has been supposed in the opossum esophageal longitudinal smooth muscle (Saha et al. 1990). This receptor has been characterized by rapid desensitization, causes contraction of longitudinal smooth muscle via PG release, and it is activated by Phe^8-d-Phe^7-BK and d-Phe^7-Hyp^8-BK (B_2 receptor antagonists).

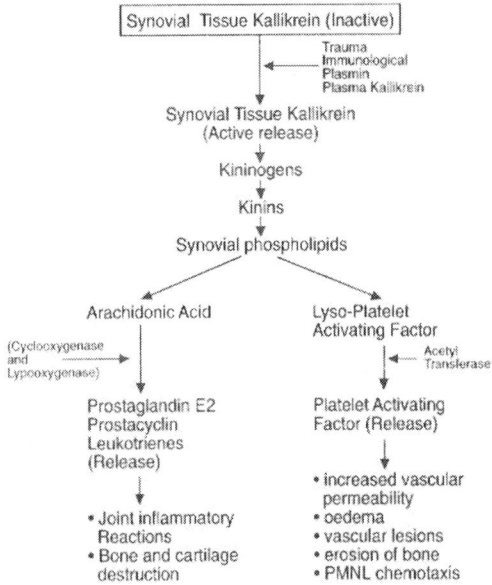

Figure 1.6. Kinin-induced release of prostaglandin E_2, prostacyclin, leukotrienes and platelet activating factor in the inflamed rheumatoid joints.

Saha et al. (1990) have suggested also the presence of B_4 receptors in the opossum esophageal longitudinal smooth muscle. The B_4 receptor shows no tachyphylaxis, its action does not involve PGs, and it is activated by B_2 receptor antagonists, [Thi^{5,8}-D-Phe^7]-BK and B6572. The pharmacological properties of BK receptors and their possible biological functions are presented in table 1.1.

Table 1.1. Biological Properties of Bradykinin Receptors

Bradykinin receptors	Functions	Antagonists
B_1 (formed by de novo synthesis in isolated aortic vascular smooth muscle and by pathological states *in vivo*)	Stimulation of smooth muscle, increased cell proliferation, increased collagen synthesis. contr-action of venous and arterial preparations *in vitro* and rela-xation of peripheral resis-tance vessels in vivo. EDRF and PGI_2 release from aortic endothelial cells.	Des-Arg^9-[Leu^8]-BK
B_2	Stimulation of rat uterus, cat and guinea-pig ileum, mediation of pain and vasodilatation, increased vascular permeability, hypotension, release of histamine and PGs, relaxation of arteries and contraction of veins, broncho-constriction, EDRF and PGI_2 release from aortic endothelial cells.	D-Arg°-[Hyp3-Thi^{5,8},D-Phe^7]-BK
B_3	Contraction of airways, opossum esophageal longitudinal with rapid de-sensitization (action involves PGs).	D-Arg[Hyp^3-Thi^5 – D-Tic$^{8-]-}$ BK
B_4	Contraction of opossum esophageal longitudinal muscle with no tach-yphylaxis (action does not involve PGs).	

It is indicated that osteoblasts are equipped with B_1, receptors mediating PGE_2, and PGI_2, formation and subsequent bone resorption (Ljunggren and Lerner 1990), whereas B_2 receptors are involved in mediating pain, increased vascular permeability, vasodilatation, oedema, and PGE_2 release from the osteoblasts (Regoli 1984). It is possible, therefore, that in areas adjacent to inflammatory processes, bone tissue may become more sensitive to kinins due to availability of an increased number of B_1 receptors in addition to B_2 receptors. In porcine cultured articular chondrocytes, kinins cause increased inositol phosphate generation, intracellular free calcium ions, and PG synthesis via activating B_2 receptors (Benton et al. 1989). The properties of BK receptors in joint inflammatory disease are presented in figure1.7. These findings strongly suggest that kinins could be considered as prime mediators in inducing significant pathological changes seen in arthritic joints, although, the functions of kinins in the contribution of bone and ca rtilage destruction in human arthritis require further investigations.

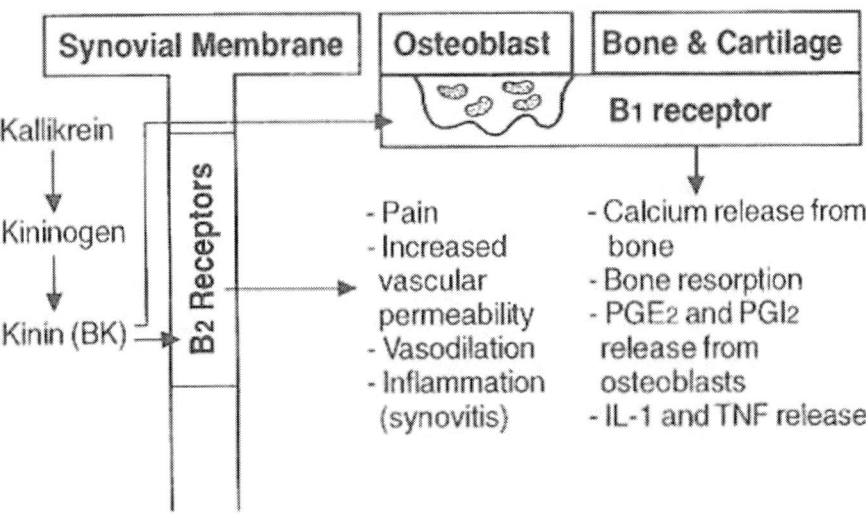

Figure 1.7. Pathogenic properties of bradykinin receptors in chronic inflammatory joint disease.

THERAPEUTIC PROSPECTS OF KININ RECEPTOR ANTAGONISTS IN RHEUMATOID ARTHRITIS

In recent years, several BK antagonists have been synthesized (Vevrek and Stewart 1985; Hock et al. 1991; Regoli et al. 1991) with major therapeutic goalsto block the pathological conditions caused by either enhanced production or inadequate metabolism of kinins. A B_2 receptor antagonist, DArg Hyp^3 DPhe^7 BK, inhibits the development of carrageenan-induced oedema in rats (Burch and DeHaas 1990). The B_1 receptor antagonist (des-Arg^9-Leu^8-BK) can inhibit des-Arg9-BK-induced release of 45 Ca from prelabelled neonatal mouse calvarial bone in vitro (Ljunggren and Lerner 1990). Highly potent BK antagonists include D-Arg (Hyp^3, D-Phe^7, Leu^8) - BK (Regoli et al. 1991) and Hoe 140 (Hock et al. 1991). These antagonists are under experimental investigation to establish the future prospects of their clinical utilities in rheumatology. It is suggested that the combinations of B_1 and B_2 antagonists with y-IFN may provide additive properties in achieving greater anti-rheumatic therapeutic values, since y-IFN causes inhibition of abnormal biochemical changes taking place in joint inflammation (Lerner et al. 1991). Wirth et al. (1992) have tested the ability of a new highly potent BK2 receptor antagonist (Hoe 140) to cause inhibition of oedema of rat paws induced by scalding and carrageenan. These investigators showed that Hoe 140 (0. I mg/kg i.v.) treatment inhibited scalding and carrageenan oedema for more than four to six hours, respectively. Furthermore, we have also demonstrated the anti-inflammatory effects of Hoe 140 (1.5 mg/ kg i.p.) treatment for nine days in chronic joint inflammatory disease in rats induced by Mycobacterial adjuvant (Sharma, unpublished observations). It is possible to suggest that the novel BK receptor antagonists could be clinically evaluated for their therapeutic potential in rheumatology and gastroenterology. Figure 1.8 represents the possible mode of kinin release, and the functions of B_1 and B_2 receptor antagonists in RA.

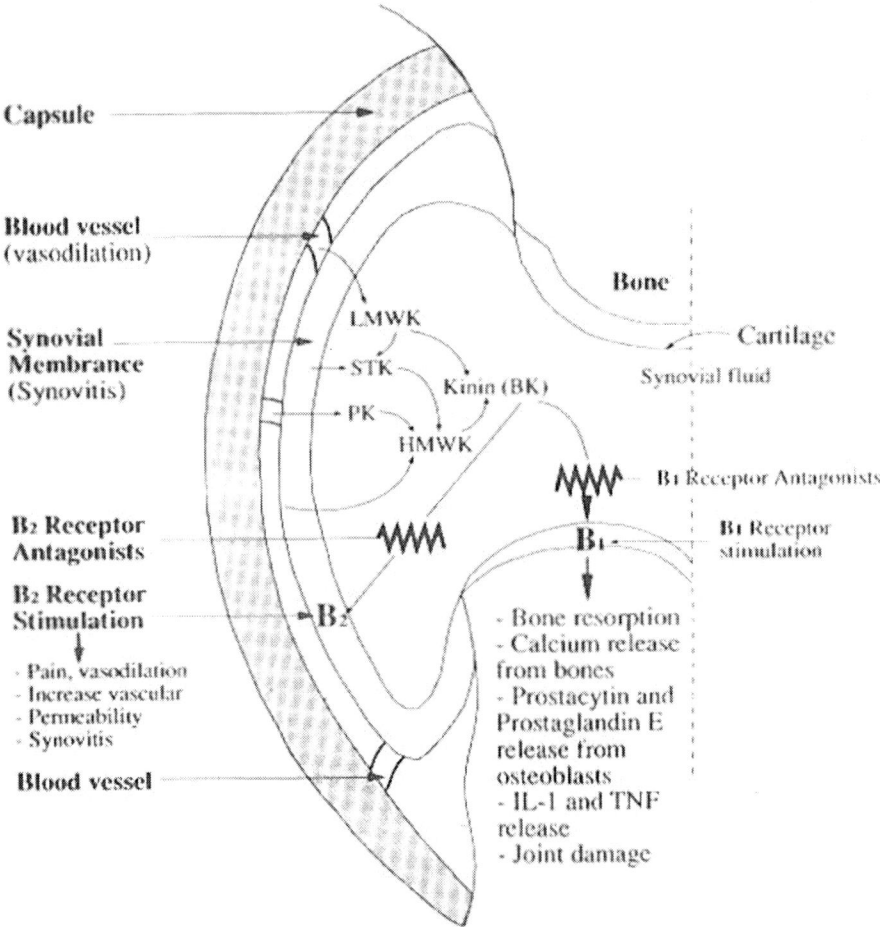

Figure1.8.The mechanism of abnormal kinin release in the synovial joints, and the blocking of bradykinin receptors with the use of specific antagonists may be anti-rheumatic agents.HMWK (high molecular weight kininogen), LMWK (low molecular weight kininogen), STK (synovial tissue kallikrein) and PK (plasma kallikrein).

REFERENCES

Abelous JE, Bardier E: Lee substances hypotensives des l'urine humaine normale. *C R Sac Biol (Paris) 1909*; 66: 511-512.

Al-Haboubi HA, Bennett D, Sharma JN, et al.: A synovial amidase acting on tissue kallikrein-selective substrate in clinical and experimental arthritis. *Adv Exp Med Biol 1986; 198B*: 405-411.

Amundsen E, Nustad K: Kinin-forming and destroying activities of cell homogenates. *I Physiol (Land.) 1965*; 179: 479-488.

Archer CB, Page CP, Morley J: Accumulation of inflammatory cells in response to intracutaneous platelet activating factor (PAF-acether) in man. *Br I Dermatol 1985*;112: 285-290.

Baker AR, Shine J: Human kidney kallikrein: cDNA cloning and sequence analysis. *DNA 1985; 4*: 445-450.

Barabe J, Droulin JN, Regoli D, et al.: Receptors for bradykinin in intestine and uterine smooth muscle. Can J Physiol *Pharmacol 1977; 55*: 920-926.

Benton HP, Jackson TR, Hanley MR: Identification of a novel inflammatory stimulant of chondrocytes. *Biochem J 1989*; 269: 861-867.

Boissonnas RA, Guttmann S, Jacquenoud PA: Synthese de la L-arginyl-L-prolyl-L-prolyl-L-glycyl-L-phenylalanyl-L-seryl-L-prolyl-L-phenylalanyl-L-arginine, un nonapeptide presentant les proprietes de la bradykinine. *Helv chim Acta 1960; 43*: 1349-1355.

Boura ALA, Svolmanis AP: Converting enzyme inhibition in the rat by captopril is accompanied by potentiation of carrageenin-induced inflammation. *Br J Pharmacol 1984; 82: 3-8.*

Bouthiller J, Deblois D, Marceau F: Studies on the induction of pharmacological responses to des-Arg9-bradykinin in vitro and vivo. *Br J Pharmacol 1987; 92: 257-264.*

Brandtzaeg P, Gautvik KM, Nustad K, et al.: Rat submandibular gland kallikreins: purification and cellular localization. *Br J Pharmacol 1976; 56: 155-167.*

Brooks PM, Dick WC, Sharma JN, et al.: Changes in plasma kininogen levels associated with rheumatoid activity. *Br J Clin Pharmacol 1974*; 1: 351P.

Burch RM, DeHaas C: A bradykinin antagonist inhibits carrageenan edema in rats. *Naunyn-Schmiedeberg's ArchPharmacol 1990 ;* 342: 189-193.

Burch RM: Kinin signal transduction: role of phosphoinositides and eicosanoids. *J Cardiov Pharmacol 1990; 15* (Suppl. 6): S44-S45.

Chao J, Swain C, Chao S, et al.: Tissue distribution and kininogen gene expression after acute phase inflammation. *Biochim Biophys Acta 1988;* 964: 329-339.

Cochrane CG, Revak SD, Wuepper KD: Activation of Hageman factor in solid and fluid phages. *J Exp Med 1973;* 138: 1564-1583.

Conklin BR, Burch RM, Steranka LR, et al.: Distinct bradykinin receptors mediate stimulation of prostaglandin synthesis by endothelial cells and fibroblasts. *J Pharmacol Exp Ther 1988;* 244: 646-649.

Corthorn J, Imanari T, Yoshida H, et al.: Isolation of prokallikrein from human urine. *Adv Exp Med Biol 1979;* 120B: 575-579.

Couture R, Mizrahi J, Regoli R, et al.: Peptides and the human colon: an in vitro pharmacological study. *Can J Physiol Pharmacol 1982*; 59: 957-970.

Danis VA, March LM, Nelson DS, et al.: Interleukin-1 secretion by peripheral blood monocytes and synovial machrophages from patients with rheumatoid arthritis. *J Rheumatol 1987;* 14: 33-39.

Davidson EM, Rae SA, Smith MJH: Leukotrine B 4 in synovial fluid. *J Ph arm Pharmacol 1982;* 34: 410.

Deleuran BW, Chu C-Q, Field M, et al.: Localization of tumor necrosis factor receptors in the synovial tissue and cartilage-pannus junction in patients with rheumatoid arthritis. *Arthritis Rheum 1992*; 35: 1170-1178.

Digby M, Zhang XY, Richards RI: Human prostate specific antigen (PSA) gene: structure and linkage to the kallikreinlike gene. hGk-1. *Nucleic Acids Res 1989*; 17: 2137.

Drinkwater CC, Evans BA, Richards RI: Kallikreins, Kinins and growth factor biosynthesis. *TIES 1988; 13*:169-172.

D'orleans-Juste P, de Nucci G, Vane JR: Kinins act on B1 or B2 receptors to release conjointly endothelium-derived relaxing factor and prostacyclin from bovine aortic endothelial cells. *Br J Pharmacol 1989*; 96: 920-926.

Elliott DF, Lewis GP, Horton EW: The structure of bradykinin-a plasma kinin from ox blood. *Biochem Biophys Res Commun 1960*; 3: 87-91.

Enjyoji K, Kato H, Hayashi I, et al.: Purification and characterization of rat T -kininogens isolated from plasma of adjuvant-treated rats. Identification of three types of kininogens. *J Biol Chern 1988*; 263: 973-979.

Epstein WV, Melmon KL, Tan M, et al.: Kinin generation caused by IgG-rheumatoid factor complex. J Clin Invest 1968; 47: 30-32.

Erdos EG: Kininages.In: Erdos EG (Ed.): Bradykinin, kallidin and kallikrein. Springer-*Verlag Berlin 1979*; pp.427-487.

Erdos EC: Some old and some new ideas on kinin metabolism. *J Cardiov Pharmacol 1990*; 15 (Suppl. 6): S20-S24.

Erdos EC, Wohler IM, Levine MI, et al: Carboxypeptidase in blood and other fluids. Values in human blood in normal and pathological conditions. *Clin Chim Acta 1965*; 11: 39-43.

Evans BA, Drinkwater CC, Richards RI: Mouse glandular kallikrein genes: structure and partial sequence analysis of the kallikrein gene locus. *J Biol Chern 1987*: 262: 8027-8034.

Evans BA, Yun ZX, Close JA, et al.: Structure and chromosomallocalization of the human renal kallikrein gene. *Biochemistry 1988*; 27: 3124-3129.

Farmer SG, Burch RH, Meeker SA, et al.: Evidence for a pulmonary B3 bradykinin receptor. *Molec Pharmacol 1989*; 36: 1-8.

Farmer SG, McMillan BA, Meeker SN, et al.: Induction of vascular smooth muscle bradykinin Bl' receptors in vitro during antigen arthritis. *Agents Actions 1991a*; 34:191-193.

Farmer SG, Burch Rm, Kyle DM, et al.: D-Arg[Hyp^{3}Thi^5-D- Tic^7 - Tic^8]-bradykinin, a potent antagonist of smooth muscle BK2 receptors and BK3 receptors. *Br J Pharmacol 1991b*; 102: 785-787.

Fiedler F, Werle E: Two prekallikreins from porcine pancreas. Hoppe-Seyler's Z. *Physiol ; 348: 1087-1089.*

Figueroa CD, MacIver AG, Bhoola KD: Identification of tissue kallikrein in human polymorphonuclear leucocytes. *Br J Haematol 1989*; 72: 321-328.

Figueroa CD, Bhoola KD: Leukocyte tissue kallikrein: an acute phase signal for inflammation. In: Fritz H, Schmid TI, Dietze G (Eds.): The kallikrein-kinin system in Health and Disease. Limbach-Verlag Braunschweig, Germany 1989;pp.311-320.

Frey EK: Zusammenhange zwischen Herzarbeit und Nierentatigkeit. Langenbeck's Arch Klin Chir 1926; 142: 663-669.

Frey EK, Kraut H, Schultz F: Tiber eine neue innersekretorische Funktion des Pankreas. Naunyn-Schmiedeberg's Arch Exp Pathol Pharmacol1930; 158: 334- 347.

Frey EK, Werle E: Kallikrein im inneren und auJ3eren Pankreassekret. Klin Wschr 1933; 12: 600.

Freay A, Johns A, Adam DJ, et al.: Bradykinin and inositiol 1.4.5-triphosphate-stimulated calcium release from intracellular stores in cultured bovine endothelial cells.Pfliigers Arch 1989; 414: 377-384.

Gustafson GT, Lerner U: Bradykinin stimulates bone resorption and lysosomal enzyme release in cultured mouse calvaria. Biochem J 1984; 219: 329-332.

Hara S, Kudo I, Chang HW, et al.: Purification and characterization of extracellular phospholipase A2 from human synovial fluid in rheumatoid arthritis. J Biochem 1989; 105: 395-399.

Harvey W, Bennett A: Prostaglandins and the mechanism of bone resorption. In: Prostaglandins in Bone Resorption. Florida: CRC Press 1988; pp. 43-46.

Higgs GA, Vane JR, Hart FD, et al.: Effects of anti-inflammatory drugs on prostaglandin in rheumatoid arthritis. In: Robinson HJ, Vane JR (Eds.): Prostaglandin Synthetase Inhibitors. New York: Raven Press 1974; 165-173.

Hock FJ, With K, Albus U, et al.: Hoe 140a new potent and long acting bradykinin antagonist: in vitro studies. Br J Pharmacol1991; 102: 769-773.

Hojima Y, Cochraine CG, Wiggins RC, et al.: In vitro activation of the contact system (Hageman factor) system of plasma by heparin and chondroitin sulfate E. Blood 1984;63: 1453-1459.

Howard EF, Thompson YG, Lapp CA, et al.: Reduction of T-kininogen messenger RNA levels by dexamethasone in the adjuvant-treated rat. Life Sci 1990; 46: 411-417.

Jacobsen S: Separation of two different substrates for plasma kinin-forming enzyme. Nature 1966; 210: 98-99.

Jasani MK, Katori M, Lewis GP: Intracellular enzymes and kinin enzymes in synovial fluid in joint diseases. Ann Rheym Dis 1969; 28: 497-512.

Jin LS, Seeds E, Page CP, et al.: Inhibition of bradykinininduced bronchoconstriction in the guinea-pig by a synthetic B_2 receptor antagonist. Br J Pharmacol 1989; 97: 598-602.

Kaplan AP, Reddigaris S, Brunnee T, et al.: Studies of the activation and inhibition of the plasma kallikrein-kinin system. Agents Actions 1992; 38 (Suppl. III): 317-328.

Keele CA, Eisen V: Plasma kinin-formation in rheumatoid arthritis. Adv Exp Med Biol 1970; 8: 471-475.

Kellermann J, Thelen C, Lottspeich F, et al.: Arrangement of the disulphide bridges in human low-Mr kininogen. Biochem J 1987; 247: 15-21.

Kitamura N, Kitagawa H, Fukushima D, et al.: Structural organization of the human kininogen gene and a model for its evaluation. J Biol Chern 1985; 260: 8610-8617.

Kokobu T, Kato I, Nishimura K, et al.: Angiotensin I-converting enzyme in human urine. Clin Chim Acta 1978; 89: 375-379.

Larrick JW, Kunkel SL: The role of tumor necrosis factor and interleukin-1 in immunoinflammatory response. Pharmaceutical Res 1988: 5: 129-139.

Lerner UH, Ljunggren O, Ransjo M, et al.: Inhibitory effects of y-interferon bradykinin-induced bone resorption and prostaglandin formation in cultured mouse calvarial bones. Agents Actions 1991; 32: 305-311.

Lerner UH, Ransjo M, Ljunggren O: Bradykinin stimulates production of prostaglandin E_2 and prostacyclin in murine osteoblasts. Bone and Miner-al1989; 5: 139-154.

Lerner UH, Jones IL, Gustafson GT: Bradykinin, a new potential mediator of inflammation-induced bone resorption. Arthritis Rheum 1987; 30: 530-540.

Ljunggren O, Rosenquist J, Ransjo M, et al.: Bradykinin stimulated prostaglandin E_2 formation in isolated human osteoblast-like cells. Biosc Res 1990; 10: 121-128.

Ljunggran O, Lerner UH: Evidence for BKj bradykinin receptor-mediated prostaglandin formation in osteoblasts and subsequent enhancement of bone resorption. Br J Pharmacol 1990; 101: 382-386.

Llona I, vavrek R, Stewart J, et al.: Identification of preand-postsynaptic bradykinin receptor sites in the vas deferens: evidence for structural prerequisites. J Pharmacol Exp Ther 1987; 241: 608-614.

Mandle R Jr, Colman RW, Kaplan AP: Indentification of prekallikrein and HMW-kininogen as a circulating complex in human plasma. Proc Natl Acad Sci (USA) 1976; 73: 4179-4183.

Mandle R Jr, Kaplan AP: Hageman factor substrates. II. Human plasma prekallikrein. Mechanism of activation by Hageman factor and participation of Hageman factor dependent fibrinolysis. J Biol Chem 1977; 252: 6097-6104.

Marceau F, Barabe J, St Pierre S, et al.: Kinin receptors in experimental inflammation. Can J Physiol Pharmacol 1980;58: 536-542.

Mason AJ, Avans BA, Cox DR, et al.: Structure of mouse kallikrein gene family suggests a role in specific processing of biological active peptides. Nature 1983; 303: 300-307.

Matsas R, Proud D, Nustad K, et al.: Rapid purification of a prekallikrein from rat pancreas. Anal Biochem 1981; 113: 264-270.

Meier HL, Pierce JV, Colman RW, et al.: Activation and function of human Hageman factor. The role of high molecular weight kininogen and prekallikrein. J Clin Invest 1977; 60: 18-31.

Melmon KL, Webster WC, Goldfinger SE, et al.: The presence of a kinin in inflammatory synovial effusions from arthritides of varying etiologies. Arth Rheum 1967; 10: 13-20.

Morris BJ: hGK-1: a kallikrein gene expressed in human prostate. Clin Exp Pharmacol Physiol 1989; 16: 345-351.

Muller-Esterl W: Kininogens, kinins, and kinships. J Cardiov Pharmacol1990; 15 (Suppl. 6): Sl-S6.

Nagase H, Cawston TE, De Silva M, et al.: Identification of plasma kallikrein as an activator of latent collagenase in rheumatoid synovial fluid. Biochim Biophys Acta 1982;702: 133-142.

Nouri AME, Panayi GS, Goodman SM: Cytokines and the chronic inflammation of rheumatic disease. I. The presence of interleukin-1 in synovial fluid. Clin Exp Immunol 1984;55: 295-302.

Nustad K, Vaaje K, Pierce JV: Synthesis ofkallikreins by rat kidney slices. Br J Pharmacol1975; 53: 229-234.

Okamoto H, Greenonaum LM: Isolation properties of two rat plasma T-kininogens. Adv Exp Med Biol 1986; 198: 69-75.

Pettipher ER, Higgs GA, Henderson BN: PAF-acether in chronic arthritis. Agents Actions 1987; 21: 98-103.

Pierce JV, Guimaraes JA: Further characterization of highly purified human plasma kininogens. In: PISANO II, AUSTEN KF (Eds.): Chemistry and Biology of the kallikrein-kinin system in Health and Disease. U.S. Government Printing Office. Washington, D.C. 1977: pp.121-127.

Plevin R, Owen J: Multiple B_2 kinin receptors in mammalian tissues. TIPS 1988; 58: 536-542.

Proud D, Baumgarten CR, Nacleiro RM, et al.: Kinin metabolism in human nasal secretions during experimentally-induced allergic rhinitis. J Immunol1987; 138:428-434.

Ratnoff OD, Davie JW, Mallet DL: Studies on the action of Hageman factor. Evidence that activated Hageman factor in turn activates plasma thromboplastin antecedent. J Clin Invest 1961; 40: 803-819.

Regoli D, Rhaleb NE, Tousignant C, et al.: New highly potent bradykinin B_2 receptor antagonists. Agents Actions 1991; 34: 138-141.

Regoli D: Neurohumoral regulation of precapillary vessel: the kallikrein-kinins system. J Cardiov Pharmaco 1984; 6: S401-S412.

Regoli D, Marceau F, Lavigne J: Induction of B_1 receptors for kinins in the rabbit by a bacteriallipopolysaccharide. Eur J Pharmacol1991; 71: 105-115.

Regoli D, Rhaleb NE, Drapeau G, et al.: Basic pharmacology of kinins: pharmacological receptors and other mechanisms. Adv Exp Med Biol 1989; 247A: 399-407.

Regoli D, Barabe S: Pharmacology of bradykinin and related kinins. Pharmacol Rev 1980; 31: 1-46.

Richards RI, Catanzaro DF, Mason AJ, et al.: Mouse glandular kallikrein genes: nucleotide sequence of cloned cDNA coding for a member of the kallikrein arginyl esteropeptidase group of serine proteases. J Biol Chern 1982; 257:2758-2761.

Saha JK, Sengupta JN, Goyal RK: Effect of bradykinin on opossum esophageal longitudinal smooth muscle: evidence for novel bradykinin receptors. J Pharmacol Exp Ther 1990; 252: 1012-1020.

Schachter M, Uchida Y, Longride DJ, et al.: New synthetic antagonists of bradykinin. Br J Pharmacol 1987; 92: 851-855.

Schachter M: kallikreins (kininogenase)-a group of serine proteases with bioregulatory actions. Pharmacol Rev 1980: 31: 1-17.

Schedlich LJ, Bennetts BH, Morris BJ: Primary structure of a human glandular kallikrein gene. DNA 1987; 6:429-437.

Schedlich LJ, Catanzaro DF, Morris BJ: Kallikrein genes: cloning in man and expression in rat renal hypertension. J Hypertension 1988; 6 (Suppl. 4): S395-S398.

Schini VB, Boulanger C, Regoli D, et al.: Bradykinin stimulates the production of cyclic GMP via activation of B_2 kinin receptors in cultured porcine aortic endothelial cells. J Pharmacol Exp Ther 1990; 252: 581-585.

Seidah NG, Ladenheim R, Mbikay M, et al.: The cDNA structure of rat plasma kallikrein. DNA 1989; 8:563-574.

Sharma JN: The kinin system and prostaglandins in the intestine. Pharmacol Toxicol1988; 63: 310-316.

Sharma JN: The role of the kallikrein-kinin system in joint inflammatory disease. Pharmacol Res 1991a; 23: 105-112.

Sharma JN: The role of kinin system in joint inflammatory disease. Eur J Rheumatol Inflammation 1991b; 11:30-37.

Sharma JN: Pro-inflammatory actions of the platelet activating factor: relevance to rheumatoid arthritis. Exp Pathol l991c; 43: 47-50.

Sharma JN: Involvement of the kinin-forming system in the physiopathology of rheumatoid inflammation. Agents Actions 1992; 38 (suppl. III): 343-361.

Sharma JN: Therapeutic prospects of bradykinin receptor antagonists. Gen Pharmacol1993; 24: 267-274.

Sharma JN, Buchanan WW: Kinin system in clinical and experimental rheumatoid inflammation: short review. Curr Med Res Opin 1979; 6: 314-321.

Sharma JN, Mohsin SSJ: The role of chemical mediators in the pathogenesis of inflammation with emphasis on the kinin system. Exp Pathol l990; 38: 73-96.

Sharma JN, Stewart JM, Mohsin SSJ, et al.: Influence of a kinin antagonist on acute hypotensive responses induced by bradykinin and captopril in spontaneously hypertensive rats. Agents Actions 1992; 38 (Suppl. III):258-269.

Sharma JN, Zeitlin IJ, Deodhar SD, et al.: Detection of kallikrein-like activity in inflamed synovial tissue. Arch Int Pharmacodyn Ther 1983; 262: 279-286.

Sharma JN, Zeitlin IJ, Brooks PM, et al.: A novel relationship between plasma kininogen and rheumatoid disease. Agents Actions 1976; 6: 148-153.

Sharma JN, Zeitlin IJ, Buchanan WW, et al.: The action of aspirin on plasma kininogen and other proteins in rheumatoid patients: relationship to disease activity. Clin Exp Pharmacol Physiol l980; 7: 347-353.

Sharma JN, Zeitlin IJ, Mackenzie JF, et al.: Plasma kinin-precursor levels in clinical intestinal inflammation. Fundamental Clin Pharmacoll988; 2: 399-403.

Sheikh IA, Kaplan AP: Studies of the digestion of bradykinin, lysylbradykinin, and des-arg^9 bradykinin by angiotensin converting enzyme. Biocnem Pharmacol 1986; 35: 1951-1956.

Silverberg M, Diehl S: The autoactivation of factor XII (Hageman factor) induced by low-M heparin and dextran sulfate. Biochem J 1987; 248: 715-720.

Skidel RA, Schultz WW, Tam LT, et al.: Human renal angiotensin-I converting enzyme and its helper enzyme.Kidney Int 1987; 31 (Suppl. 20): 45-48.

Suzuki M, Ito A, Mori Y, et al.: Kallikrein in synovial fluid of patients with rheumatoid arthritis. Biochem Med Metab Biol 1987; 37: 177-183.

Thompson RE, Mandle R Jr, Kaplan AP: Association of factor XI and high molecular weight kininogen in human plasma. J Clin Invest 1977: 60: 1376-1380.

Tiffany CW, Burch RM: Bradykinin stimulates tumor necrosis factor and interleukin-l release from macrophages. FEB 1989; 247: 189-192.

Ura N, Carretero OA, Erdos EG: Role of renal endopeptidase 24.11 in kinin metabolism in vitro and in vivo.Kidney Int 1987; 32: 507-513.

Vevrek RJ, Stewart JM: Competitive antagonists of bradykinin. Peptides 1985; 6: 161-164.

Werle E, Gotze W, Keppler A: Uber die Wirkung des Kallikreins auf den isolierten Darm und tiber eine neue Darmkontrahierende Substanz. Biochem Z 1937; 289:217-233.

Werle E, Berek U: Zur Kenntnis des Kallikreins. Z angew Chern. 1948; 60A: 53.

Werle E, Maier L, Ringelmann E: Hemmung von Proteinasen durch Kallikrein-Inaktivatoren. Naturwissenschaften 1953; 39: 328.

Whalley ET, Clegg S, Stewart JM, et al.: The effect of kinin agonists and antagonists on the pain response of the human blister base. Naunyn-Schiedeberg's Arch Pharmacol 1987a;336: 652-655.

Chapter 2

Interrelationship Between the Kallikrein-Kinin System and Hypertension

INTRODUCTION

The blood pressure (BP)-lowering effect of the kallikrein-kinin system (KKS) has been described for more than six decades (Frey, 1926). It is now widely believed that the KKS is involved in controlling BP. Exogenously administered kinins cause hypotension, natriuresis, arterial vasodilatation, increased renal blood flow and fall in peripheral resistance (de Freitas et al., 1964; Willis et al., 1969; Adetuyibi and Mills, 1972; Nasjletti et al., 1978; Mills, 1982). Thus, it is conceivable that reduced activity of the KKS could result in sodium retention, arterial vasoconstriction, raised peripheral resistance, increased vascular or plasma volume, and production of high BP (hypertension). Hence, reduced kinin-generation in the blood stream is thought to play an important role in the development of hypertension. In this regard, it has been demonstrated that the urinary kallikrein excretion is diminished in clinical and experimental hypertension (Margolius et al., 1971; Adetuyibi and Mills, 1972; Croxatto and San Martin, 1970; Lechi et al., 1978). Furthermore, kallikrein excretion in the urine is viewed as an index of the activity of KKS in the renal system. This review is intended to discuss the significant role of KKS in hypertension.

THE COMPONENTS OF THE KALLIKREIN-KININ SYSTEM

Vasoactive polypeptides, kinins, are released in the blood stream from precursors, kininogens, by the enzymatic actions of a group of serine proteases known as kallikreins (Figure2.1). Kinins are straight chain peptides which resemble bradykinin (BK) (Arg^1-Pro^2-Pro^3)-Gly^4-Phe^5-Ser^6-Pro^7-Phe^8-Arg^9) in structure and in pharmacological actions (Sharma and Buchanan, 1979; Schachter, 1980).

Kininogens

Two kallikrein substrates, low molecular weight (LMW) and high molecular weight (HWM) kininogens, have been isolated from bovine plasma (Komiya et al., 1974). They differ in molecular weights (HMW-76,000; LMW-48,000), and in their susceptibility to plasma and tissue kallikreins. The HMW kininogen is the main substrate for plasma kallikrein, and LMW kininogen is the most suitable substrate for tissue kallikrein. Two kininogens with different molecular weights (HMW120,000; LMW-78,000) have also been isolated from human plasma (Jacobsen, 1966; Nagasawa and Nakayasu, 1975). The presence of a third form of human kininogen of about 200,000 daltons has been demonstrated (Pierce and Guimaraes, 1975).

The deficiency of HMW kininogen appears to be the source of the multiple defects such as repaired clotting, kinin-release, and surface-activated fibrinolysis in plasma. The HMW kininogen is also known as a "Fitzgerald factor", because its absence was found first in the Fitzgerald family (Saito et al., 1974; Colman et al., 1975; Wuepper et al., 1975; Lacombe et al., 1975). Saito et al., (1975) have reported that purified preparations of "Fitzgerald factor" isolated from normal plasma contain HMW kininogen, however, the plasma from Mr. Fitzgerald contained about 50% of the amount of kininogen found in normal plasma which is of the LMW form. It seems, therefore, HMW is essential not only in the kinin-formation, but also in the regulation of blood-coagulation pathway. This defect has been reversed by the treatment with purified HMW kininogen (Wuepper et al., 1975; Lacombe et al., 1975; Colman et al., 1975). Further, Hageman factor (HF) activates prekallikrein (inactive) to kallikrein (active), which is dependent on HMW kininogen. Thus, HMW could serve as a cofactor in the initiation of blood coagulation and the inactivation of kinin-generation (Kaplan et al., 1981).

Kallikreins

Kinin forming enzymes, kallikreins, have been divided into two groups; plasma and tissue or glandular. They differ mainly in molecular weight, biological functions, physiochemical and immunological properties, and on the basis of their distribution in the body.

Plasma kallikrein

The plasma kallikrein is present in the circulation in an inactive form known as prekallikrein or Fletcher factor. It has been described that a plasma designated Fletcher trait deficiency possessed a reduced rate of surface-mediated coagulation (prolonged partial thromboplastin time) which approached normal when the incubation time with kaolin is increased. (Hathway and Alsever, 1970). Prekallikrein is activated by HF (Kaplan and Austen, 1971). Plasma kallikrein has also been shown to activate inactivated HF to active HF in the fluid phase (Cochrane et al., 1973).

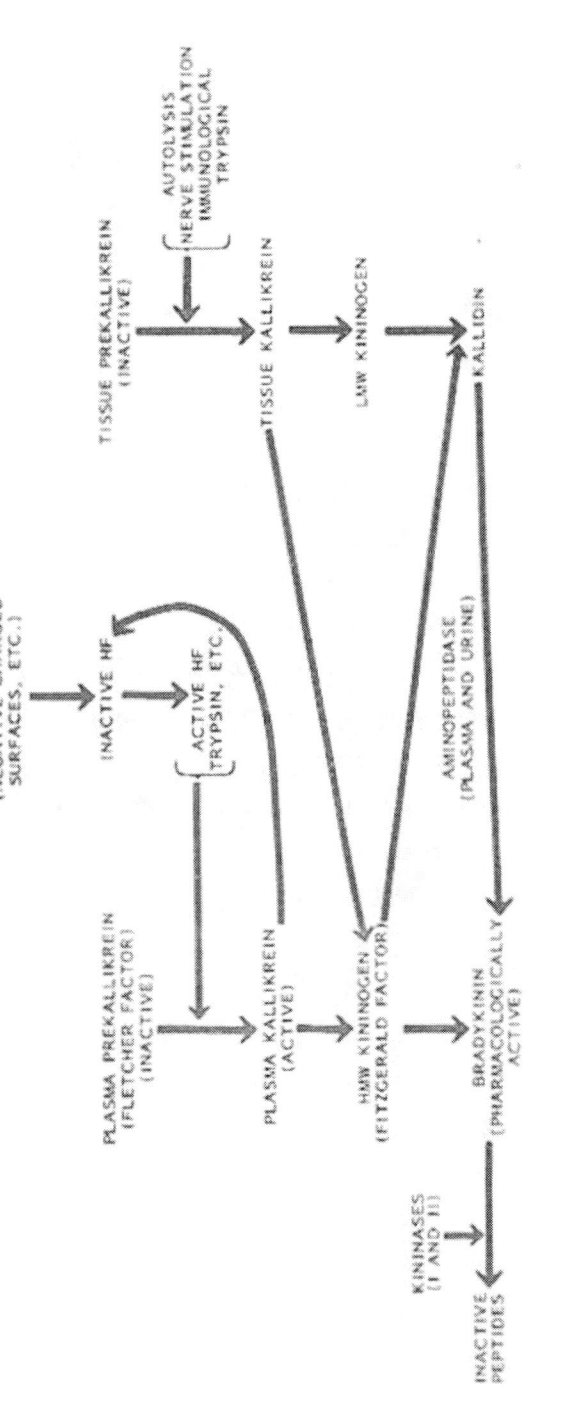

Figure 2.1. Scheme of the components of the kinin-forming and inactivating system.

Kaplan et al., (1977) suggested the conversion of a small amount of prekallikrein to kallikrein by activated HF is necessary prior to feedback activation of HF. This finding has further demonstrated that plasma kallikrein does not only liberate kinins, but it is also required for the regulation of normal circulatory homeostasis. A genetic defect resulting in prolonged blood-clotting time (Fletcher disease) has been corrected successfully with plasma prekallikrein (Wuepper, 1973).

Tissue kallikrein

Tissue kallikreins are present in the kidney, pancreas, intestine, salivary gland, bronchoalveolar lavage fluid of asthmatic patients and synovial tissue (Nustad et al., 1975; Fiedler et al., 1970; Zeitlin, 1972; Bhoola et al., 1965; Christiansen et al., 1987; Sharma et al., 1983a). However, the presence of tissue kallikreins in the plasma has also been reported (Nustad et al., 1979; Rabito et al., 1979; Lawton et al., 1981; Rabito et al., 1982). The value of these observations remains unclear. Although, the release of submandibular gland kallikrein into the circulation has been indicated after sympathetic nervous system stimulation, which may cause reactive vasodilation in the rat submandibular gland (Rabito et al., 1983). Tissue kallikreins have similar physiochemical properties, and these enzymes are immunologically identical within the same species (Fiedler, 1979), although, the factors which determine tissue kallikrein secretion are not well defined, and could exhibit tissue as well as species differences. It has been reported that the salivary secretion of kallikrein in the rat is regulated by the sympathetic and parasympathetic nervous systems, although the stimulation of sympathetic produces an increased secretion of kallikrein than the stimulation of parasympathetic system (Beilenson et al., 1968; Ørstavik and Gautvik, 1977; Rabito et al., 1983). On the other hand, α -adrenergic stimulation appeared to inhibit urinary kallikrein excretion from the kidney of the dog and the rat (Olsen, 1980; 1982). In the kidney, tissue kallikrein is synthesized in the distal tubular cells (Ørstaviket al., 1976). It has been suggested that part of the kallikrein excreted in the urine could be of plasma origin (Fink et al., 1980). Although the urinary kallikrein appears to be secreted in the distal segments of the nephron (Scicli et al., 1976). The urinary excretion of kallikrein reflects the activity of the enzyme in the rat kidney (Marin-Grez et al., 1982). The renal kallikrein has been suggested to regulate BP and its possible involvement in the physiopathology of hypertension (Carreterro and Scicli, 1981; Ørstavik, 1981, Sharma, 1984; Sharma and Fernandez, 1982). Furthermore, tissue kallikreins are implicated in a variety of physiological actions, including salt and water excretion, and activation of both striopeptigen and prorenin, as well as release of lysylbradykinin (kallidin) from kininogens. Several agents that non-specifically block serine proteases, including kallikreins, have been reviewed by Vogel (1979). A recent study has provided new data on the specificity of tissue kallikreins and its involvement in enkephalin biosynthesis(Prado et al., 1983)

Kininases

When a kinin is incubated with blood or with a tissue homogenate, it is rapidly cleaved to inactive peptides. Therefore, kinin inactivating enzymes are collectively known as kininases.

Kininase I (carboxypeptidase N) is present in the plasma of man and animals that cleaves basic C-terminal amino acids, including Arg9 of BK (Erdos and Sloane, 1962). This enzyme has been purified from human plasma (Erdos et al., 1967; Oshima et al., 1974). Whereas, Erdos and Yang (1966, 1967) first detected an enzyme in the kidney cortex and subsequently in the plasma (Yang and Erdos, 1967) which inactivates BK by cleaving the C-terminal of the nonapeptide. This kininase was named as kininase II (peptidyldipeptide hydrolase) or angiotensin I-converting enzyme (ACE). At present kinanase II (ACE) inhibitors are clinically more important in the treatment of hypertension.

INTERACTIONS WITH OTHER ENDOGENOUS AGENTS

Renin-angiotensin system

It has been suggested that the rennin-angiotensin system (RAS) and KKS act as opposing forces in the regulation of BP (Vinci et a!., 1979). Under certain situations, the inhibition of a vasodilator system (KKS) occurring during the activation of a vasoconstrictor system (RAS) might function together in control or increase of BP. The inactive renin is activated in vitro by plasma and tissue kallikreins (Sealey et al., 1978; Derkx et al., 1979). Although, it has been reported that the inactive renin separated from active renin could not be activated by tissue kallikrein, however, after acid treatment, the inactive renin was activated in the presence of tissue kallikrein (Yokosawa et al., 1979) This finding was confirmed when Hiwada et al., (1983) reported that tissue kallikrein does not directly activate inactive renin but participates in the activation process of inactive renin. An increased urinary kallikrein excretion has been observed in dogs after intra-arterial infusions of angiotensin II (MacFarlane et al., 1974). Mills et al., (1976) suggested that under situations of raised renin angiotensin production, the renal KKS might also be activated to antagonize raised vasoconstriction of renal vasoculatures. Indeed, kinase II (ACE) is known for the conversion of angiotensin I into the potent vasoconstrictor angiotensin II, as well as responsible for the biodegradation of BK, a potent vasodilator agent (Erdos and Skidgel, 1985). The multihormonal regulation of renal kallikrein and its possible interactions with the renin-angiotensin-aldosterone system, the corticotropin-glucocorticoid system, antidiuretic hormone, catecholamine and prostaglandins (PC) have been discussed in an excellent review by Martin-Grez (1982). However, there was no correlation between renal tissue kallikrein and plasma renin activity in either two-kidney or one-kidney renal hypertension (Carreterro et al., 1974).

Prostaglandins

PGE possesses a wide range of pharmacological actions. It is synthesized by vascular tissue, and participates in regulation of vascular tone, and also acts as a local vasoactive agent in the kidney through influencing local blood flow, salt and water excretion (Bunting et al., 1976; Gryglewski et al., 1976; Vane and McGiff, 1975). Nonetheless, there is considerable evidence to suggest the pharmacological interactions between BK and PGs. BK-mediated production of PGs has been observed in a variety of tissue such as the kidney (McGiff et al.,

1972), spleen (Ferreira et al., 1971), and the lung (Palmer et al., 1973). Furthermore, intrarenal arterial infusions of BK into the canine kidney caused release of PGE-like agents. In the rat, it has been reported that administration of tissue kallikrein inhibitor Trasylol, produced reduction in PGE, and kallikrein concentration in the urine (Nasjletti et al., 1978). In this way, alterations in KKS might have profound effects on PGS concentrations in the renal circulation (Colina-Chourie et al., 1976), therefore, PGS could contribute to the actions of BK on salt and water excretion (McGiff et al., 1975). Intraperitoneal administration of PGE_2 can produce reduction in plasma kininogen levels in the rat (Sharma and Zeitlin, 1982; Murakami et al., 1982). It is suggested that PGE_2, but not PGF_2, might produce kinins by activating plasma pre-kallikrein to kallikrein (Sharma and Zeitlin, 1982). Also, the duration of hypotensive action of BK in Dahl rats is inhibited by PGs synthetase inhibitor such as indomethacin (Sharma et al., 1984a). This reduction in the duration of the hypotensive effect of BK is the result from an inhibition of the cyclo-oxygenase system in the Dahl rats. It has also been reported that BK activates a phospholipase (Hong and Levine, 1976) which releases arachidonic acid and lead to increased synthesis of PGs (Dams and Bourdon, 1974).

In patients with Bartter's Syndrome, there is high plasma renin, hyperaldosteronism, hypokalemic akalosis and juxtaglomerular hyperplasia, however, in spite of the raised plasma renin, the BP remains normal (Bartter et al., 1962). Enhanced renal kallikrein and PG have been implicated in the aetiology of this syndrome. These suggestions are supported by the findings of raised PGE2 and kallikrein concentrations in the urine (Gill et al., 1976; Vinci et al., 1976; Lechi et al., 1976). In patients with Bartter's Syndrome, indomethacin and other cyclo-oxygenase inhibitors therapy caused a remarkable reduction in the plasma renin concentrations and aldosterone, PGE2 and kallikreins levels in the urine and also corrected the hypokalemic alkalosis without altering the BP (Gill et al., 1976; Haluska et al., 1977). These observations strongly suggest that PGE is involved in the renal regulation of renin and kallikrein systems. Thus, reduction in angiotensin II might cause fall in the aldosterone levels to normal so that hypokalemia could be corrected (Mills, 1979). However, Strand and Gilmore (1982) reported that PGs do not mediate the renal effects of BK in the dog.

Vasopressin

There are several reports to suggest a complex interaction between vasopressin (VP) and KKS. Kinins are powerful antagonists of the hydroosmotic effect of VP in the toad urinary bladder (Furtado, 1981; Carvounis et al., 1981), and water permeability in the renal medulla (Barroclough and Mills, 1965). These investigators also observed that this action of kinin was antagonized by anti-diuretic hormone. Kinins are known as potent activators of PG synthesis in the kidney (McGiff et al., 1972). Further, it has been reported that PGs interfere with the hydroosmotic actions of VP (Fejes-Toth et al., 1977). VP administration can cause PGE release in the rabbit kidney (Miller et al., 1986a), which might reduce the response of the collecting duct to VP (Zusman and Keiser, 1977). Fejes-Toth and Fejes-Toth (1986) provided indirect evidence to support the notion that arginine-vasopressin might activate renal KKS, but the mechanism of action and its implication in hypertension remains to be determined. Hence, it is possible to suggest that interactions between the renal KKS and renal PGs might contribute to the control of renal blood flow, and salt and water homeostasis. Recently, it has been shown that arachidonic acid stimulating PG release takes place in pre-glomerular blood vessels and hence 6-keto-PGE1α, whereas arginin-vasopressin (AVP) activates PGE_2 release from post-glomerular sites, an action shared with angiotensin II (Miller et al., 1986a; Miller et al, 1986b). It indicates that arachidonic acid and AVP differ in profile of PG release in the renal vascular compartments. Interactions between the KKS, PGs and VP might have greater physiological importance in the control and counter balance of antidiuretic hormone, however, such evidence needs to be established. In this regard, Fejes-Toth et al., (1982), and Fejes-Toth and Fejes-Toth (1986) reported that VP is a potent activator of kallikrein when given during water diuresis and the kinin released may antagonise the effect of VP thus, completing a full negative feedback system. Figure2.2 shows the KKS, renin-angiotensin, and prostaglandin systems interactions at various sites.

KALLIKREIN-KININ SYSTEM IN HYPERTENSIVE CONDITIONS

Kinins have potent vasodilator and natriuretic effects, and deficiency of KKS may participate in the genesis of hypertension. The physiopharmacological abnormality of the KKS in hypertension is based on the observations such asreduced activity of renal kallikrein, increased levels of kallikrein inhibitor, decreased synthesis of HWW and/or LMW kininogen and the presence of high concentrations of kininases e.g. II. These factors would result in subnormal kinin-generation within the renal system. The correlation between KKS and hypertension was observed by Elliott and Nuzum (1934). These investigators found that patients with essential hypertension excreted less kallikrein in the urine than normotensive individuals. This observation was ignored for 37 yrs, when Margolius and co-investigators (1971; 1974; 1972) reported reduced urinary kallikrein excretion in various types of hypertensive patients, and in rats with hypertension. Reduced urinary kallikrein excretion would suggest that hypertension might result from a defect in the kinin-generation. The pharmacological effects of kinin in relation to the regulation of BP are vasodilatation in most areas circulation, reduction in total pheripheral resistance, and regulation of sodium excretion from the kidney (Adetuyibi and Mills, 1972; de Freitas et al., 1964; Marin-Grez et al., 1982; Mills, 1982; Maxwell et al., 1962).

The injection of BK into the renal artery causes a diuresis and natriuresis by increasing renal blood flow (Webster and Gilmore, 1964). These actions of BK have been attributed to PGs release in the renal circulation (McGiff et al., 1975; McGiff et al., 1976). Nevertheless, the renal KKS has been suggested as an intrarenal hormone system that controls water and electrolyte excretion and participates in the regulation of BP (Scicli and Carretero, 1986; Carretero and Scicli, 1981). Moreover, the concentration of kallikrein present in the urine may serve as an indicator of renal activity of KKS since it originates from the kidney (Nustad, 1970; Mills, 1979), although the underlying mechanisms are poorly understood. In this regard, genetical abnormalities and the loss of renal parenchyma might be of clinical significance.

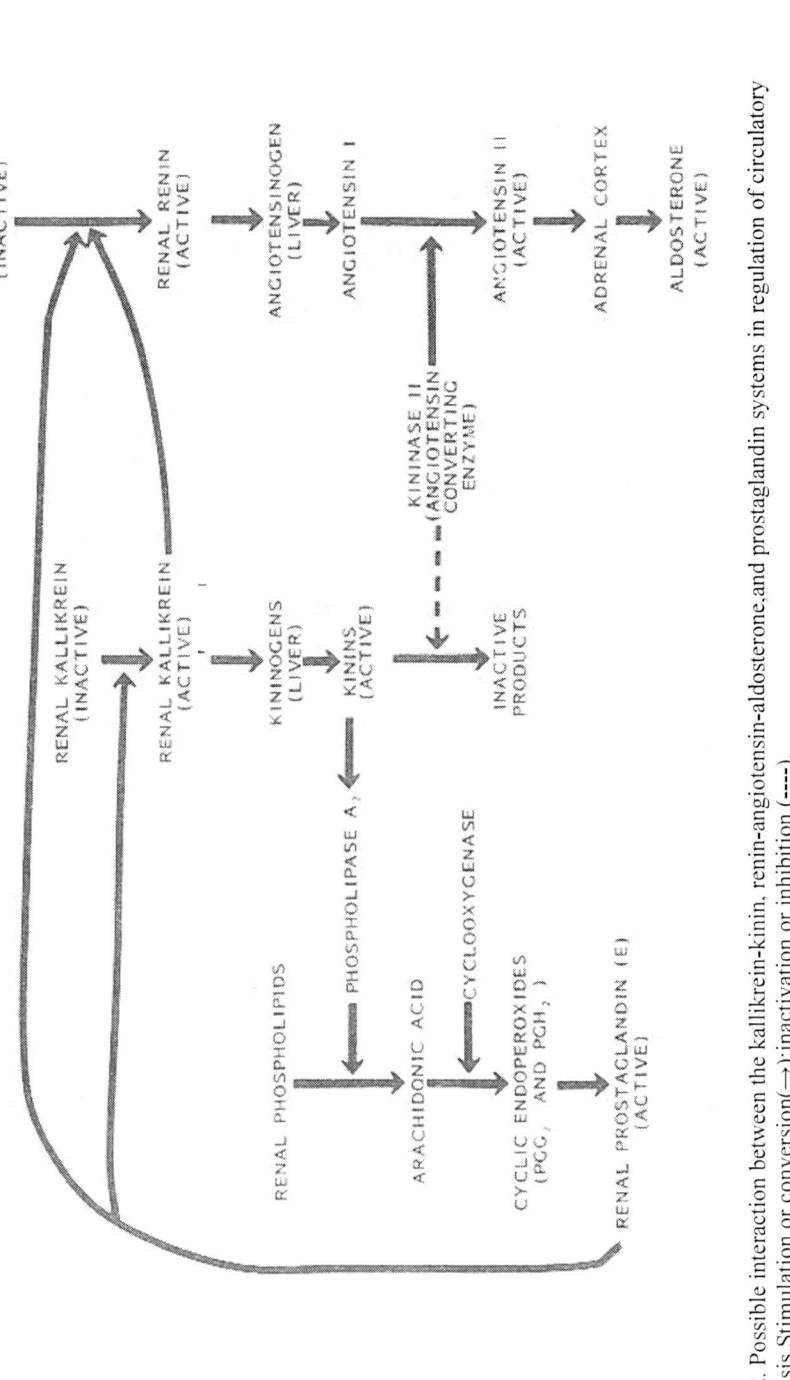

Figure2.2. Possible interaction between the kallikrein-kinin, renin-angiotensin-aldosterone,and prostaglandin systems in regulation of circulatory homeostasis.Stimulation or conversion(→);inactivation or inhibition (----).

It has been suggested that the race and sodium intake in hypertension have greater influence upon kallikrein excretion (Zinner et al., 1976, 1978; Levy et al., 1977). These investigators evaluated urinary kallikrein levels in large populations of hypertensive cases and their families. The result showed that whites excrete more kallikrein than blacks, and white hypertensives excrete less kallikrein than white normotensive individuals. All test groups had higher kallikrein execretion when kept on low sodium intake. Black hypertensives excreted less kallikrein than black normotensives during sodium reduction. Furthermore, families with reduced kallikrein excretion had higher BP than those with increased urinary kallikrein excretion. This could suggest a genetic defect in the renal kallikrein and/or the presence of higher amounts of tissue kallikrein inhibitor in certain races. In this connection, Horl et al., (1982) stated that the inhibitory effect of α-antitrypsin or kallikrein activity should be taken into account in studies related with renal kallikrein.

Alteration in KKS has also been observed in genetically salt-sensitive hypertensive rats. This experimental hypertensive model is thought to have similar pathogenic mechanism as human essential hypertension. Through selective inbreeding, Dahl and his colleagues (Dahl et al., 1962) developed two strains from Sprague–Dawley rats; they are known as Dahl salt-sensitive (DSS) hypertensive and Dahl salt-resistant (DSR) normotensive rats. It has been reported that urinary kallikrein activity is reduced in DSS hypertensive rats when compared with the DSR normotensive rats (Carretero et al., 1978). Arbeit and Serra (1985) also reported reduced urinary kallikrein excretion in DSS rat fed on 0.0064% and 0.4% sodium chloride. Although, these investigators did not report the BP of DSS rats, it is impossible to evaluate the correlation between the severity of hypertension and reduction in urinary kallikrein concentration in DSS rats. However, it has been suggested that altered sodium and water excretion due to reduced production of kinin-forming enzyme, might be the cause of hypertension in DSS rats (Sustarsic et al., 1980, 1981). A similar mechanism might also prevail in human essential hypertension. The mechanism of altered renal kallikrein activity in hypertesive patients remains unknown. It is speculated that mode of decreased kallikrein levels in hypertensive patients might be due to decrease synthesis, or an increased inhibition. Kallikrein excretion is also suppressed in renal parenchymal hypertension, experimental diabetic hypertension. hypertension after renal transplant and glucocorticoid-induced hypertension in rats (Mites et al., 1978; Hayashi et al., 1983; O'Connor et al., 1982; Handa et al., 1983). These findings further support the role of renal kallikrein in the genesis of various forms of hypertension. Furthermore, it has been found that the rate of kinin inactivation is increased in one-kidney, one clip hypertension in rats (Salgado et al., 1986), and in the hypertension caused by acute renal artery constriction in the dog (Moore Jr et al., 1984). These data indicate once again that decreased circulating kinin might potentiate the vasoconstrictor action of angiotension II, and contribute to the development of hypertension.

However, urinary kallikrein excretion is increased in desoxycorticosterone acetate (DOCA) induced hypertension in rats (Margolius et al., 1972), and in rabbits (Marchetti et al., 1984). Increased urinary kallikrein activity has also been observed in majority of hypertensive patients who have primary aldosteronism (Margolius et al., 1971, 1974). This could be possibly due to mineralocorticoid mediated regulation of renal kallikrein (Vince et al., 1979; Horwitz et al., 1978).

Investigations of the systemic changes in the KKS have provided further evidence regarding the mechanism of various hypertensive conditions. In this regard, plasma kininogen levels and a kinin potentiating factor have been found to be reduced in essential and malignant hypertensive patients (Sharma and Zeitlin, 1981; Almeida et al., 1981). It may be that the deficiency in plasma HMW kininogen might be related to decrease in liver synthesis in individuals who developed hypertension after mild exercise (James and Donaldson, 1981). Thus, it seems possible that deficient kallikrein-kininogen-kinin formation might be a significant factor in physiopathology of hypertension. Further, it is suggested that reduced concentrations of kinin-forming system might be the cause of increased arterial vascoconstriction in clinical and experimental hypertension (Sharma and Zeitlin, 1981; Sharma, 1984; Sharma and Fernandez, 1982). The kinin system also participates in the regulation of vascular reactivity by opposing the vasoconstrictor actions of vasopressor agents and enhanced adrenergic activity (Carretero and Scicli, 1981). The role of KKS in the regulation of renal physiology remains incompletely understood. It may not be possible to understand distinctly the actions of KKS in the pathogenesis of hypertension and other cardiovascular diseases, until systemic, renal, myocardial, and vascular smooth muscle responsibilities of kallikrein-kinin are investigated.

TISSUE KALLIKREIN AND KININASE II INHIBITORS AS ANTIHYPERTENSIVE AGENTS

The kallikrein might have a prime action in the regulation of systemic BP, because administration of tissue kallikrein to hypertensive patients can bring the BP at the normal levels. It has been shown that the pig pancreatic kallikrein therapy lowered the BP significantly and normalized their reduced urinary kallikrein excretion in patients with essential hypertension (Overlack et al., 1980, 1981). These data provide favourable evidence that the presence of subnormal activity of kinin-generating system might be a prominent predisposing cause in the genesis of hypertension. Since the antihypertensive mechanism(s) of pancreatic kallikrein treatment remains unknown, the possibility exists that tissue kallikrein may have independent actions in regulating arterial BP. There is, however, no direct evidence in support of this hypothesis.

Kininase II (ACE) inhibitors such as captopril, enalapril and teprotide are currently used in the treatment of both clinical and experimental hypertension (Silberbauer et al., 1982; Antonacci, 1982; Sharma et al., 1983b, 1984b; Fernandez et al.. 1983a, 1983b; Edery et al., 1981). Kininase II inhibitors might possibly lower BP by inhibiting the biodegradation of kinin as well as inhibiting angiotensin II-formation at the renin site (see Figure2.3). Katz et al., (1980) determine the inter-relationship between the changes in plasma kinin levels and BP reduction during i.v. infusions of BK and reported that increased plasma kinin levels of I to 2 ng/ml caused a significant reduction in BP(nearly 30 mm Hg). The magnitude of the increment in plasma kinin levels was similar to that observed during the administration of kininase II inhibitor (Swartz et al., 1979). Although there are methodological difficulties on the estimation of plasma kinin concentrations, these findings do suggest that circulating kinin contributes to the antihypertensive effects of kininase II inhibition.

Plasma kininogen decrease has been reported in clinical condition after administration of non-steroidal antiinflammatory agents (Sharma et al., 1976, 1980; Zeitlin et al., 1976, 1977). It is important to emphasize that inhibition of kininase leading to kinin accumulation may play a major contributing role in the mechanism of hypotensive action of teprotide, kininase

II inhibitor, in humans (Edery et al., 1981). Abnormality in the urinary kallikrein excretion has also been corrected after nifedipine, a calcium-channel blocker treatment in patients with essential hypertension (Tsunoda el al., 1986). Whereas, Sharma et al., (1984c) demonstrated differential sensitivity of DSS hypertensive and DSR normotensive rats to the hypotensive action of nifedipine. This might reflect a significantly more important role of diminished renal kallikrein-kinin activity in DSS hypertensive than DSR normotensivc rats. This possibility has yet to be examined.

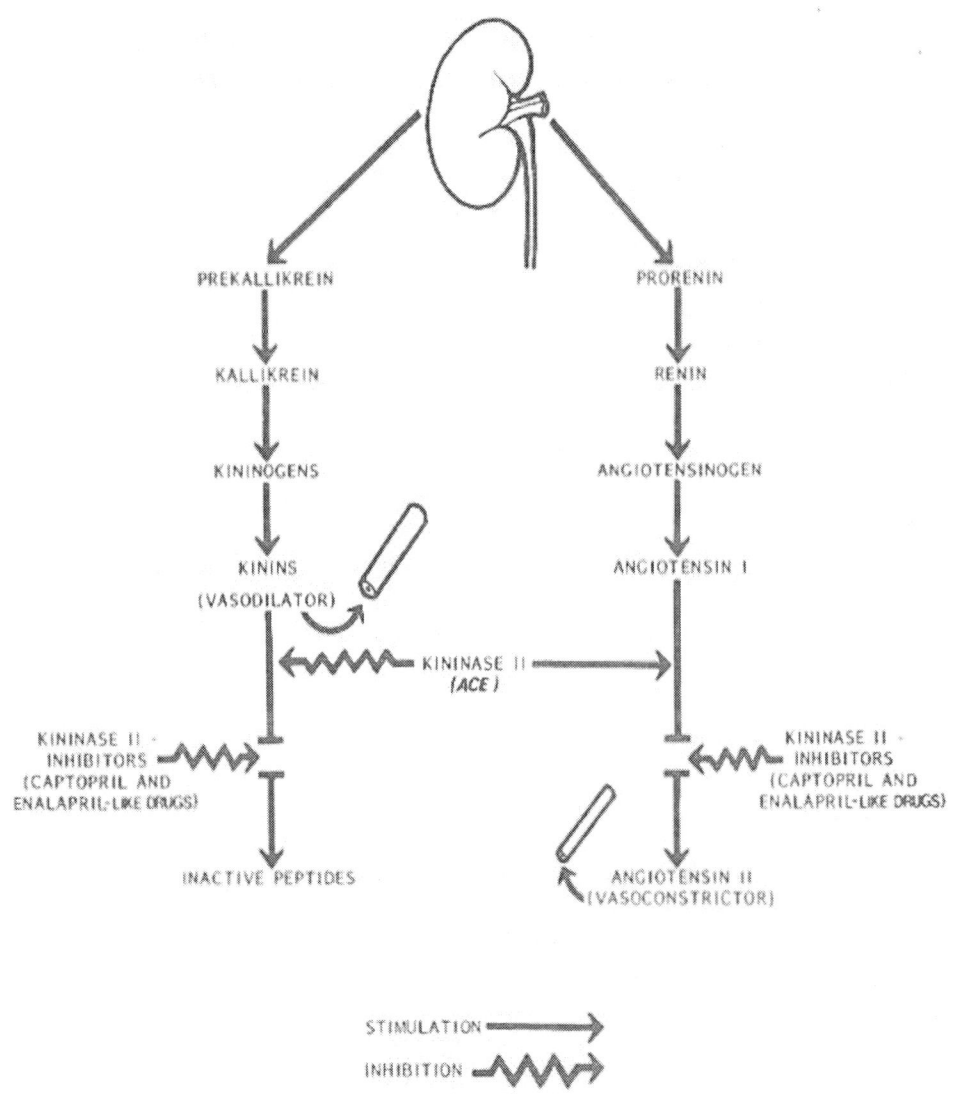

Figure 2.3. Antihypertensive effects of kininase II inhibitors (captopril and enalapril like drugs). These drugs inhibit degradation of kinins, vasodilators. In addition, these drugs block the formation of angiotensin II. The kininase II is also known as angiotensin converting enzyme.

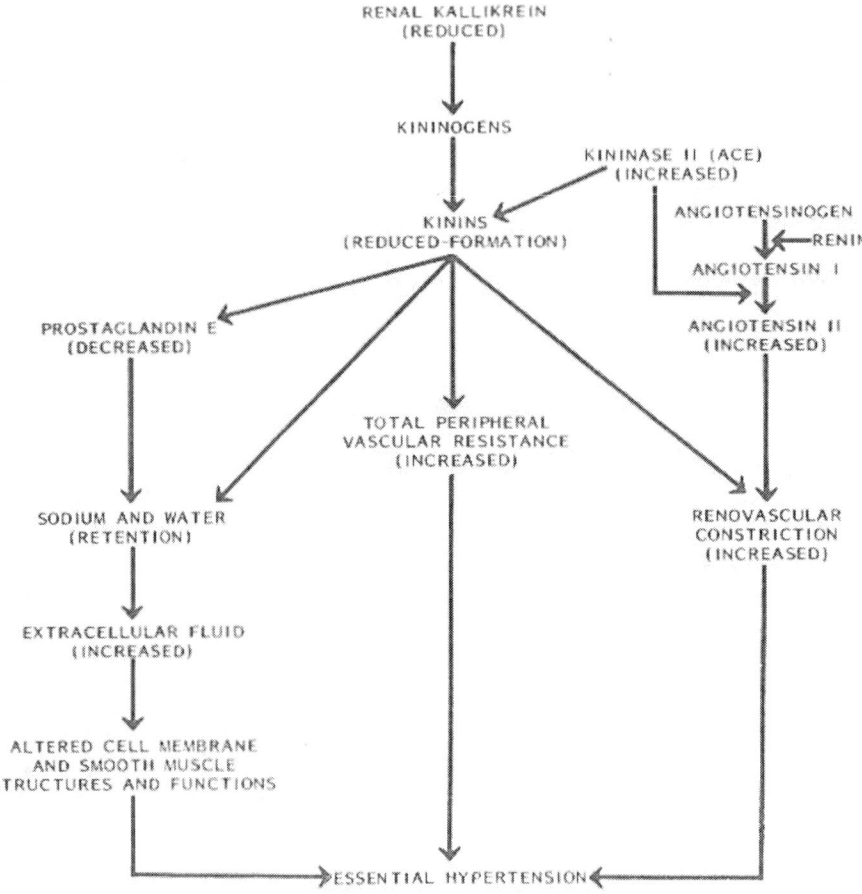

Figure 2.4. A hypothetical presentation of the involvement of the renal kallikrein-kinin, prostaglandin and renin-angiotensin systems in the physio-pathology of essential hypertension.

REFERENCES

Adetuyibi A, Mills IH: Relationship between urinary kallikrein and renal function, hypertension, and excretion of sodium and water in man. Lancet 1972; 2: 203-207.

Almeida FA, Stella RCR, Voos A, Ajzen H, Ribeiro AB, et al.: Malignant hypertension: a syndrome associated with low plasma kininogen and kinin potentiating factor. Hypertension 1981; 3: II46--II50.

Antonaccio MJ: Angiotensin converting enzyme (ACE) inhibitors. A Rev Pharmac Tox 1982; 22: 57-87.

Arbeit LA, Serra SR: Decreased total and active urinary kallikrein in normotensive Dahl slat susceptible rats. Kidney Int 1985; 28: 440-446.

Barraclough WA, Mills IH: Effect of bradykinin on renal function. Clin Sci 1965; 28: 69-74.

Bartter FC, Pronove P, Gill JR, MacCardle RC: Hyperplasia of the juxtaglomerular cortex with hyperaldo-steronism and hypokalemic alkalosis. Am J Med 1962; 33: 811-828.

Beilenson S, Schachter M, Smaje LH: Secretion of kallikrein and its role in vasodilation in the submaxillary gland. J Physiol Lond 1968; 199: 303-317.

Bhoola KD, Mordy J, Schachter M, et al.: Vasodilatation in the submaxillary gland of the cat. J Physiol Lond 1965;179: 172-184.

Bunting S, Gryglewski R, Moncada S, et al.: Arterial walls generation from prostaglandin endoperoxides a substance (prostaglandin X) which relaxes strip of mesenteric and coeliac artery and inhibits plate aggregation. Prostaglandins 1976;12: 897-913.

Carretero OA, Amin VM, Ocholik T, et al.: Urinary kallikrein in rats bred for their susceptibility and resistance to the hypertensive effect of salt. A new radio-immunoassay for its direct determination. Circulation Res 1978; 42: 727-731.

Carretero OA, Scicli AG: Possible role of kinins in circulatory homeostasis: State of the art review. Hypertension 1981; 3: 366--369.

Carretero OA, Oza NB, Schork A: Renal tissue kallikrein, plasma renin, and plasma aldosterone in renal hypertension. Acta physiol Lat Am 1974; 24: 448-452.

Carvounis CP, Carvounis G, Arbveit LA: Role of the endogenous kallikrein-kinin system modulating vassopressin-stimulated water flow and urea permeability in the toad urinary bladder. J Clin Invest 1981; 67: 1792-1796.

Christiansen SC, Proud D, Cochrane CG: Detection of tissue kallikrein in the bronchoalveolar lavage fluid of asthmatic subjects. J Clin Invest 1987; 79: 188-197.

Cochrane CG, Revak SD, Wuepper KD: Activation of Hageman factor in solid liquid phases. A critical role of kallikrein. J exp Med 1973; 138: 1564-1583.

Colina-Chourio J, McGiff JC, Miller MP, et al.: Possible influence of intrarenal generation of kinins on prostaglandin release from the rabbit perfused kidney. Br J Pharmac 1976; 58: 165-172.

Colman RW, Bagdasarian A, Talamo RC, et al.: Williams trait: human kininogen deficiency with diminished levels of palsminogen pro activator and pre-kallikrein associated with abnormalities of the Hageman factor-dependent pathways. J Clin Invest 1975; 56: 1650-1662.

Croxatto HR, Martin M: Kallikrein-like activity in the urine of renal hypertensive rats. Experientia 1970; 26: 1261-1271.

Damas J, Bourdon V: Liberation d'acide arachidonique par la bradykinine. c.r. seanc Soc Biol 1974; 168: 1445-1448.

De Freitas FM, Farraco EZ, De Azevedo DF: General circulatory alterations induced by intravenous infusion of synthetic bradykinin in man. Circulation 1964; 29: 66-70.

Derkx FHM, Tan-Tjiong HL, Manint Veld AJ, et al.: Activation of inactive plasma reinin by tissue kallikreins. J Clin Endocrinol Metab 1979; 49: 765-769.

Edery H, Rosenthal T, Amitzur G, et al.: The influence of SQ 20881 on the blood kinin system of renal hypertensive patients. Drugs Exptl Clin Res 1981; VII: 749-756.

Elliot AH, Nuzum FR: Urinary excretion of a depressor substance (kallikrein of Frey and Kraut) in arterial hypertension. Endocrinology 1934; 18: 462-474.

Erdos EG, Sloane EM: An enzyme in human plasma that inactivated bradykinin and kallidin. Biochem Pharmac 1962; 11: 585-592.

Erdos EG, Skidgel RA: Structure and functions of human angiotensin I converting enzyme (kininase II) Biochem Soc Trans 1985; 13: 42-44.

Erdos EG, Yang H. YT: Inactivation and potentation of the effects of bradykinin. In Hypotensive Peptides (Edited by Erdos EG, Back N and Sicuteri F) Springer-Verlag Berlin 1966; pp. 235-250.

Erdos EG, Yang HYT: An enzyme in microsomal fraction of kidney that inactivates bradykinin. Life Sci 1967; 6: 569-574.

Erdos EG, Yang HYT, Tague LL, et al.: Carboxypeptidase in blood and other fluids III. The esterase activity of the enzyme. Biochem Pharmac 1967; 16: 1287-1297.

Fejes-Toth AN, Fejes-Totah G: Urinary kinin excretion following alterations of vasopressin levels in man and rat. Renal Physiol 1986; 9: 302-307.

Fejes-Toth G, Magyar A, Walter J: Renal response to vasopressin after inhibition of prostaglandin synthesis. Am J Physiol 1977; 232: F416-F423.

Fejes-Toth G, Zahajszky T, Filep J: Effect of vasopressin on the renal kallikrein-kinin system. Agents Actions (Suppl.) 1982; 9: 491-495.

Fernandez PG, Sharma JN, Kim BK, et al.: Left ventricular regression and blood pressure control of Dahl (D) rat with MK-42 1 (an angiotensin I converting enzyme inhibitor, CEI) and hydrochlorothiazide (HTZ) Clin Res 1983a; 31: 332A (Abst).

Fernandez PG, Kim BK, Sharma JN, et al.: Left ventricular regression (LVR) in association with blood pressure control in the Dahl model of hypertensive that (DS and DR) treated with enalapril maleate (MK-42l, an angiotensin converting enzyme inhibitor) or hydrochlorothiazide (HTZ). Clin Invest Med 1983b; 6: (Suppl 2), 55 (Abst.).

Ferreira SH, Moncada S, Vane JR: Indomethacin and aspirin abolish prostaglandin release from the spleen. Nature 1971; 231: 237-239.

Fiedler F: Enzymology of glandular kallikreins. In Handbook of Experimental Pharmacology (Edited by Erdos EG) Springer-Verlag, Berlin 1979; pp 103-161.

Fiedler F, Muller C, Warle E: Purification of prekallikrein B from pig pancreas with p-nitrophenyl-pguanidimobenzoate. FEBS Lett 1970; 24: 41-44.

Fink E, Geiger R, Witte J, et al.: Biochemical, pharmacological, and functional aspects of glandular kallikreims. In Enzyme Release of Vasoactive Peptides (Edited by Gross F and Vogel G) Raven Press, New York 1980; pp 101-115.

Frey EK: Zusammenhange Zwischen, et al: Langenbeck's Arch Klin Chir 1926;142: 663-669.

Furtado MRF: Inhibition of the permeability response to vasopressin and oxytocin in the toad bladder effects of bradykinin, kallidin, eleodoisin and physalaemin. J Membr Bioi 1981; 4: 165-168.

Gill JR, Frolich JC, Bowden RE, et al.: Bartter's Syndrome: a disorder characterized by high urinary prostaglandins and a dependence of hyperreninemia on prostaglandin synthesis. Am J Med 1976; 61: 43-51.

Gryglewski RJ, Bunting S, Moncada S: Arterial walls are protected against deposition of platelet thrombi by a substance (prostaglandin X) which they make from prostaglandin endoperoxides. Prostaglandins 1976; 12: 685-714.

Halushka PV, Wohltman H, Privitero PJ, et al.: Bartter's Syndrome: urinary prostaglandin E-like material and kallikrein; indomethacin effects. Ann Inter Med 1977; 87: 281-286.

Handa M, Kondo K, Suzuki H: Urinary prostaglandin E_2 and kallikrein excretion in glucocorticoid hypertension in rats. Clin Sci 1983; 65: 37-42.

Hathaway WE, Alsever J: The relation of "Fletcher factor" to factors XI and XII. Hr. J Haemat 1970;18:161-169.

Hiwada K, Matsumoto C, Kokubu T: Role of glandular kallikrein in the activation process of human plasma inactive renin. Hypertension 1983; 5: 191-197.

Hoyashi M, Senba S, Saito I, et al.: Changes in blood pressure, urinary kallikrein, and urinary prostaglandin Ez in rats with streptozotocin-induced diabetes. Naunyn-Schmiedebergs Arch. Pharmac 1983; 322: 290-294.

Hong SL, Levine L: Stimulation of prostaglandin synthesis by bradykinin and thrombin and their mechanisms of action on MC5-5 fibroblasts. J bioi Chem 1976; 251: 5814-5816.

Horwitz D, Margolius HS, Keiser HR: Effect of dietary potassium and race on urinary excretion on kallikrein and aldosterone in man. J Clin Endocrinol Metab 1978; 47: 269-299.

Hrol WH, Schafer RM, Heidland A: Role of a-antitrypsin in padutin (kallikrein) inactivation. Eur. J Clin Pharmac 1982; 22: 541-544.

Jacobsen S: Substrate for plasma kinin-forming enzymes in human, dog and rabbit plasma. Hr. J Pharmac 1966; 26: 403-411.

James FW, Donaldson VH: Decreased exercise tolerance and hypertension in severe hereditary deficiency of plasma kininogens. Lancet 1981; 1: 889.

Kahl LK, Heine M, Tassinar L: Role of genetic factors in susceptibility to experimental to experimental hypertension due to chronic excess salt ingestion.Nature 1962; 194: 480-482.

Kaplan AP, Austen KF: A prealbumin activator of prekallikrein II. Derivation of activators of prekallikrein from active Hageman factory by digestion with plasmin. J expo Med 1971;133: 696-712.

Kaplan AP, Silverberg M, Dunn JT, et al.: Mechanisms for Hageman factor activation and role of HMW kininogen as a coagulation cofactor. Ann NY Acad Sci 1981; 370: 253-260.

Kaplan AP, Meiler HL, Yecies D, et al.: Hageman factor and its substrates: the role of factor XI, prekallikrein, and plasminogen proactivator in coagulation, fibrinolysis and kinin generation. In Chemistry and Biology of the Kallikrein-Kinin System in Health and Disease (Edited by Pisano JJ and Austen KF) U.S Government Printing Office Washington D.C 1977; pp. 237-254.

Katz J, Williams GH, Hollenberg NK: Plasma concentration and the depressor response to bradykinin infusion. Life Sri 1980; 27: 573-576.

Komiya M, Kato H, Suzuki T: Structural comparison of high molecular weight and low molecular weight kininogen. J. Biochem. Tokyo 1974; 76: 833-845.

Lacombe MJ, Varet B, Levy JP: A hitherto undescribed plasma factor acting at the contact phase of blood coagulation (Flaujeac factor) case report and coagulation studies. Blood 1975; 46: 761-768.

Lawton WJ, Proud D, French ME, et al.: Characterization and origin of immunoreactive glandular kallikrein in rat plasma. Hiochem Pharmac 1981; 30: 1731-1737.

Lechi A, Covi G, Lechi C, et al.: Urinary kallikrein excretion and plasma renin activity in patients with essential hypertension and primary aldosteronism. Clin SciMolec Med 1978; 55: 51-55.

Lechi A, Covi G, Lechi C, et al.: Urinary kallikrein excretion in Bartter's syndrome. J Clin Endocr Metab 1976; 43: 1175-1178.

Levy SB, Lilley JJ, Frigon RP: Urinary kallikrein and plasma renin activity as determinants of renal blood flow; the influence of race and dietary sodium intake. J Clin Invest 1977; 60: 129-138.

MacFarlane NAA, Mills IH, Wraight EP: Changes in kallikrein excretion during arterial infusion of angiotensin. J Endocr 1974; 61: 72P.

Margolius HS, Geller R, deJong W, et al.: Altered urinary kallikrein excretion in rat with hypertension. Circulation Res 1972; 30: 358-362.

Margolius HS, Geller R, Pisano JJ, et al.: Altered urinary kallikrein excretion in human hypertension. Lancet 1971; 2: 1063-1065.

Margolius HS, Horwitz D, Pisano JJ, et al.: Urinary kallikrein excretion in hypertensive man: relationships to sodium intake and sodiumretaining steroids. Circulation Res 1974; 35: 820-825.

Marchetti J, Imbert-Teboul M, Alhenc-Gelas F, et al.: Kallikrein along the rabbit microdissected nephron: a micromethod for its measurement, effect ofadrenalectomy and DOCA treatment. Pfiiigers Arch. ges Physiol 1984; 401: 27-33.

Marin-Grez M: Multihormone regulation of renal kallikrein. Biochem Pharmac 1982; 31: 3941-3947.

Marin-Grez M, Schaechtelin G, Bonner G: Relationship between the renal kallikrein activity and the urinary excretion of kallikrein in rats. Experientia 1982; 38: 941-943.

Maxwell GM, Elliott RB, Kneebone GM: Effect of bradykinin on systemic and coronary vascular bed on intact dog. Circulation Res 1962; 10: 359-365.

Moore Jr J, Gagnon J A, Verma PR., Sander SE, et al.: Plasma kinin levels in acute renovascular hypertension in dogs. Renal Physiol 1984; 7: 102-114.

Murakami E, Hiwada K, Kokubu T: Effect of prostaglandins on renin substrate production by the liver. Clin Sci 1980; 59: 137s-139s.

McGiff JC, Terragno NA, Malik KU, et al.: Release of a prostaglandin E-like substance from canine kidney by bradykinin: comparison with eledoisin. Circulation Res 1972; 31: 36-43.

McGiff JC, Itskovitz HD, Terragno NA: The action of bradykinin and eledoisin in the canine isolated kidney; relationship to prostaglandins. Clin Sci Molec Med 1975; 49: 125-131.

McGiff JC, Itskovitz HD, Terrango A, et al.: Modulation and mediation of the renal kallikrein-kinin system by prostaglandins. Fedn Proc Fedn Am Socs expo Biol 1976; 35: 175-180.

Miller MJS, Westlin WF, McNeill H, et al.: Renal prostaglandin efflux induced by vasopressin, dDA VP and arachidonic acid: contrasting profile and sites of release. Clin expo Pharmac Physiol 1986a;13: 577-584.

Mills IH: Kallikrein, kininogen and kinin in control of blood pressure. Nephron 1979; 23: 61-71.

Mills IH: The renal kallikrein-kinin system and sodium excretion. Q. J expo Physiol 1982; 67: 393-399.

Mills IH, MacFarlane NAA, Adetuyibi A: On the role of kallikrein in the renal adaptation to intra-arterial infusion of angiotensin II. Excerpta Med Int Congr 1976; Ser No 256: 586 (Abst.).

Miller MJS, Carrara MC, Westlin WF, et al.: (l986b) Compartmental prostaglandin release by angiotensin II and arginine-vasopressin in rabbit isolated perfused kidneys. Eur. J Pharmac 1986b; 120: 43-50.

Mitas JA, Levy SB, Holle R, et al.: Urinary kallikrein activity in the hypertension of renal parachymal disease. New Engl. J Med 1978; 299: 162-165.

Nagasawa S, Nakayasu T: Enzymatic and chemical cleavages of human kininogens. Life Sci 1975; 16: 791-792.

Nasjletti A, Colina-Chourio J, McGiff JC: Disappearance of bradykinin in the renal circulation of dogs. Circulation Res 1975; 37: 59-65.

Nasjletti A, McGiff JC, Colina-Chourio J: Interrelationships of the renal kallikrein-kinin system and renal prostaglandins in the conscious rat. Circulation Res 1978; 43: 799-807.

Nustad K: Relationship between kidney and urinary kininogenases. Br J Pharmac 1970; 39: 73-86.

Nustad K, Gautvik K, Ørstavik T: Radioimmunoassay of rat submandibular gland kallikrein and the detection of immuno-reactive antigen in blood. In The Kinins II, Biochemistry, Pathophysiology and Clinical Aspects (Edited by Fujii S, Moriya H and Suzuki T) Plenum Press, New York 1979; pp 225-234.

Nustad K, Vaaje K, Pierce JV: Synthesis of kallikrein by rat kidney slices. Br J Pharmac 1975; 53: 229-234.

O'Connor DT, Barg AP, Amend W, et al.: Urinary kallikrein excretion after transplantation:relationship to hypertension, graft source and renal function. Am J Med 1982; 73: 475-481.

Olsen UB: Clonidine decreases rat urine kallikrein excretion by a-adrenergic receptor stimulation. Eur. J Pharmac 1982; 79: 311-314.

Olsen UB: Changes of urinary kallikrein and kinin excretions induced by adrenalin infusion in conscious dogs. Scand. J Clin Lab Invest 1980; 40: 173-178.

Oshima G, Kato J, Erdos EG: Subunits of human plasma carboxypeptidase N (kininase I; anaphylatoxin inactivator). Biochim. biophys Acta 1974; 365: 344-348.

Østravik TB: The kallikrein-kinin system in exocrine organs. J. Histochem. Cytochem 1981; 28: 881-889.

Ørstavik TB, Gautvik KM: Regulation of salivary kallikrein secretion in thesubmandibular gland. Acta physiol scand 1977; 100: 33-44.

Ørstavik T. B, Nustad K, Brandtzaeg P, et al.: Cellular orginine of urinary kallikreins. J. Histochem Cytochem 1976; 24: 1037-1039.

Overlack A, Stumpe KO, Ressel C, et al.: Decreased urinary kallikrein activity and elevated blood pressure normalized by orally applied kallikrein in essential hypertension. Klin. Wsch 1980; 58: 37-40.

Overlack A, Stumpe KO, Kollock R, et al.: Antihypertensive effect of orally administered glandular kallikrein in essential hypertension. Hypertension 1981; 3: 118-121.

Palmer MA, Piper PJ, Vane JR: Release of rabbit aorta contracting substances (RCS) and prostaglandins induced by chemical or mechanical stimulation of guinea pig lungs. Br. J Pharmac 1973; 49: 226-242.

Pierce JV, Guimaraes JA: Further characterization of highly purified human plasma kininogen. Life Sci 1975; 16: 790-791.

Prado ES, Carvalho LPD, Araujo-Viel MS, et al.: A met-enkephalin-containingpeptide, Bam 22P, as a novel substrate for glandular kallikreins. Biochem. biophys. Res Commun 1983; 1l2: 366-371.

Rabito SF, Ørstavik TB, Scicli AG, et al.: Role of the autonomic nervous system in the release of rat submandibular gland kallikrein into the circulation. Circulation Res 1983; 52: 635-641.

Rabito SF, Scicli AG, Kher V, et al.: Glandular kallikrein in plasma and urine: evaluation of a direct RIA for its determination In The Kinins II, Biochemistry, Pathophysiology and Clinical Aspects (Edited by Fujii S, Moriya H and Suzuki T) 1979; pp 127-142.Plenum Press, New York.

Rabito SF, Scicli AG, Kher V, et al.: Immunoreactive glandular kallikrein in rat plasma: a radioimmunoassay for its determination. Am. J Physiol 1982; 242: H602-H610.

Saito H, Ratnoff OD, Donaldson VH: Defective aclivation of clotting, fibrinolytic, and permeability enhancing system in human Fletcher trait plasma. Circulation Res 1974; 34: 641-651.

Saito H, Ratnoff OD, Waldmann R, et al.: Fitzgerald trait. Deficiency of a hitherto unrecognized agent, Fitzgerald factor, participating in surface mediated reactions of clotting, fibrinolysis, generation of kinins, and the property of diluted plasma enhancing vascular permeability (PF/dil). J Clin Invest 1975; 55: 1082-1089.

Salgado MCO, Rabito SF, Carretero OA: Blood kinin in one-kidney, one clip hyertensive rats. Hypertension 1986; 8: 1110-1113.

Schachter M: Kallikrein (kininogenases) a group of serine pro teases with biological actions. Pharmac. Rev 1980; 31: 1-17.

Scicli AG, Carretero OA: Renal kallikreinkinin system. Kidney Int 1986; 29: 120-130.

Scicli AG, Carretero OA, Hampton A, et al.: Site of kininogenase secretion in the dog nephron. Am. J Physiol 1976; 230: 533-536.

Sealey JE, Atlas SA, Laragh JH, et al.: Human urinary kallikrein converts inactive to active renin and is a possible physiological activator of renin. Nature 1978; 275: 144-145.

Sharma JN: Kinin-forming system in the genesis of hypertension. Agents Actions 1984; 14: 200-205.

Sharma JN, Buchanan WW: Kinin system in clinical and experimental rheumatoid inflammation. Curro Med Res Optimum 1979; 6: 314-321.

Sharma JN, Zeitlin IJ, Brooks PM, et al.: A novel relationship between plasma kininogen and rheumatoid disease. Agents Actions 1976; 6: 148-153.

Sharma JN, Zeitlin IJ, Brooks PM, et al.: The action of asprin on plasma kininogen and other proteins in rheumatoid patients: relationship to disease activity. Clin expo Pharmac Physiol 1980; 7: 347-354.

Sharma JN, Zeitlin IJ: Altered plasma kininogen in clinical hypertension. Lancet 1981; 1: 1259-1260.

Sharma JN, Zeitlin IJ: Reduced plasma kininogen concentrated by prostaglandin E2 in rats. Eur. J Pharmac 1982; 83: 119-121.

Sharma JN, Zeitlin IJ, Deodhar SD, et al.: Detection of kallikrein-like activity in inflamed synovial tissue. Arch. into Pharmacody. Ther 1983a; 262: 279-286.

Sharma JN, Fernandez PG: Pharmacological abnormality of kallikrein-kinin system in hypertension. Med Hypoth 1982; 9: 379-384.

Sharma JN, Fernandez PG, Kim BK, et al.: Cardiac regression and blood pressure control in the Dahl rat treated with enalpril maleate (MK 421, an angiotensin converting enzyme inhibitor) and hydrochlorothiazide. J Hypertension 1983b; 1: 251-256.

Sharma JN, Fernandez PG, Triggle CR: The effect of indomethacin on the duration of the hypotensive action of bradykinin in Dahl salt-resistant rats: role of cyclo-oxygenase inhibition. Prost. Leukotri Med 1984a; 14: 131-135.

Sharma JN, Fernandez PG, Kim BK, et al.: Systolic blood pressure responses to enalapril maleate (MK 421, an angiotensin converting enzyme inhibitor) and hydrochlothiazide in conscious Dahl saltsensitive (S) and salt-resistant (R) rats. Can. J Physiol Pharmac 1984b; 62: 846-849.

Sharma JN, Fernandez PG, Laher I, et al.: Defferential sensitivity of Dahl salt-sensitive and salt-resistant rats to the hypotensive action of acute nifedipine administration. Can. J Physiol Pharmac 1984c; 62: 241-243.

Silberbauer K, Stanek B, Temple H: Acute hypotensive effect of captopril in man modified by prostaglandin synthesis inhibition. Br. J Clin Pharmac 1982; 14: 87S-93S.

Sustarsic DL, McPartland RP, Rapp JP: Total and kallikrein arginine esterase activities in the urine of salt-hypertensive susceptible and resistant rats. Hypertension 1980; 2: 813-820.

Sustarsic DL, McPartland RP, Rapp JF: Developmental patterns of blood pressure and urinary protein, kallikrein, and prostaglandin E2 in Dahl salthypertensive susceptible rats. J Lab Cli. Med 1981; 98; 599-606.

Swartz SL, Williams GH, Hollenberg NK, et al.: Converting enzyme inhibition in essential hypertension: the hypotensive response does not reflect only reduced angiotensin II formation. Hypertension 1979; 1: 106-111.

Tsunoda K, Abe K, Ornata K, et al.: Hypotensive and natriuretic effects of nifedipine in essential hypertension. Role of renal kallikrein-kinin-prostaglandin and renin-angiotensinaldosterone systems. J Clin Hypertension 1986; 2: 263-270.

Vane JR, McGriff JC: Possible contributions of endogenous prostaglandins to the control of blood pressure. Circulation Res 1975; 36-37 (Suppl I) 163-175.

Vinci JM, Telles DA, Bowden RW, et al.: The kallikrein-kinin system (KKS) in Bartter's syndrome (BS) and its response to prostaglandin synthesis inhibition (PGSI). Clin Res 1976; 24: 414A.

Vinci JM, Zusman RM, Izzo JL, et al.: Human urinary and plasma kinins. Relationship to plasma sodium-retaining steroids and plasma renin activity. Circulation Res 1979; 44: 228-237.

Vinci JM, Zusman RM, Izzo JL, et al.: Human urinary and plasma kinins: relationship to sodium retaining steroids and plasma renin activity. Circulation Res 1979; 44: 228-237.

Vogel R: Kallikrein inhibitors. In Handbook of Experimental Pharmacology (Edited by Erdos G) Springer-Verlag, Berlin, Heidelberg, New York. Pp 1979; 163-225.

Webster ME, Gilmore JP: Influence of kallidin-10 on renal function. Am. J Physiol 1964; 206: 714-718.

Willis LR, Luden JH, Hook JB, et al: Mechanism of natriuretic action of bradykinin. Am. J Physiol 1969; 217: 1-5.

Wuepper KD, Miller KR, Lacombe MJ: Flaujeac trait deficiency of human plasma kininogen. J Clin Invest 1975; 56: 1663-1672.

Wuepper KD: Prekallikrein deficiency in man. J expo Med 1973; 138: 1345-1355.

Yang HYT, Erdos EG: Second kininase in human blood plasma. Nature 1967; 215: 1402-1403.

Yokosawa N, Takahashi N, Inagami T, et al.: Isolation of completely inactive plasma prorenin and its activation by kallikreins. Biochim. Biophys. Acta 1979; 569: 211-215.

Zeitlin IJ: Rat intestinal kallikrein. Adv. expo Med biol 1972; 21: 289-296.

Zeitlin IJ, Sharma JN, Brooks PM, et al.: Raised plasma kininogen levels in rheumatoid arthritis-response to therapy with non-steroidal antiinflammatory drugs. Adv. expo Med Biol 1976; 70: 335-343.

Zeitlin IJ, Sharma JN, Brooks PM, et al.: An effect of indomethacin on raised plasma kininogen levels in rheumatoid patients. In Chemistry and Biology of the Kallikrein-Kinin System in Health and Disease (Edited by Pisano JJ and Austen KF) US Government Printing Office, Washington DC. 1977 pp 483-486.

Zinner SH, Margolius HS, Rosener B, et al.: Stability of blood pressure rank and urinary kallikrein concentration in childhood: an eight-year follow-up. Circulation 1978; 58: 908-915.

Zinner SH, Margolius HS, Rosner B, et al.: Familiar aggregation of urinary kallikrein concentration in childhood. Am. J Epidemiol 1976; 104: 124-132.

Zusman RM, Keiser HR: Prostaglandin E2 biosynthesis by rabbit renomedullary interstitial cells in tissue culture. Mechanism of stimulation by angiotensin II, bradykinin, and arginine vasopressin. J Clin Invest 1977; 60: 215-233.

Chapter 3

The Role of Chemical Mediators in the Pathogenesis of Inflammation with Emphasis on the Kinin System

SUMMARY

In recent years numerous agents have been recognized as inflammatory mediators. In this review, however, we discuss only those having direct relevance to human inflammatory diseases (see table 3.1). These mediators are clinically important due to their proinflammatory properties such as vasodilation, increased vascular permeability, pain and chemotaxis. They may lead to the fifth cardinal sign, loss of function in inflammatory diseases. Agonists and non-specific antagonists are used as pharmacological tools to investigate the inflammatory role of PGs, LTs, PAP. IL-I. histamine, complement, SP, PMN-leukocytes, and kallikrein-kininogen-kinin systems. Unfortunately, no compound is known which concurrently abolishes all actions and interactions of inflammatory mediators. Therefore it would be highly useful to promote efforts in developing selective and competitive antagonists against pro-inflammatory actions of these chemical mediators. This may help to a better understanding of the pathogenesis of inflammatory reactions, and it may also be useful for the therapy of inflammatory diseases.

INTRODUCTION

Inflammation is a complex sequence of events termed as phlogosis by the Greeks and as inflammatio by the Romans. The four cardinal signs of inflammation including redness (rubor), swelling (tumor), pain (dolor), and heat (calor) were described by Celsus in A. D. 178. It is purported that Galen (A. D. 130-200) added loss of function (functio laesa) as fifth cardinal symptom (Rather 1971). The major contribution of inflammatory mediators in the genesis of inflammatory diseases is recognized via three convincing lines of investigation: by endogenous agents administered exogenously by release of chemical substances in various types of inflammatory processes, and by the special antagonizing action of anti-inflammatory drugs. The mediators are products of arachidonic acid metabolites (prostaglandins and leukotrienes), histamine, serotonin, substance P, components of the kallikrein-kinin system, leukokinin, interleukins, and the complement system. Hageman factor (HF), lysosomal constituents and endothelial derived-factors. These endogenous agents are implicated in the response of organisms to noxious stimuli.

Although extensive in vitro investigations implicate these mediators and modulators in inflammatory reactions, relatively few in vivo studies demonstrate their specific pathophysiological roles and pharmacological mechanisms. However, it seems that the actions of these mediators during the early phase of local inflammatory reactions contribute to the destruction of noxious substance. Nonetheless, sustained release at levels above the physiological requirement may lead to production of anaphylactic shock as well as joint and bowel inflammatory diseases (Sharma 1988 a; Sharma et al. 1988). This paper is intended to critically review the mediators of inflammation with special emphasis on the kallikrein-kinin system and arachidonic acid metabolites in chronic inflammatory conditions.

ARACHIDONIC ACID METABOLITES

Arachidonic acid (AA) can be metabolized into a spectrum of biologically active eicosanoids via the lipooxygenase, cyclooxygenase and cytochrome P450-dependent monooxygenase pathways. Prostaglandins (PGs) constitute a family of 20-carbon polyunsaturated acids whose initial synthesis involves the release of the precursor from phospholipids of the cell membrane due to the action of an enzyme known as phospholipase A_2 (Flower and Blackwell 1976). The cyclooxygenase pathway converts AA into transient endoperoxidase, e.g. PGH_2, or PGG_2- PGH_2 is converted by enzymatically-catalyzed reactions into several biologically active products.

These products are known as PGD_2, PGE_2, PGF_2', thromboxane A_2 (TXA_2) and prostacyclin (PGI_2) (Hamberg et al. 1975; Hamberg and Samuelsson 1973). The lipooxygenase pathway converts AA into 5-hydroperoxyeicosatetraenoic acid (5-HPETE) and 5-monohydroxyeicosatetraenoic acid (5-HETE). They are produced along with leukotrienes (LTs) (Murphy et al. 1979). Most recently cytochrome P450-dependent epoxygenase has been established as a pathway which metabolizes AA into pharmacologically active agents termed epoxides and diols (Caroll et al. 1987). The pharmacologically active products of AA metabolites are summarized in Figure 3.1.

Table 3.1. Survey of Mediator's Effects

Mediators	Proinflama-tory effects	Mediation of pain	Induction of fever	Vascular permeability changes	Oedema formation	Vascular tone	Platelet aggregation	Chemotactic properties	Stimulation of other mediators	Smooth muscle contraction
Arachidonic acid metabolites										
PGE2	+	+	+							+
PGE1	+	+	+							+
TXB2	+	?	?	?	?	+	+	+		
PGI2	+					+		?		+
LTB4	+	+		+				+		+
LTC4		+		+	+		+			+
LTD4	+			+	+					+
LTE4				+	+					+
Serotonin	+			+	+	+			+	+
Histamin	+	+		+		+				+
Interleukin-I	+		+	+(via PMNs)			+(in vivo)			+
Platelet activating factor (PAF)	+			+	+			+ (in vitro)	+	+

Table 3.1.(Continued)

Mediators	Proinflama-tory effects	Mediation of pain	Induction of fever	Vascular permeability changes	Oedema formation	Vascular tone	Platelet aggregation	Chemotactic properties	Stimulation of other mediators	Smooth muscle contraction
Complement system: C5a&C5a des Arg.	+			+				+		?
C3a				+		+			+	
Kinin system	+	+		+	+	+			+	+
Substance P	+	+		+		+			+	+

Each of the cells (platelets, macrophages, lymphocytes, and neutrophils) of acute and chronic inflammationis capable of transforming AA into biologically active compounds, e.g. PGs, PGI_2, TXA_2 and LTs (Movat 1985). The ability of various cells to produce the metabolites of AA cannot be considered in detail; however, a few examples of the complexities are examined as potential cellular sources of PGs and LTs at the site of inflammation. PGD_2 and LTs are the prime products of AA in the mast cells (Lewis and Austen 1981). Polymorphonuclear (PMN) neutrophils are able to generate metabolites of AA such as LTB_4 (Payan et al. 1984). It is demonstrated that AA stimulates human PMN degranulation with cytosolic free calcium and protein kinase C appearing to be two components of the signal transduction system coupled to the activation pathway (Smith et al. 1987).

During inflammatory reactions phospholipase A_2, is released from leukocytes, which may release AA from membrane bound phospholipids to produce various PGs (Johnston et al. 1979).

The source of high PGE_2 level probably are macrophages or synoviocytes type A with their release stimulated by interleukin-1 in synovial fluid obtained from rheumatoid patients (Daymond and Rowell 1988).

Products of the cyclooxygenase pathway. e.g. PGE_2 and PGI_2 play a central role in the expression of inflammatory response by acting as mediators in producing pain, fever, increased vascular permeability and oedema (Zeitlin 1981: Larsen and Henson 1983; Lewis 1983) and as mediators of several types of lymphocytic and phagocytic cell function (Davis et al. 1984). Indeed, the mode of action of non-steroidal anti-inflammatory drugs (NSAIDs) is currently accepted to bedue to inhibition of biosynthesis of these products (Ferreira and Vane 1979; Sharma and Buchanan 1980).

Using 85Sr-microspheres to measure skin blood flow in the guinea pig, rat and rabbit, a positive correlation is observed between the degree of hyperemia produced by PGs and the degree of the increased vascular permeability in the presence of histamine, serotonin or kinin (Johnston et al. 1976; Williams and Peck 1977). These investigators suggest that PGs may directly mimic the hyperemia of the inflammatory process and modulate the changes in vascular permeability caused by other inflammatory mediators. Thus, the most important action of PGE_2 and PGI_2 in inflammation is the induction of vasodilation and enhancing blood flow. In addition, PGs are capable of inducing most of the signs (for review see Weissmann 1980), and their raised concentrations are observed in various inflammatory diseases. Elevated levels of PGE_2 are detected consistently in the inflamed rectal mucosa and colonic venous plasma of patients with ulcerative colitis (Harris et al. 1978; Gould et al. 1977; Pacheco et al. 1987), as well as in a guinea pig model of immune colitis (Norris et al. 1982). In rats PGE_2 and PGF_2 treatment produces inflammatory bowel disease characterized by severe diarrhoea, passage of blood and loss of body weight (Sharma 1983).

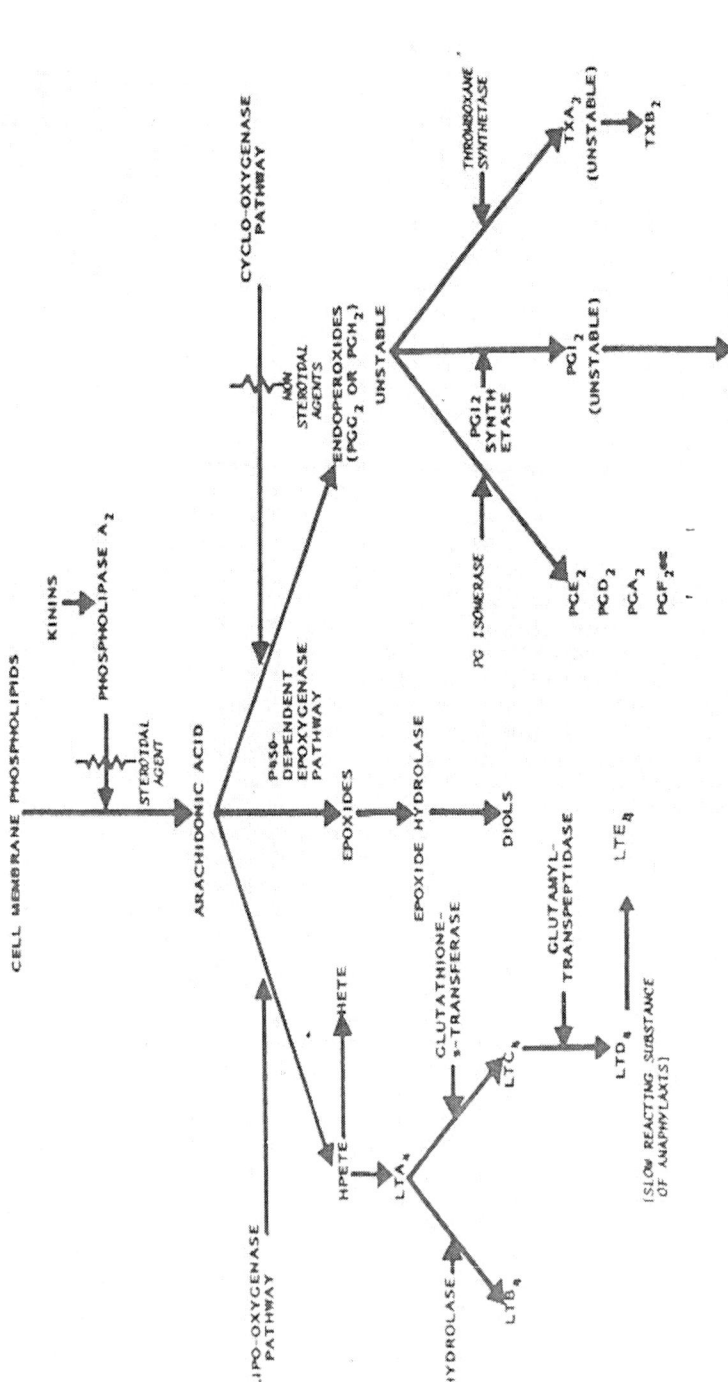

Figure 3.1.A schematic presentation of the release of inflammatory mediators from 3 main pathways of arachidonic acid metabolism. Stimulation or conversion (→): inactivation or inhibition (⤳).

Prostaglandins are detected in human synovial fluids collected from inflamed joints, and concentrations are reduced after treatment with NSAIDs (Higgs et al. 1974; Robinson and Levine 1974). Tissue cultures taken from rheumatoid synovitis are able to generate PGs, too (Robinson et al. 1975; Struge et al. 1978). Furthermore, synovial effusions from rheumatoid joints are reported to contain TXB_2 and 6-keto-PGF_1 (the stable product of PGI_2) (Brodie et al. 1980; Salmon et al.1983). It is demonstrated that the injection of AA into the hind limb of rat induces a rapid and severe inflammation which is inhibited by corticosteroids but not by aspirin-like drugs (Dimarline et al. 1987 a). The role of thromboxanes in inflammation is poorly understood. While TXA_2 is a vasoconstrictor and an aggregator of platelets (Moncada and Vane 1979) TXB_2, is found to have chemotactic action on leukocytes (Kitchen et al. 1978). It seems probable; therefore, that thromboxane may antagonize the actions of PGI_2 in reducing platelets aggregation in an inflamed area. Further studies on the effects of TXB_2, in a chronic inflammatory model may help usunderstand the significance of this agent in inflammation.

The leukotrienes released from many cells following both non-immunological and immunological stimuli, have a wide spectrum of biological activity (Voelker et al. 1982; Lewis and Austen 1981). Leukotrienes B_4, C_4 are active at sub-nanogram concentrations which can account for some of the clinical symptoms associated with inflammatory diseases (Ford-Hutchinson and Letts 1986; Smith et al. 1980; Samuelsson 1983; Smith 1981). Increase in vascular permeability induced by LTB_4 is mediated by polymorphonuclear leukocytes (PMNLs) as observed by Bjork et al. (1982). This mechanism enhances the tissue damage when complement activation induces intravascular neutrophil aggregation caused by LTB_4 (Ringertz et al. 1982). Further, LTB_4 produces hyperalgesia which is dependent on PMNLs (Levine et al. 1984), and is potently chemotactic toward PMNL in rabbits (Bray et al. 1981; Higgs et al. 1981) and in man (Camp et al. 1983; Soter et al. 1983). LTB_4 and PGE_2 are demonstrated in the inflamed skin of the rabbit after, intradermal injection of AA (Aked and Foster 1987) where both these eicosanoids are rapidly synthesized.

In the synovial fluid of patients with gout (RAE et al. 1982) or rheumatoid arthritis (Davidson et al. 1982) high concentrations of LTB_4 are measured. —LTC_4, LTD_4 and LTE_4 are shown to induce whealing and prolonged flares in human skin, whereas LTB_4 causes a time-dependent induration (Lewis et al. 1982). LTB_4 is implicated in the pathogenesis of bowel inflammation in man (Sharon and Stenson 1984; Lauritsen et al. 1986) and in experimentally induced colitis in animals (Sharon and Stenson 1985; Zipser et al) 1987).

Recently, Lauritsen et al. (1987) observed significantly raised concentrations of PGE_2 and LTB_4 in the rectal dialysates of patients with relapsing ulcerative proctitis. Vitamin E administration, however, fails to alter the PGE_2 and LTH_2 levels in these patients. Both lipooxygenase and cyclooxygenase products of AA metabolism are implicated in acute and chronic inflammatory conditions including rheumatoid arthritis (Davidson 1983). An enormous research effort is aimed towards the discovery and development of LTs biosynthetic antagonists. The next few years should indicate whether these agents will have therapeutic value in inflammatory diseases.

HISTAMINE

Since the discovery of histamine by Sir Henry Dale at the beginning of this century the multiple functions of this amine as a chemical mediator during immunological release from the mast cells have been progressively revealed. The action of histamine is mediated via distinct subclasses of receptors, the H_1, H_2 (Black et al. 1972) and H_3 (Arrang et al. 1987; Ishikawa and Sperelakis 1987) receptors.

Histamine release from mast cells and basophil leukocytes is due to the interactions of an antigen with membrane bound immunoglobulin gamma E (IgE) antibody. IgE is secreted by plasma cells in response to the first appearance of an antigen. The IgE becomes fixed to receptors on the surface of mast cells. When the antigen is again encountered, epitopes on an antigen molecule are bound by two adjacent IgE molecules.

The bridging of the IgE molecule initiates a process whereby the mast cell is degranulated, and its chemical mediators of inflammation are released (Lewis and Austen 1981; Tang 1980). Histamine is a potent vasodilator as well as an agent increasing vascular permeability, and it can effectively cause pain and itch (Rocha E Silva 1978).

However, it has a very short lasting effect. Moreover, while histamine induces increase in vascular permeability, it is less potent than Platelet Activating Factor (PAF) (Humphrey et al. 1984). These authors demonstrate both an immediate and a prolonged vascular leakage lasting up to 1 h. PAF known as acetyl glyceryl ether phosphorylcholine (AGEPC) is 1,000 to 10,000 fold more potent than histamine in producing the immediate vascular permeability, and this is not PMNdependent, despite the leukotactic effect of AGEPC. This substance is present in many tissues and is released in most types of inflammation. H2-receptors subserving the vasoactive actions of histamine are reported to be present in the synovial vasculature of canine (Grennan et al. 1977). It is also shown that cimetidine (H_2-receptor antagonist), but not mepyramine (H_1-receptor antagonist) significantly reduces paw swelling during adjuvant-induced arthritis in rats (A_1-Haboubi and Zeitlin 1982, 1983). These findings may suggest that the production of adjuvant arthritis may be mediated by the pro-inflammatory effect of histamine on H_2-receptors. Studies on the release of biologically active agents during carrageenan inflammation revealed that histamine, kinins and PGE_2 are released sequentially (Willis 1969) whereas Capasso et al. (1975) observed a large amount of histamine in carrageenan induced pleural inflammation. Furthermore, the possible involvement of histamine H_2-receptor activation is indicated in the genesis of carrageenan-induced rat paw inflammation (Al-Haboubi and Zeitlin 1983). It is of great interest to note that histamine is not only a pro-inflammatory agent, but also an anti-inflammatory substance in higher doses (2-10 mg/kg) (SAEKI et al. 1976). These investigations suggest that histamine may inhibit the development of adjuvant arthritis by an immunosuppressive mechanism through activation of H_2,-receptors on lymphoid cells. Nevertheless, mast cells are found in high amount in rheumatoid synovial membrane (Norton and Ziff 1966), and histamine and its converting enzyme (histidine decarboxylase) are formed in the inflamed synovial membrane (Roth et al. 1964). Histamine content is found to be raised in colonic tissue taken from the guinea pig model of immune colitis (Norris et al. 1982). It is concluded that measurement of both histamine and its metabolites may be essential to the understanding of the role of histamine in pathological states (Green et al. 1987), just as measurement of the metabolites of other biogenic amines is critical to understanding their functions in diseases.

The role of newly discovered H3-receptors of histamine in the pathophysiology of inflammation remains to be elucidated. It would not be surprising to find that this inflammatory mediator could modulate immunity, since histaminergic receptors are non-randomly distributed on lymphocytes (cp. review by Melmon and Khan 1987).

INTERLEUKIN-1

Interleukin-1 (IL-1) is a group of proteins derived from monocytes, macrophages and synovial cells which mediate important regulatory functions between leukocytes in the immune system. It can produce a variety of reactions that are observed in the genesis of acute as well as chronic inflammation (Dinarello 1984; Miossec 1987). IL-1 is implicated in immunological reactions. In these reactions it is known as lymphocyte activating factor (LAF) whereas in fever it is defined as endogenous pyrogen (EP). IL-1 is also shown to be involved in inflammatory reactions particularly in mediating endotoxin-induced inflammation, disseminated intravascular coagulation and certain phenomena of gram negative sepsis. There are many reports on IL-1 and tumor necrosis factor (TNF) in the literature, among others, concerning their synergistic action. The role in inflammation is reviewed extensively by Cybulsky et al. (1988). It is suggested that IL-I stimulates synthesis of PGs, collagenase, plasminogen activator, proteoglycanase, bone reabsorption (Benjamin et al. 1985) and cartilage erosion or degradation, too (O'Byme et al. 1987; Arner et al. 1987). The isolation of an IL-I-like factor in joint effusions from patients with rheumatoid arthritis (Nouri et al. 1984; Wood et al. 1983) and in macrophages of rats with adjuvant arthritis (Dimartino et al. 1987) suggests its role in the initiation of destruction of connective tissue and cartilage seen in rheumatic diseases. Raineord (1987) demonstrated that NSAIDs may cause reduction in IL-1 levels of the porcine synovial tissue. Furthermore, the generation of AA metabolites may be modulated or mediated via IL-1 within the synovial tissue. Moreover, the addition of human IL-I to cultured rheumatoid synovial cells cause dose-related increase in PGE formation (Taylor et al. 1988).

Recently it has been reported that IL-1 treatment causes activation of phospholipase A_2, (an enzyme involved in PGs production) in rabbit chondrocytes (Chang et al. 1986: Gilman et al. 1987). These authors propose that the activation of phospholipase A_2 is the main action of IL-1 in inducing inflammatory responses. Kaushansky et al. (1988) showed that IL-I stimulates fibroblasts to synthesize macrophage and granulocyte colony-stimulating factors which may be the mechanisms of the haematopoietic response to inflammation. Recently attention is paid to a more specific interaction with IL-I using IL-I analogues, specific anti-IL-1 receptors or IL-I inhibitors (see review by Martin and Resch 1988).

Platelet Activating Factor (PAL) or Acetyl Glyceryl Ether Phosphoryl Choline (AGEPC)

For several years AGEPC has been known as a chemical mediator which can induce release from platelets. It is characterized and named as PAF by Benveniste et al. (1972). The properties of the PAF released in vitro, and in vivo are compatible with an ether phospholipid (Benveniste et al. 1977). Subsequently PAF is synthesized and found to be an endogenous, phospholipid which is identified as 1-O-alkyl-2-sn-glycerol-3-phosphocholine having biological activity similar to naturally generated PAF (Demopoulos et al. 1979; Snyder 1985).

PAF is considered as a potent mediator in both allergy and inflammatory responses. It is synthesized by a variety of cell types including platelets, macrophages, leukocytes and endothelial cells (Braquet et al. 1987).

The intradermal injection of PAF into the rat is followed by increased vascular permeability, oedema, vascular lesion, and thrombosis (Martins et al. 1987; Pirotzky et al. 1984). Similar proinflammatory actions of PAF are noticed in the rabbit (Humphrey et al. 1982, 1984). Intradermal administration of PAF to humans can induce a biphasic inflammatory response characterized by acute and late-onset components (Archer et al. 1984). PAF causes PMNL chemotaxis and degranulation in vitro (Gortzl et al. 1980), and when injected into human skin it produces accumulation of PMNL and mononuclear cells (Archer et al. 1985).

High concentration of PAF is present in the synovial fluid of adjuvant-induced arthritis in the rabbit (Pettipher et al. 1987) causing joint inflammation and leukocyte infiltration. Therefore, it is possible that PAF may play an important role in attracting inflammatory cells into the clinical arthritic joint with erosion and swelling being produced. Hence, the experimental model of antigen-induced arthritis in the rabbit is an appropriate model to search for the role of PAF in the pathogenesis of erosion of bone and cartilage observed in rheumatoid arthritis (Sharma 1977; Sharma and Sharma 1977; Dumond. and Glynn 1962). It is suggested that PAF is involved in the genesis of inflammatory skin disorders, such as psoriasis; PAF is detected in psoriatic scales (Ramesha et al. 1987: Mallet and Cunningham 1985) and is responsible for the maintenance of the pathological process. Furthermore, the synthesis of PAF initially involves the activation of phospholipase A_2, resulting in the formation of lyso-PAF from membrane phospholipids (Albert and Snyder 1983). This enzyme is responsible for the release of PGs and LTs which are powerful inflammatory mediators.

Indeed, it is possible that the release of PAF could be accompanied by PGs, LTs, IL-1 and kinins production at the inflammatory site. In the anaphylactic phase of allergic air pouch inflammation in rats, lyso-PAF concentrations in the pouch fluid are significantly raised as compared to normal rats (Watanabe el al. 1987). This suggests that PAF might play a relevant role in causing allergic inflammation. Furthermore, topical application of PAF, LTB_4, or substance P causes leukocyte migration and leukocyte-dependent extravasation of macromolecules in the rabbit and in the hamster (Thureson-Klein et al. 1987). These authors stated that substance P is proved to act as an effective pro-inflammatory substance in the golden hamster cheek pouch preparation.

In recent years, numerous PAF antagonists were described (for review see Braquet et al. 1987). In this regard, these antagonists are classified into two groups. Firstly, the nonspecific inhibitors of PAF effects, which include drugs which interfere with intracellular calcium activities, modulation of cyclic nucleotides and phosphocholine esterase inhibitors (Issekutz and Szpejda 1986; Coeffier et al. 1986). Secondly, the specific inhibitors of PAF which are compounds derived from chemical modification of the PAF structure (Braquet et al. 1987). The clinical significance of these PAF antagonists has yet to be evaluated in chronic inflammatory diseases. E.g. rheumatoid arihritis.

COMPLEMENT SYSTEM

The complement system consists of 9 major components (C1 to C9) of plasma proteins which mediate cell membrane damage and cell lysis. Products of complement activation are responsible for increasing vascular permeability, enhancing phagocytosis, migration of PMNLS, damaging cell membrane and releasing several proinflammatory agents (histamine, PGs, LTs and kinins) (Regal et al. 1983; Regal and Bell 1987 Zeitlin and Grennan 1976; Regal 1987; Mullereberhard 1968).

The activation of the complement system can be brought about by two mechanisms: the classical and alternative or properdin pathways. The classical pathway is a complex of three subunits, Clq, C Ir „ and Cls, which are bound in the form of the macromolecule, CI, in the presence of calcium ions (Lepow et al. 1963). It has natural substrates termed as C4 and C2. Activation of CI by the antigen-antibody complex promotes its conversion into a proteolytic enzyme (CI) which reacts with two substrates (C4 and C2) to produce C42 (also called C3 convertase) (Mullereberhard et al. 1967). C3 convertase is an important enzyme, because it can cleave the third component (C3) into two critical fragments, C3a and C3b. In this way C3a is released into circulation, and C3b forms C423. Further, C423 reacts with C5 to produce C5a and C5b. C5b reacts with C6 and C7 to produce another complex termed C567. Additional binding of C567 with C8 and C9 produces C5b - 9 (lytic agent) (Hugli and Morgan 1984).

On the other hand, the alternative pathway is activated by polysaccharides produced by yeast or bacteria and during episodes of endotoxemia (Whaley et al. 1979).

C5a is known to induce histamine release from rat, guinea-pig and human basophils (Regal et al. 1983). In addition, Golden et al. (1987) have shown that C5a administration into a cutaneous basophil-rich site in the guinea-pig can induce a local anaphylactic-type reaction characterized by increased vascular permeability and basophil degranulation. Furthermore, it is suggested that C5a induces the degranulation of both basophils and mast cells in the guinea-pig. Chemotactic activity of C567 and 5a is found in synovial effusions of joint inflammatory disease (Ward and Zvaifler 1971). Depressed activities of CI, C4, C2 and C3 are reported in the systemic circulation of patients with rheumatoid arthritis (Rynes et al. 1974). These findings support that the activation of the classical complement pathway is responsible for chronic inflammation.

COMPLEMENT DERIVED MEDIATORS OR ANAPHYLATOXINS (C3A, C5A AND C4A)

C3a, C5a and C4a are a family of bioactive factors derived from precursor molecules of the complement system. These agents have common biological activities, namely, contraction of smooth muscle, enhancement of vascular permeability and induction of release of vasoamines (Hugli 1982). C5a is thought to be the most potent anaphylatoxin playing an important role in the activation of the alternative pathway (Yancey 1988).

It is reported that des Arg form of C5a, i.e. C5a des Arg is likely to be the relevant C5a derived inflammatory glycopeptide in vivo (Swerlick et al. 1988). These authors propose that

C5a des Arg is a potent mediator of cutaneous inflammation and may function as the physiologically relevant C5 derived anaphylatoxin in the human skin based on their in vivo studies. During the past years considerable effort has been devoted towards gaining a better understanding of the role of the anaphylatoxins, C3a, C5a and C4a in the pathophysiology of various diseases (Vogt 1986). Elevated levels of C3a in granulocytopenia, C3a and C5a in microvascular leukocyte sequestration (Chenoweth 1986) and C5a mediated leukocyte sequestration in adult respiratory distress syndrome (Hammerschmidt et al. 1980) are some examples. Other conditions in which intravascular complement activation can result in anaphylatoxin productions are infusion of radiographic contrast media, high doses of drugs like penicillin, sulphonamides, and serum sickness (Lawley et al. 1984). The development of molecular genetic techniques may permit further detailed investigations on the initiation and regulation of complement production during homeostasis and inflammatory diseases (Perlmutter and Colten 1988).

SEROTONIN (5-HYDROXYTRYPTAMINE)

Serotonin (5-hydroxytryptamine, 5-1-HT) is an endogenous biogenic amine produced through tryptophan metabolism and stored primarily in the gastrointestinal tract, nervous system, and platelets. Release of 5-HT is shown to induce vasodilation and increased vascular permeability in human cutaneous microcirculation (Oyvin and Shegel 1965), and it produces inflammatory reactions after administration in the human skin (Geaves and Shuster 1967). 5-HT is found in the exudates during the early phase of experimental inflammation (DI Rosa et al. 1971).

Although 5-HT participates in anaphylactic reactions in certain animal species, its involvement is, however, questionable in human inflammatory diseases (Arrigoni Martelli 1977). Furthermore, serotonin-induced blood vessel alterations are not antagonized by aspirin, and pure serotonin antagonists are not anti-inflammatory agents (Weissmann 1982). Thus, serotonin may have some role in the acute phase of inflammation in experimental models, but not in clinical inflammatory disorders.

KALLIKREIN-KININ SYSTEM

Kinins, vasoactive polypeptides, are released into the circulation from precursors, kininogen, by the enzymatic action of a group of serine proteases termed kallikreins. Figure3.2 illustrates the kinin forming and its inactivating pathways. Kinins are short-chain peptides (9 or 10 amino acids) which resemble bradykinin in structure and in their pharmacological, physiological and pathological aspects (Sharma. and Buchanan 1979; Margolius 1980; Schachter 1980; Regoli and Barabe 1980, Eisen 1980).

Kallikreins are classified into two groups: plasma and tissue/glandular kallikreins. These two enzymes differ in their molecular weights, biological functions, physico-chemical and immunological properties and their distribution in the body. The plasma kallikrein is present in the circulation in an inactive form called prekallikrein or Fletcher factor. Plasma, lacking prekailikrein (designated Fletcher trait deficiency) possesses a reduced rate of surface-mediated coagulation (prolonged partial thromboplastin time) which approaches normal values when the incubation time with kaolin is increased (Hathway and Alsever 1970). Prekallikrein is activated by HF (Kaplan and Austen 1971). Plasma kallikrein also activates the inactivated HF in the fluid phase (Cochrane et al. 1973). Kaplan and Austen (1971) suggested that the conversion of a small amount of prekallikrein to kallikrein by activated HF is necessary prior to feedback activation of HF. This finding further demonstrates that plasma kallikrein does not only liberate kinins, but also may be required for the regulation of normal circulatory homeostasis. A genetic defect resulting in prolonged blood-clotting time (Fletcher disease) has successfully been corrected with plasma prekallikrein (Wuepper 1973), however, such individuals do not suffer from a haemorrhagic tendency or any other recognizable pathologic process.

Tissue kallikreins are present in the kidney, pancreas, intestine, salivary glands, bronchoalveolar lavage fluid of asthmatic patients and synovial membranes (Bhoola et al. 1965; Fiedler et al, 1970; Zeitlin 1971; Nustadt et al. 1975; Sharma et al. 1983; Christiansen et al. 1987). However, the presence of tissue kallikreins in the plasma is also reported (Nustadt et al. 1979; Rabito et al. 1979); Lawton et al. 1981; Rabito et al. 1982). The significance of this observation' still remains unclear. The release of submandibular gland kallikrein into the circulation is detected after sympathetic nerve stimulation, which may cause reactive vasodilation in the rat submandibular gland (Rabito et al. 1983). Tissue kallikreins have similar physicochemical properties, and these enzymes are immunologically identical within the same species (Fiedler 1979). The factors which determine tissue kallikrein secretion are not well defined, and could exhibit tissue as well as species differences. The salivary secretion of kallikrein in rat is regulated by the sympathetic and parasympathetic nervous systems; secretion of kallikrein produced by sympathetic stimulation is higher than by parasynthetic stimulation (Beilenson et al. 1968; Ostravik and Gautvik 1977; Rabito et al. 1983).

On the other hand; alpha-adrenergic stimulation appears to inhibit urinary kallikrein excretion from the kidney of dog and rat (Olsen 1980, 1982). In the kidney, tissue kallikrein is synthesized in the distal tubular cells (Fing et al. 1980). It was suggested that a part of the kallikrein excreted in the urine could be of plasma origin (Ostravik et al. 1976), but this seems unlikely since urinary kallikrein appears to be secreted in the distal segments of the nephron (Scicli et al. 1976). The urinary excretion of kallikrein reflects the activity of the enzyme in the rat kidney (MartinGrez et al. 1982). The renal kallikrein is suggested to regulate blood pressure, and it is probably involved in the pathogenesis of hypertension (Carretero and Scicli 1981; Sharma 1984, 1988 b; Scicli and Carretero 1986). Two kallikreins are found in the small intestine of rat with molecular weights of 33,000 and 35,000 (Moriwaki 1980), while a kallikrein with a molecular-weight of 33,000 is demonstrated in the whole length of the bowel.

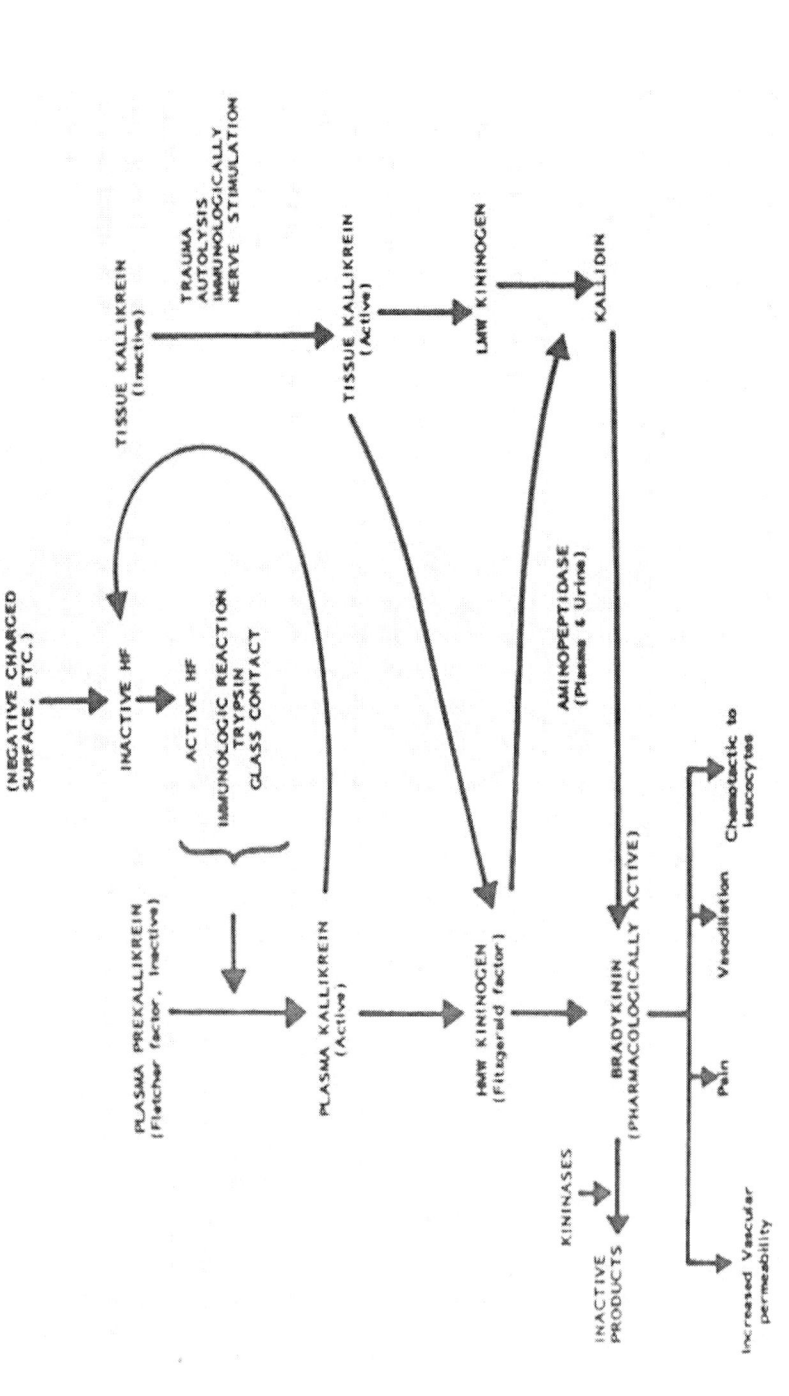

Figure 3.2. The mode of kinin-generation and its inactivation in the body.

This latter kallikrein differs from plasma kallikrein and has inhibitor and substrate specificities of a glandular kallikrein (Zeitlin 1971). The tissue kallikrein from inflamed synovial membranes may originate from plasma (Al- Haboubi et al. 1986). Therefore it may be suggested that plasma kallikrein is the major source of kinin-forming enzyme under inflammatory conditions.

Two kinin-forming substrates, low molecular weight (LMW) and high molecular weight (HMW) kininogens are isolated from bovine plasma (Komiya et al. 1974). They differ in molecular weights (HMW = 76,000; LMW 48,000), and in their susceptibility to plasma and tissue kallikreins. HMW kininogen is the main substrate for plasma kallikrein, and LMW kininogen is the most suitable substrate for tissue kallikrein. Two kininogen with different molecular weights (HMW = 120,000; LMW = 78,000) are also isolated from human plasma (Jacobsen 1966; Nagayasu and Nagasawa 1979). The presence of a third form of human kininogen of about 200.000 daltons is demonstrated (Pierce and Gulmaraes 1975). T-kininogen is only dicovered in rat plasma but not in human plasma (Okamoto and Greenbaum 1983). Deficiency of HMW kininogen appears to be the source of multiple defects such as impaired clotting, kinin release, and surface activated fibrinolysis in plasma. HMW kininogen is also known as a "Fitzgerald factor", because its absence was first found in the Fitzgerald family (Saito et al. 1974; Lutcher 1976; Donaldson et al. 1976, 1977), Saito and his coworkers (1975) report that purified preparations of "Fitzgerald factor" isolated from normal plasma contain HMW kininogen, however, the plasma from Mr. Fitzgerald contained about 50% of the amount of kininogen found in normal plasma which is of the LMW form. Therefore HMW kininogen is essential not only in the kinin-formation, but also in the regulation of a blood-coagulation pathway. This defect is reversed by the treatment with purified HMW kininogen (Colman et al. 1975; Lacombe et al. 1975; Wuepper et al. 1975). Corresponding to the Fletcher trait no discernible pathologic syndrome is associated with HMW kininogen deficiency. Furthermore, HE activates prekallikrein to kallikrein, which is dependent on HMW kininogen. Thus, HMW kininogen could serve as a cofactor in the initiation of blood coagulation and the activation of kinin-generation (Kaplan et al. 1981), particularly by forming a complex with factor XI, thus mediating its binding to negatively charged surfaces.

Kinins are rapidly cleaved to inactive peptides when incubated with blood or with tissue homogenate. Therefore, kinin inactivating enzymes are collectively termed kininases. Kininase I (carboxypeptidase N) is present in the plasma of man and animals that cleaves C-terminal amino acids, including Arg^9 of BK (Erdos et al. 1967; Oshima et al. 1974). Erdos and Young (1967a, 1967b) first detected another enzyme in the kidney cortex and subsequently in the plasma which activates BK by cleaving the C-terminal of the nonapeptide. This is named kininase II (peptidyldipeptide hydrolase) or angiotensin I converting enzyme.

The most prominent actions of kinins are those that resemble the cardinal features of inflammation, including vasodilation, increased vascular permeability, stimulation of pain receptors and swelling (Sharma and Buchanan 1979; Eisen 1980; Zeitlin and Grennan 1976). Kallikrein can cause neutrophil chemotaxis which is partially complement dependent and thereby contributes to tissue inflammation (Kaplan et al. 1982).

PGE series and PGI_2 potentiate the inflammatory and nociceptive (pain) responses produced by BK (William and Morley 1973: Ferreira et al. 1973; Prasad et al. 1982; Vane 1976; Hori et al. 1986; Ikeda et al. 1975). Katori and coworkers (Katori et al. 1979, 1982;

Uchida et al. 1982, 1983; Hori et al. 1988) demonstrated the significant role of plasma kallikrein-kinin system, PG and histamine in the accumulation of pleural fluid during carrageenan and kaolin-induced pleurisy in the rat. BK release is found to be a prime factor for plasma exudation during the entire course of this pleural inflammation.

High concentrations of plasma kinin precursor (kininogen) are detected in rats 48h after laparotomy, nephrectomy and intramuscular administration of acetic acid and croton oil (Zach and Werle 1973). Similar results are obtained in the plasma of rats after subcutaneous injection of turpentine (Borges and Gordon 1976). An increased plasma kininogen is noted under chronic inflammatory conditions in adjuvant-induced arthritis ofrat (Van Arman and Nuss 1969; Reis et al. 1982). T-kininogen (different from HMW and LMW kininogens) is discovered in rat plasma (Okamoto and Greenbaum 1983). T-kininogen is found to be raised in adjuvant arthritis of rats, while the plasma levels of HMW and LMW kininogens are not modified (Greenbaum 1984). To gain further knowledge regarding the significance of T-kininogen in inflammation, carrageenan paw edema is produced in T-kininogen-deficient strain rats (B/N-Katholiek) and in normal strain rats (B/N-ketasdato) by OH-ISHI et al. (1987). The authors report that the time course of the inflammatory reactions in these two strains of rats is absolutely different. Normal rats show a peak swelling at 3-5 h after carrageenan, but B/N-Katholiek rats fail to develop inflammation even after 24 h. It is suggested that BK formation from HMW kininogen is responsible for inflammatory reactions in normal rats (Oh-Ishi et al. 1987). On the other hand, raised T-kininogen is unable to release BK in the B/N-Katholiek rat (contains only T-kininogen). Therefore it is possible to suggest that T-kinin released from the precursor, T-kininogen, could be devoid of proinflammatory actions, and/or raised T-kininogen has undiscovered properties in inflammation. In dog knee joints, injections of BK produce acute inflammatory reactions characterized by pain and swelling (Van Arman and Carlson 1970; Ferreira et al. 1974).

Kinin-forming components are significantly raised in colonic tissue of patients with inflamed gut (Zeitlin and Smith 1973). We observed raised plasma kininogen levels in the peripheral blood of patients with inflammatory bowel diseases compared to concentrations found in normal subjects (Sharma 1976). Raised kinin-forming activity in human colon may account for inflammatory intestinal conditions. It is possible that infiltration into the intestinal fluid of increased levels of plasma kallikrein and kininogen may occur in intestinal inflammation (Fasth et al. 1978). Hence, abnormal release of kinin may be responsible for inflammatory bowel diseases in human.

Kinin formation is also suggested as aetiological factor in the pathogenesis of inflamed rheumatoid joints (Melmon et al. 1967). Synovial exudates of patients with rheumatoid and gouty arthritis contain kinin, kallikrein and kininogens (Melmon; et al. 1967; Eisen 1970; Keele and Eisen 1970; Sawai et al. 1979: Katori et al. 1982). The components of the kinin-forming system found in the synovial fluid are originating from plasma (Jasani et al. 1969). Rheumatoid patients removed from therapy or given placebo have high levels of plasma kininogen (Brooks et al. 1974; Sharma et al. 1976, 1980). The raised plasma kininogen found in rheumatoid patients may be due to augmented synthesis compensating for a chronically increased rate of kinin-generation within the inflamed joints (Zeitlin et N. 1976, 1977). In the synovial membrane of dog BK increases the blood flow (Dick et al. 1976) and the permeability in very small concentrations (Grennan et al. 1977). BK has a pain producing action which is potentiated by PGE_2 (Ferreira et al. 1974). We observed highly appreciable levels of kallikrein-like activity in inflamed synovial tissues taken from rheumatoid patients, arthritic dogs and adjuvant arthritic rats (Sharma et al. 1983; Al-Haboubi et. al. 1986). The mode of activation of inactive synovial kallikrein may be mediated via PGs and IgE mediated immune reaction. PGs are capable of producing inflammatory reactions (Kaley and Weiner 1971). These PGs have been reported to stimulate renal tissue kallikrein release, while PGs synthetase inhibitors can antagonize it (Mills 1979; Nasjletti and Malik 1979). High amounts of PGE are detected in the rheumatoid synovial fluid as well (Higgs et al. 1974). Kallikrein-like activity can be produced by human basophils as a direct result of IgE-mediated immune reaction, thus providing a main link between reactions of immediate hypersensitivity and the tissue kininforming system (Newball et al. 1979). Nonetheless, BK evokes the release of labeled AA, PGE and PGF from synovial fibroblasts pre-labeled with 3H-AA (Newcombe et al. 1977). These interactions between the BK, PGs and PGI_2 may represent significant factors in the inflammatory processes of rheumatoid synovial tissues (see Figure 3.3).

However, the significant role of kinins in tissue injury and in inflammation is reviewed by Marceau et al. (1983). Nevertheless, definite evidence of kinins' involvement in inflammation is uncertain, since appropriate effective antagonists have not been available. Three years ago a number of kinin antagonists were synthesized (Vavrek and Steward 1985). The compound B3824 is a potent antagonist of BK-induced vascular permeability in rabbit skin (Schachter et al. 1987). It is known that the kinin receptor mediating pain on the human blister base is of the B_2 type (Whalley et al. 1987). These investigators note that B_2 receptor antagonists (D-Arg-Arg-Pro-Hyp-TGly-Thi-Ser-D-Phe-Thi-Arg-TFA) and (D-Pro-Phe-Arg-heptylamide) cause significant antagonism of BK-induced pain responses at doses which have no effect against those produced by 5-HT or potassium chloride.

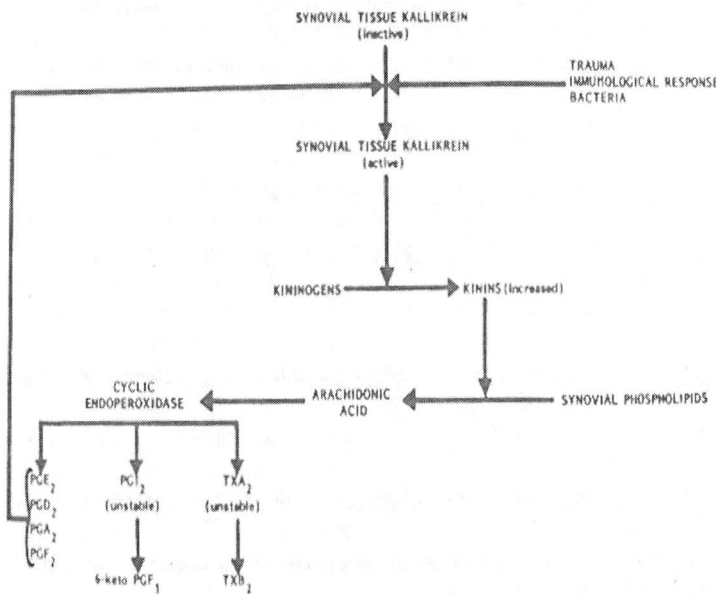

Figure 3.3. A model for the interaction of the kallikrein-kinin system and the prostaglandins in the joint inflammatory diseases. According to this concept, the development of rheumatoid arthritis may be the consequence of an abnormality in synovial tissue induced by a defect in the kallikrein-kinin formation, which may induce release of proinflammatory agents from arachidonic acid.

These observations lead to the suggestion that the use of specific BK antagonists is promising in experimental and/or clinical inflammations. Indeed, BK can cause increased vascular permeability and rhinitis without releasing mast cell mediators in healthy subjects after administration to the nasal mucosa (Proud et al. 1988; Naclerio et al. 1988). These observations suggest that kinins can contribute to the induction of human inflammatory diseases of the upper respiratory tract. Generally, the hypothesis is supported that the kinin-system is directly involved in the pathogenesis of inflammatory disorders. Rapid advancement in radioenzymatic assays may provide in the near future additional evidence that kinins are products of inflamed tissues where they are acting as local inflammatory hormones.

SUBSTANCE P

Substance P (SP) is an 11-amino acid peptide, which has a blood pressure lowering effect as well as potent vasodilating properties (Von Euler and Gaddum 1931; Von Euler 1936). It is more effective than histamine, kinin and PGE_2, as vasodilating compound (Hortnagl et al. 1984). SP can cause smooth muscle contraction as well as enhance activities of mast cells, PMNs, T-lymphocytes, and macrophages (Pernow 1983; Marasco et al. 1981; Payan et al. 1984; Hartung and Toyka 1983). It is known to be a mediator of painful sensory stimuli via the stimulation of nocieeptice C fibers (Otsuka and Konishi 1976). When released from these fibers it may cause vasodilation, fluid extravasation and neurogenic inflammatory reactions (Lembeck and Holzer- 1979: Lembeck et al. 1981). Tissot et al. (1988) demonstrated a detectable release of SP-like compound in the inflammatory pleural exudates induced by intrapleural injection of either calcium pyrophosphate or carrageenan in rats. It is suggested that SP is involved in inflammatory response either directly or via causing the release of other mediators or acting on nociceptive fibers and causing vascular changes. Blisters of inflammatory dermatoses show raised levels of SP-immunoreactive activity (Wallengren et al. 986). Devilller et al. (1986) reported highly raised levels of tachykinin-like activity in inflammatory joint fluids. These findings suggest that neurogenic pathways may play a role in the pathogenesis of rheumatoid arthritis. It is of interest to indicate that SP can cause leukocyte migration and leukocyte dependent extravasation of macromolecules in rabbit and hamster (Thureson-Klein et al. 1987). Furthermore, by the golden hamster cheek pouch preparation SP is shown to be a more effective pro-inflammatory agent than PAF, or LTB.

POLYMORPHONUCLEAR LEUKOCYTE DERIVED SUBSTANCES

PMN-leukocytes contain a number of components which can cause vascular injury and endothelial cell detachment in vitro and in vivo. PMN-derived factors are the most important mediators in producing vascular alterations in the microcirculation in acute inflammatory conditions, either induced naturally or experimentally (Movat 1985). Lysosomes and proteases are the prime constituents of PMNs which can degrade basement membrane at low pH in vitro (Cochrane and Aikin 1966). The acid proteases are capable of degrading various proteins present within the digestive vacuoles, e.g. hydrolysis of kininogen producing kinin-like agents (Wasi et al. 1966). The kinin produced by leukokininogenases (acid proteases such as cathepsin D) is designated as leukokinin (high weight, pharmacological active peptide) (Greenbaum 1977). It is suggested that leukokininogenases and neutral proteases originating from the PMN cells are fundamental catalysts of the inflammatory-like agents observed in chronic inflammation. An elastase-like enzyme has potential pathogenetical significance. This enzyme is found in PMN lysosomes ofrabbit (Cotter and Robinson 1980). and in human PMNs ; it comprises the main neutral protease activity. However, inflammatory microvascular injury, including increased vascular permeability, microhaemorrhage and microthrombosis, are usually associated with inflammatory reactions elicited by immune complexes or bacteria both in man and experimental animals.

In experimental models no such injury can be induced in animals rendered neutropenic, implicating an important role of neutrophil derived factors such as lysosomal proteinases (elastase, collagenase, cathepsin C) and oxygen radicals (Carp and Janoff 1983; Fantone and Ward 1982). Movat (1985) stresses that the PMN-derived factors are the most important mediators in bringing about the vascular changes in microcirculation during acute inflammatory reaction. At least three mediators (PAF, IL-1 and activated complement) can induce microvascular injury via neutrophil leukocytes by initiating their migration and eliciting their degranulation. Isszauzz (1984) emphasizes the PMN-induced vasopermeability and the mediator's responsibility in causing plasma protein leakage. Probably, PAF acts as a mediator because it is produced by PMNs and causes directly an increase in vascular permeability (Humphrey et al. 1982, 1984). PMN dependent PAF release may also be due to platelets in an early acute inflammation (Issekutz et al. 1983).

Leukotriene B_4 and PAF stimulate PMN-leukocyte chemotaxis through endothelial cell monolayers (EC);however, LTC_4 and D_4 are inactive, and LTA_2 is weakly active (Hopkins et al. 1984). Angiotensin II and histamine stimulate the generation of a neutrophil chemoattractant by EC, too (Farber et al. 1985, 1986), and these actions are antagonized by lipooxygenase inhibitors. Activated PMN-leukocytes cause detachment of EC monolayers by releasing elastase from PMN leukocytes (Smedley et al. 1986; Harlan et al. 1981). αl-protease inhibitor can protect normal PMN-leukocytes from elastase by oxidant mechanisms. However, nonoxidant mechanisms may also be existing because PMN-leukocytes can also be protected from elastase in patients with chronic granulomatous disease (Weiss et al. 1986). EC lysis may be seen after release of oxygen radicals by PMN-leukocytes (Sacks et al. 1978), which can be potentiated by the presence of platelet products (Boogaerts et al. 1982). Furthermore, a PMN-leukocyte product known as hydrogen peroxide can stimulate PGI_2 release from EC (Harlan and Callahan 1984). The importance of EC in the regulation of inflammation and immunity is critically evaluated by Cotran (1987) and Jaffe (1988).

REFERENCES

- An effect of indomethacin on raised plasma kininogen in rheumatoid patients. In: Pisano JJ, Austen KF (eds) Chemistry and biology of kallikrein-kinin system in health and disease; US Government Printing Office, Washington DC. 1977; pp. 483-486.
- An enzyme in microsomal fraction in kidney that inactivates bradykinin. Life Sci. 1967a; 6: 569-574.
- Clonidine decreases rat urine kallikrein excretion by ~-adrenergic receptor stimulation. Eur. J. Pharmac. 1982; 79: 311-315.

- Does vitamin E supplementation modulate in vivo arachidonate metabolism in human inflammation" Pharmac. Toxicol. 1987; 61: 246-249.
- Kinetics of prostaglandins production in various inflammatory lesions measured in draining lymph. Am. J Pathol 1979: 95: 225-238.
- Kinin system in clinical and experimental rheumatoid inflammation. Curr. Med. Res. Opin. 1979; 6: 314- 321.
- Kinins in physiology and pathology. TIPS 1980; 1: 212-215.
- Metabolism of arachidonic acid in acetic acid colitis in rat: Similarity to human inflammatory bowel disease. Gastroenterology 1985; 88: 55-63.
- Potentiation of prostaglandins of the nociceptive activity of bradykinin in the dog knee joint. Br. J Pharmac 1974; 50: 461 p.
- Preparation of substance P. Scand. Arch. Physiol. 1936; 73: 142- 144.
- Re-appraisal of the role of histamine in carrageenan-induced paw oedema. Eur. J Pharmac 1983; 88:169-176.
- Second kininase in human blood plasma. Nature 1967b; 215: 1402-1403.
- The biochemistry of inflammation: rheumatoid arthritis and anti-inflammatory drugs. Eur. J. Rheumatol Inflamm 1982; 5: 366-381.
- T-kinin and T-kininogen. children of new technology. Biochem. Pharmac1984; 33: 2943-2944.

Ability of prostaglandins to induce acute inflammatory bowel disease in the rat: a preliminary report. J, Med. 1983; 14: 157-160.

Aked DM, Foster SJ: Leukotriene B4 and prostaglandin E2 mediate the inflammatory response of rabbit skin to intradermal arachidonic acid. Br. 1. Pharmac 1987; 92: 545-552.

Albert DH, Snyder F: Biosynthesis of l-alkyl-2-acetyl-sn-glycero-3-phosphocholine (platelet-activating factor) from l-alkyl-2-acyl-sn-glycero-3-phosphocholine by rat alveolar macrophages. Phospholipase A2 and inophore stimulation. J Biol Chern 1983; 258: 97-102.

Al-Haboubi HA, Bennett D, Sharma JN, et al.: A synovial amidase acting on tissue kallikrein-selective substrate in clinical and experimental arthritis. Adv. Exp. Med. Biol 1986; 198B: 405-411.

Arachidonate metabolites in inflammation. Clin. Rheumat. Dis. 1981; 7: 781-798.

Archer CB, Page CP, Paul W, et al.: Inflammatory characteristics of platelet activating factor (PAF-acether) in human skin. Br. J Dermatol 1984; 110: 45-50.

Arner EC, Darnell LR, Pratta MA, et al.: Effect of amiintlammatory drugs on human interleukin-I-induced cartilage degradation. Agents Actions 1987; 17: 334-336.

Arrang JM, Garbarg M, Lecomte JM, et al.:Highly potent and selective]igands for histamine Hrreceptors. Nature 1987; 327: 117-123.

Arrigoni-Martelli E: lntlammation and anti-intlammatories spectrum publication, New York 1977; pp 55-63.

Bebveniste J, Camussi J, Polonsky J: Platelet activating factor. Monogr. Allergy 1977; l2: 138- 142.

Beilenson S, Schachter M, Smaje LH: Sccretion of kallikrein and its role in vasodilation in submaxillary gland J. Physiol. (Lond) 1968; 199: 303-317.

Bell RL: Mediators of C5a-induced bronchoconstriction in guinea-pig Int. Arch. Allergys Appl. Immun 1987; 84: 414-423.

Benjamin WR, Lomedico PT, Killian PL: Interleukin-1. In: Bailey MD, ed.; Annual reports in medicinal chemistry. Academic Press, London 1985; pp 173-183.

Bhoola KD, Morely J, Schachter M, et al.: Vasodilatation in the sub-maxillary gland of the cat. J Physiol (Lond) 1965; 179: 172-184.

Bjork J, Hedqvist P, Arfors KE: Increase in vascular permeability by leukotriene B4 and the role of polymorphonuclear leukocytes, Inflammation 1982; 6: 189-200.

Black JW, Duncan WAM, Durant CJ, et al.: Definition and antagonism of histamine Hz receptors. Nature 1972; 236: 385-390,

Boogaerts MA, Yamada O, Jacos HS, et al.: Enhancement of granulocyte endothelia] cell adherence and granulocyte induced cytotoxicity by platelet release products. Proc, Natl. Acad. Sci 1982; 79: 7019-7023.

Borges DR, Gordon AH: Kininogen and kinogenase synth~sis by the liver of norma] and injured rats. J Pharm Phamac 1976; 28: 44-48.

Braquet P, Touqui L, Shen TY, et al.: Perspectives in plate]et-activatingfactor research.Pharmac. Rev 1987: 39: 97-145.

Bray MA, Cunningham FM, Ford-Hutchinson AW, et al.: Leukotriene B4: an inflammatory mcdiator ill vivo, Prostaglandins 1981; 22: 213-???

Brodie MJ, Hensby CN, Parke A, et al.: Is prostacyclin the major pro-intlammatory prostanoid in joinI fluid') Life Sci 1980; 27: 603-608.

Brooks PM, Dick WC, Sharma JN, et al.: Changes in plasma kininogen levels associated with rheumatoid activity. Br. J Clin Pharmac 1974; 1: 351 p.

Buchanan WW: Some modern aspects of the mode of action of non-steroidal anti-inflammatory drugs. Pharmacotherapeutica 1980; 2: 387-396.

Camp RDR, Coutti AA, Creaves MW, et al.: Responses of human skin to intradermal injection of leukotrienes C4, D4 and B4, Br. J Pharmac 1983; 80: 497-502.

Capasso F, Dunni CJ, Yamamoto S, et al.: Further studies on carrageenan-induced pleurisy in rats. J Pathol 1975; 116: 117-128.

Carp H, Janoff A: Modulation of inflammatory cell protease tissue anti protease interactions at sites of intlammation by leukocyte-derived oxidants. Adv. Inflam Res 1983; 5: 173-201.

Carretero OA, Scicli AG: The possible role of kinins in circulatory homeostasis, Hypertension 1981; 3: (Suppl1): 4-12.

Carroli MA, Schwartzman M, Capdevila J, et al.: Vasoactivity of arachidonic acid epoxides, Eur. J Pharmac 1987; 138: 281-283.

Center DM, Rounds S: Bovine and human endothelial cell production of neutrophil chemoattractant activity in response to components of the angiotensin system. Circulation Res 1985; 57: 898-902.

Chang J, Gilman SC, Lewis AJ: Inter]eukin-I activates phospholipase Az inrabbit chondrocytes: a possible signal for IL-action. J Immunol 1986; 136: 1283-1287.

Changes in biochemical parameters associated with experimental arthritis in rabbits. Biomedicine 1977; 27: 252-255.

-Chemistry and reaction mechanisms of complement. Adv. lmmunol. 1968; 8: 1-80.

Chenoweth DE: Anaphylatoxin formation in eXlracorporeal circuits. Complement 1986; 3: 152-168.

Christiansen SC, Proud D, Cochrane CG, et al.: Detection of tissue kallikrein in the bronchoalveo]ar lavage tluid of asthmatic subjects. J Clin Invest 1987; 79: 188-197.

Cochrane CG, Aikin BS: Polymorphonuclear leukocytes in immunological reactions: the destruction of the basement membrane in vivo and in vitro. J Exp Med 1966; 124: 733-752.

Coeffier E, Borrel MC, Lefort J, et al.: Effects of PAF-acether and structural analogues on platelet activation and bronchoconstriction in guinea pigs. Eur. J Pharmacol 1986; 131: 179-188.

Colman RW, Bagdasarian A, Taloma RC, et al.: William trait: human kininogen deficiency with diminished levels of plasminogen proactivator and pre-kallikrein associated with abnormalities of the Hageman factor-dependent pathways. J Clin Invest 1975; 56: 1650-1662.

Cotran RS: New roles for the endothelium in inflammation and immunity Am. J Pathol 1987; 129: 407-413.

Cotter TG, Robinson GB: Purification and characterization of an elastase like enzyme from rabbit polymorphonuclear leukocytes. Biochim. Biophys. Acta 1980; 615: 414-425.

Could SR, Brash AR, Conolly ME, et al.: Increased prostaglandin production in ulcerative colitis. Lancet 1977; II: 98.

Cybulsky MI, Chan MKW, Movat HZ: Acute inflammation and microthrombosis induced by endotoxin, interJeukin-I, and tumor necrosis factor and their implication in gram-negative infection. Lab. Invest. 1988; 58: 365-378.

Davidson EM: Leukotriene B4' a mediator of inflammation present in the synovial fluid in rheumatoid arthritis. Ann. Rheum Dis 1983; 42: 677-679.

Davies P, Bailey PJ, Goldenberg M, et al.: The role of arachidonic acid oxygenation products in pain and inflammation. Ann. Rev. Immunol 1984; 2: 335-357.

Davudsibme EM, Rae SA, Smith MJH: Leukotriene B4 in synovial fluid J. Pharm. Pharmac 1982; 34: 410.

Daymond TJ, Rowell FJ: Reduction of prostaglandin E2 concentrations in synovial fluid of patients suffering from rheumatoid arthritis following tiaprofenic acid or indomethacin treatment. Drugs 1988; 35 (Suppl I): 4-8.

Demopoulos CA, Pinckard RN, Hanahan DJ: Platelet-activating factor: evidence for 1-0-alkyl-2-acetylsn-glyceryl-3-phosphorylcholine as the active component (A new class of lipid chemical mediators). Comm. J Biol Chem. 1979; 254: 9355-9358.

Deodhar SD, Buchanan WW: Detection of kallikrein-like activity in inflamed synovial tissue. Arch Int Pharmacodyn Ther 1983; 262: 279-286.

Devillier P, Weil B, Renoux M, et al.: Elevated levels of tachykinin-like immunoreactivity in joint fluids from patients with inflammatory rheumatic diseases. N. Engl. J Med 1986; 314: 1323.

Dick WC, Grennan DM, Zeitlin IJ: Studies on the relative effects of prostaglandins, bradykinin, 5-hydroxytryptamine and histamine on the synovial microcirculation in dogs. Br. J Pharmac 1976; 56: 313- 316.

Dick WC: A novel relationship between plasma kininogen and rheumatoid disease. Agents Actions 1976; 6: 148-153.

Dimartino MJ, Campbell GK, Wolff CE, et al.: The pharmacology of arachidonic acid induced rat paw edema. Agents Actions. 1987a; 21: 303-305.

Dinarello CA: Interleukin-l. Rev. Infect Dis 1984; 6: 51-55.

Dirosa M, Giroud JP, Willoghby DA: Studies on the mediators of the acute inflammatory response induced in rats in different sites by carageenan and turpentine. J Pathol 1971; 104: 15-29.

Donaldson VH, Glueck IH, Miller MA, et al.: Kininogen deficiency in Fitzgerald trait; role of high molecular weight kininogen in clotting and fibrinolysis. J Lab Clin Med 1976; 87: 327- 337.

Drazen JM, Figueiredo JC, Corey EJ: A review of recent contributions'on biologically active products of arachidonate conversion. Int. J Immunopharmac 1982; 4: 85-90.

Dumonde DC, Clynn LE: The production of arthritis in rabbits by an immunological reaction to fibrin, Br. J Exp Pathol 1962; 43: 373-383.

Eisen V: Formation and function of kinins. Rheumatology 1970; 3: 103-168.

Erdos EG, Sloane EM: An enzyme in human plasma that inactivated bradykinin and kallidin. Biochem Pharmac 1962; 11: 585-592.

Fantone JC, Ward PA: Role of oxygen-derived free radicals and metabolites in leukocyte dependent inflammatory reactions. Am. J Pathol 1982; 107: 395-418.

Farber HW, Weller PF, Rounds S, et al.: Generation of lipid neutrophil chemoattractant activity by histamine-stimulated cultured endothelial cells. J Immunol. 1986; 137: 2918-2924.

Fasth S, Hulten L, Johnson BJ, et al.: Mobilization of colonic kallikrein following pelvic nervc stimulation in the atropinized cat. J. Physiol. (London) 1978; 285: 471-478.

Ferreira SH, Moncada S, Vane JR: Prostaglandins, aspirin-like drugs and the oedema of inflammation. Nature 1973; 246: 217-219.

Fiedler F: Enzymology of glandular kallikrein. In: ERDOS, E G. (cd.), Handbook of experimentall'hannacoiogy. Springer-Verlag, Berlin, New York 1979; pp 102-161.

Fing E, Geiger R, Witte J, et al.: Biochemical, pharmacological and functional aspects of glandular kallikreins. In: Gross F, Vogei G (eds), Enzyme release of vasoactive peptides. Raven Press, New York, 1980; pp. 101-115.

Flower RJ, Blackwell GJ: The importance of phospholipase A2 in prostaglandin biosynthesis. Biochem Pharmac 1976; 25: 285291.

Ford-Hutchinson A, Letts G: Biological actions of leukotrienes: state of the art lecture. Hypertension 19S6: 8 (suppl II): II-44-1I-49.

Ford-Hutchinson AW, Bray MA: Leukotriene B_4: a potential mediator of inflammation. J Pharmac 1980; 32: 517-518.

Geaves M, Shuster S: Responses of skin blood vessels to bradykinin. histamine and S-hydroxytriptamine. J Physiol (London) 1967; 193: 255-267.

Ghebrehiwet B: Interaction of the clotting, kinin-forming, complement, and fibrinolytic pathways in inflammation. Ann. N. Y. Acad. Sci 1982; 389: 25-38.

Gilman SC, Berner PR, Chang J: Phospholipase A2 activation by interleukinl; release and metabolism of arachidonic acid by ILl-stimulated rabbit chondrocytes. Agents Actions 1987; 21: 34S- 347.

Goetzl E, Derian CK, Tauber AIV, et al.: Novel effect of 1-0-hexadecyl-2-acetyl-sn-glycero-3-phosphorylcholine mediators of human leukocyte function: delineation of the specific roles of the acyl substituents. Biochem. Biophys Res Commun 1980; 94: 881-888.

Golden HW, Iacuzio DA, Otterness IG: Inhibition of CSa-induced basophil degranulation by disodium chromoglycate. Agents Actions. 1987; 17: 271-274.

Goldman DW, Goetzl EJ: Biochemical and cellular characteristics of the regulation of human leukozyte function by lipoxygenase products of arachidonic acid. In: Chakrin LW, Bailey DM (eds), The leukotrienes: Chemistry and biology. Academic Press, New York 1984; pp. 231-245.

Green JP, Prell GD, Khanelwal JK, et al.: Aspects of histamine metabolism. Agents Actions 1987; 22: 1-15.

Greenbaum LM: Cellular kininogenases and leukokinins. In: Pisano JJ, Austen KF (eds). J Chemistry and biology of the kallikrein-kinin system in health and disease. U. S. Govt. Printing Office, Washington DC. 1977; pp.455-469.

Grennan DM, Mitchell W, Miller W, et al.: The effects of prostaglandin El' bradykinin and histamine on canine synovial permeability. Br. J Pharmac 1977; 60: 251-254.

Grennan DM: The role of inflammatory mediators in joint inflammation. In: Buchanan WW, Dick WC (eds), Recent advances in rheumatology, Churchill Livingstone, Edinburgh 1976; pp 195-212.

Hammerschmidt DE, Weaver LJ, Hudson LD, et al.: Association of complement activation and elevated plasma-C5a with adult respiratory distress syndrome. Pathophysiological relevance and possible prognostic value. Lancet 1980; I: 497-499.

Hamreg M, Samuelsson B: Detection and isolation of an endoperoxide intermediate in prostaglandin biosynthesis. Proc Natl Acad-Sci. USA 1973; 70: 899-903.

Hardy TM, Casey FB, Chakrin LW: C5a-induced histamine release. Int. Archs. Allergy Appl Immun 1983; 72: 362-365.

Harlan JM, Callahan KS: Role of hydrogen peroxide in the neutrophil mediated release of prostaglandin from cultured endothelial cells. J Clin Invest 1984; 74:442-448.

Harris D, Smith PR, Swan CHJ: Venous prostaglandin-like activity in diarrhoel states. Gut. 1978; 19: 1057-1058.

Hartung HP, Toyka KV: Activation of macrophages by substance P; Induction of oxidative burst and thromboxane release. Eur. J Pharmacol. 1983; 89: 301-305.

Hathway WE, Alsever J: The relation of "Fletcher factor" to factor XI and XII. Br. J. Haemtol. 1970; 18: 161-169.

Henson PM, Cochrana CG: Leucocyte dependent histamine release from rabbit platelets. J Exp Med 1972; 136: 1356-1377.

Higgs GA, Salmon JA, Spayne JA: The inflammatory effects of hydroperoxy and hydroxy acid products of arachidonate lipooxygenase in rabbit skin. Br. J Pharmac 1981; 74: 429-433.

Holzer P: Substance P as neurogenic mediator of antidromic vasodilation and neurogenic plasma extravasation. Arch. Pharmacol 1979; 310: 175-183.

Hopkins NK, Schaub RG, Gorman RR: Acetyly glyceryl ether phosphorylcholine (PAF-acetherl and leukotriene B_4-mediated neutrophil chemotaxis through an intact endothelial cell monolayer. Biochim. Biophys. Acta 1984; 865: 30- 36.

Hori Y, Jyoyama H, Yamada K, et al.: Interaction of endogenous kinins and prostaglandins in the plasma exudation of kaolin· induced pleurisy in rats. Adv. Exp. Med Biol, in press 1988

Hortnagi H, Singer EA, Lenz K, et al.: Involvement of substance P in the pathogenesis of cardiovascular complications in hepatic failure. In: Kleinberger G, Ferenci P, Riederer P, Thaler H (eds). Advances in hepatic encephalopathy and urea cycle diseases. Karger. Basel. 1984; pp. 731-739.

Hugli TE: The structural basis for anaphylatoxin and chemotactic fractions of C3a. C4a and C5a. CRC Critical Rev. Immunol 1982; 1: 321-366.

Humphrey DM, Hanahan DJ, Pinckard RN: Induction of leukocytic infiltrates in rabbit skin by acetyl glyceryl ether phosphorylcholine. Lab. Invest. 1982; 47: 227-234. .

Humphrey DM, Hanahan DJ, Pinckard RN: Induction of leukocytic infiltrates in rabbit skin by acetyl ether phosphorylcholine. Lab. Invest 1982; 47: 227-234.

Ikeda AK, Tanaka K, Katori M: Potentiation of bradykinin-induced vascular permeability increase by prostaglandin E_2 and arachidonic acid in rabbit skin. Prostaglandins 1975; 10: 747-758.

Interrelationship between th kallikrein-kinin system and hypertension. A review. Gen. Pharmac. 1988b; 19: 177-187. .

Ishikawa S, Sperelakis N: A novel class (H_3) of histamine receptors on perivascular nerve terminals. Nature 1987; 327: 158- 160.

Issekutz AC: Role of polymorphonuclear leukocytes in the vascular responses of acute inflammation. Lab. Invest 1984; 50: 605-607.

Jacobsens M: Substrate for plasma kinin-forming enzyme in human, dog, and rabbit plasma. Br. J. Pharmac 1966; 26: 403-411.

Jaffa EA: Endothelial cells. In: Gallin JI, Goldstein IM, Snyderman R (eds), Inflammation: Basic principles and clinical correlates. Raven Press, New York 1988; p. 559-576.

Jasani MK, Katori M, Lewis GP: Intracellular enzymes and kinin enzymes in synovial fluid in joint diseases. Ann. Rheum. Dis 1969; 28: 497-511.

Johnson WJ, Votta B, Hanna N: Effect of antiarthritic drugs on the enhanced interleukin-l (11.-1) production by macrophages from adjuvant-induced arthritis (AA) rats. Agents Actions 1987b; 21: 348-350.

Johnston MG, Hay JB, Movat HZ: The modulation of enhanced vascularpermeability by prostaglandins through alterations in blood flow (hyperemia). Agents Actions 1976; 6: 705-711.

Kaley G, Weiner R: Prostaglandin E,: a potential mediator of the inflammatory response. Ann. N. Y. Acad. Sci 1971: 180: 338-350.

Kaplan AP, Austen KF: A prealbumin activator of prekallikrein II. Derivation of activators of prekallikrein from active Hageman factor by digestion with plasmin. J. Exp. Med. 1971; 133: 696- 712.

Katori M, Harada Y, Uchida Y, et al.: Potentiation of bradykinin-induced nociceptive response by arachidonate metabolites in dogs. Eur. J Phamac 1986; 132: 47-52.

Katori M, Uchida Y, Oh-Ishi S, et al.: Involvement of plasma kallikreinkinin system in rat carrageenin-induced pleurisy. Eur. J. Rheumatol Infl 1979; 2: 217-219.

Kaushansky K, Lin N, Adamson JW: Interleukin-I stimulates fibroblast to synthesize granulocytemacrophage and granulocyte colony stimulating factors. Mechanism for the hematopoietic response to inflammation. Jl Clin. Invest 1988; 81: 92-97.

Keele CA, Eisen V: Plasma kinin formation in rheumatoid arthritis. Adv. Exp. Med. Biol 1970; 8: 471-475.

Killen PD, Harker IA, Striker GI, et al.: Neutrophil mediated endothelial injury in "ilro mechanisms of cell detachment. J Clin Invest 1981; 68: 1394-1403.

Kinin-forming system in the genesis of hypertension. Agents Actions 1984; 14: 200-205.

Kitchen EA, Boot JR, Dawsan W: Chemotactic activity of thromboxane B_2 prostaglandins and their metabolites for polymorphonuclear leukocytes. Prostaglandins 1978; 16: 239-244.

Kleniewski J, Saito H, Sayed JK: Prekallikrein deficiency in a kindred with kininogen deficiency and Fitzgerald trait clotting defect. Evidence that high molecular weight kininogen and prekallikrein exist as a complex in normal human plasma. J Clin Invest 1977; 60: 571-583.

Komiya M, Kato H, Suzuki T: Structural comparison of high molecular weight and low molecular weight kininogens. J Biochem 1974; 76: 833-845.

Lacombe MJ, Varet B, Levy JP: A hitherto undescribed plasma factor acting at the contact phase of blood coagulation (Flaujeac factor): case report and coagulation studies. Blood 1975; 46: 761-768.

Larsen GL, Henson PM: Mediators of inflammation. Ann. Rev. Immunol 1983; 1: 335-359.

Lauritsen K, Laursen LS, Bukhave K, et al.: Effects of topical 5-amino-salicylic acid and prednisolone on prostaglandin E_2 and leukotriene B_4 levels determined by equilibrium in vivo dialysis of rectum in relapsing ulcerative colitis. Gastroenterology 1986; 91: 837-844.

Lawley TJ, Bielory L, Gscon P, et al.: A prospective and sequential study of serum sickness in man. N. Eng. J Med 1984; 31: 1407-1410.

Lembeck F, Donnerer J, Colpaert FC: Increase in substance P in primary afferent nerves during pain. Neuropcptides 1981; 1:175- 81.

Lepow IH, Naff GB, Todd EW, et al.: Chromatographic resolution of the first component of human complement into three as;tivities. J Exp Med 1963; 117: 983-1008.

Levine JD, Lau W, Kwiat G, et al.: Leukotriene B_4 produces hyperalgesia that is dependent on polymorphonuclear leukocytes. Science 1984; 225: 743-745.

Lewis GP: Iinmunoregulatory activity of metabolites of arachidonic acid and their role in inflammation. Br. Med Bull. 1983; 39: 243-248.

Lewis RA, Austen F: Mediation of local homeostasis and inflammation by leukotrienes and other mast celldependent compounds. Nature 1981; 293: 103-108.

Lewton WJ, Proud D, French ME, et al.: Characterization and origin of immunoreactive glandular kallikrein in rat plasma. Pharmac 198 I; 30: 1731-1737.

Lutcher Cl: Reid trait: a new expression of high molecular weight kininogen deficiency. Clin Res 1976; 24: 440A.

Mackenzie JF, Russel RI: Plasma kinin-precursor levels in clinical intestinal inflammation Fundamental Clin Pharmacol 1988; in press.

Mallet AI, Cunningham FM: Structural identification of platelet activating factor in psoriatic scale. Biochem. Biophys Ress Commun 1985; 126: 192-198.

Marasco WA, Showell HJ, Becker EL: Substance P binds to the formylpeptide chemotaxis receptor on the rabbit neutrophil. Biochem. Biophys. Res Commun 1981; 99: 1065- 1072.

Marceau F, Lussier A, Regoli D, et al.: Pharmacology of kin ins : Their relevance to tissue injury and inflammation. Gen. Pharmac 1983; 14: 209-229.

Margolius HS: Pharmacological prospects in the kallikrein-kinin system. TIPS 1980; 1: 293-295.

Martin M, Resch K: Interleukin-I: more than a mediator between leukocytes. Trends in Pharmacological Sciences 1988; 9: 171-177.

Martin-Grez M, Schaechtelin G, Bonner G, et al.: Renal kallikrein activity and urinary kallikrein excretion in rats with experimental renal hypertension. Clin Sci 1982; 63: 349-354.

Martins MA, Silva PMR, Neto HCF, et al.: Interactions between local inflammatory and systemic haematologic effects of P AF-acether in the rat. Eur. J Pharmac 1987; 142: 353-360.

McManus LM, Hanahan DJ, Pinckard RN: Morphologic basis of increased vascular permeability induced by acetylglyceryl ether phosphorylcholine. Lab Invest 1984; 50: 16-25.

Meiler HL, Yecies D, Heck LW: Hageman factor and its substrates: the role of factor XI, prekallikrein and plasminogen proactivator In coagulation, fibrinolysis, and kinin generation. In: Pisano JJ, Austen KF (eds), Chemistry and biology of the kallikrein-kinin system in health and disease, US Govt. Printing Office, Washington DC. 1977; 237-254.

Melmon KL, Khan M: Histamine and its lymphocyte-selective derivatives as immune modulators. TIPS 1987; 8: 437-441.

Miller KR, Lacombe MJ: Flaujeac trait: deficiency of human plasma kininogen. J Clin Invest 1975; 56: 1663-1672.

Mills IH: Kallikrein, kininogen and kinins in control of blood pressure. Nephron 1979; 23: 61-71.

Miossec P: The role of interleukin-1 in the pathogenesis of rheumatoid arthritis. Clin. Exp. Rheumatol 1987; 5: 305-308.

Moncada S, Vane JR: Pharmacology and endogenous roles of prostaglandin endoperoxides thromboxane A_2 and prostacyclin. Pharmac Rev 1979; 30: 293-331.

Morgan EL: Mechanisms of leukocyte regulation by complement derivedfactors. Contemp. Topics Immunobiol 1984; 14: 109-154.

Moriwaki C, Fujimori H, Toyono Y, et al.: Studies on kallikreins V. Purification and characterization of rats intestinal kallikrein. Chern. Pharm Bull 1980; 28: 3612-3620.

Morley J, MacDonald DM: Accumulation of inflammatory cells in response to intracutaneous platelet activating factor (PAF-acether) in man. Br. J. Dermatol 1985; 112: 285-290.

Movat HZ: The inflammatory reaction, Elsevier Science Publishers, Amsterdam, New York, Oxford 1985; pp. 77-160.

Muller C, Werle C, Werle E: Purification of prekaJlikrein from pig pancreas with p-nitrophenyl-p-guanidinobenzoale. FEBS. LeU. 1970; 24: 41-44.

Muller-Eberhard HJ, Polley MJ, Calcott MA: Formation and functional significance of a molecular complex derived from the second and the fourth component of human complement. J. Exp. Med 1967; 125: 359-380.

Murphy RC, Hammerstorm S, Samuelsson B: Leukotriene C: a slow reacting substance from murine mastocytoma cells. Proc. Natl Acad Sci USA 1979; 76: U275-U279.

Naclerio RM, Proud D, Lichtenstein L, et al.: Kinins are generated during experimental Rhinovirus colds. J, Infect. Dis 1988; 157: 133-142.

NagayasuT, Nagasawa S: Studies of human kininogen. Isolation. characterization, and cleavage by plasma kallikrein of high molecular weight (HMW) kininogen. J Biochem 1979; 85: 249-258.

Nasjletti A, Malik KU: Relationship between the kallikrein-kinin and prostaglandin system. Life Sci 1979; 25: 99-110.

Newball HH, Berninger RW, Talamo RC, et al.: Anaphylactic release of a basophil kallikrein-like activity. J Clin Invest 1979; 64: 457-456.

Newcombe DS, Fahey JY, Ishikawa Y: Hydrocortisone inhibition of the bradykinin activation of human synovial fibroblasts. Prostaglandins 1977; 13: 235-244.

Norris AA, Lewis AJ, Zeitlin IJ: Changes in colonic tissue levels of inflammatory mediators in guinea pig model of immune colitis. Agents Actions 1982; 12: 243-246.

Norton WL, Ziff M: Electron microsopical observation on the rheumatoid synovial membrane. Arthr. Rheum 1966; 9: 589-610.

Nouri AME, Panayi GS, Goodman SM: Cytokines and the chronic inflammation of rheumatic disease.

Nuss GW: Plasma bradykininogen levels in adjuvant arthritis and carrageenin inflammation. J Pathol 1969; 99: 245-250.

Nustad K, Brandtzaeg P, Pierce JV: Cellular origin of urinary kallikreins. J Histo Chem Cytochem 1976; 24: 1037-1039.

Nustad K, Gautvik KM, Østravik TB: Radio-immunoassay of rat submandibular gland kallikrein and the detection of immuno-reactive antigen in blood. Adv. Exp. Med. Biol 1979; 120B: 225-234.

O'Byrne EM, Schroder HC, Stefano C, et al.: Catabolism and interleukin-I regulation of cartilage and chondrocyte metabolism. Agents Actions 1987; 21: 341-344.

Oh-Ishi S, Hayashi I, Utsunomiya I, et al.: Role of kallikrein-kinin system in acute inflammation: studies on high-and low-molecular weight kininogens-deficient rats (B/N-Katholiek strain). Agents Actions 1987; 21: 384-386.

Okamoto H, Greenbaum LM: Kininogen substrates for trypsin and cathepsin D in human, rabbit and rat plasma. Life Sci 1983; 32: 2007-2013.

Olsen UB: Changes in urinary kallikrein and kinin excretions induced by adrenal in infusion in conscious dogs. J Clin Lab Invest 1980; 40: 173-178.

Oshima G, Kato J, Erdos EG: Sub-units of human plasma carboxypeptidase N (Kininase I; anaphylatoxin inactivator). Biochem. Biophys Acta 1974; 365: 344-348.

Østravik TB, Gautvik KM: Regulation of salivary kallikrein secretion in the rat submandibular gland. Acta Physiol Scand 1977; 100: 33-44.

Otsuka M, Konishi S: Substance P and excitatory transmitter of primary sensory neurons. Cold Spring Harbor Symp. Quant Biol 1976;40: 135-143.

Oyvin IA, Shegel SN: Changes in skin blood flow and capillary permeability in man and animals following 5-hydroxytryptamine (serotonin) injections. Arch. Int. Pharmacodyn. Ther 1965; 153: 226- 231.

Pacheco S , Hiller K, Smith C: Increased arachidonic acid levels and phospholipids of human colonic mucosa in inflammatory bowel disease. Clin. Sci 1987; 73: 361-364.

Payan DG, Brewster DR, Missirian-Bastion A, et al.: Substance P recognition by a subset of human T lymphocytes. J Clin Invest 1984; 74: 1532-1539.

Peck MJ: Role of prostaglandin mediated vasodilation in inflammation. Nature 1977; 270: 530-532.

Perlmutter DH, Colten HR: Complement: molecular genetics. In: Gallin JI, Goldstein IM, Snyderman R (eds), Inflammation: basic principle and clinical correlates. Raven Press, New York 1988; pp. 75-88.

Pernow B: Substance P. Pharmacol. Rev. 1983; 35: 85-141.

Pettipher ER, Higgs GA, Henderson B: PAF-acether in chronic arthritis, Agents Actions 1987; 21: 98-103.

Pierce JV, Guimaraes JA: Further characterization of highly purifted human plasma kininogen. Life Sci 1975: 16: 790-791.

Pirotzky E, Page CP, Roubin R, et al.: PAF-acether-induced plasma exudation in rat skin is independent of platelets and neutrophils. Microcirc. Endothel. Lymphatics 1984; 1:107-122.

Prasad CM, Adamski SW, Svensjo E, et al: Pharmacological Modification of edema produced by combined infusions of prostaglandin E, and bradykinin in canine forelimbs. J Pharmac Exp Ther 1982; 220: 293-298.

Proud D, Reynolds Cj, Lacapra S, et al.: Nasal provocation with bradykinin induces sympstoms of rhinitis and a sore throat. Am. Rev Respir Dis 1988; 137: 613-616.

Rabito SF, Østravik TB, Scicli AG, et al.: Role of the autonomic nervous system in the release of rat submandibular gland kallikrein into the circulation. Circ Res 1983; 52: 635-641.

Rae SA, Davidson EM, Smith MJH: Leukotriene B_4, an inflammatory mediator in gout. Lancet 1982; II: 1122-1124.

Rainford KD: Effects of antiinflammatory drugs on the release from porcine synovial tissue in viira of interleukinl like cartilase degrading activity. Agents Actions 1987; 21: 337-340.

Ramesha CS, Soter N, Pickett WC: Identification and quantitation of PAF from psoriatic scales. Agents Actions 1987; 21: 382-383.

Rather LJ: Disturbance of function (functio laesa): The legendary fifth cardinal sign of inflammation, added by Galen to the four cardinal signs of a Celsus. Bull. N. Y. Acad. Med. 1971; 47: 303-322.

Regal JF.: Mediators of C5a-induced bronchoconstriction. Agents Actions 1987; 21: 362-365.

Regoli D, Barabe J: Pharmacology of bradykinin and related kinins. Pharmacol. Rev. 1980; 32: 1-46.

Reis ML, Leme J, Sudo LS: Plasma "kininogen" levels in rat with adjuvant arthritis. Agents Action 1982; 9 (Suppl): 368- 378.

Revak SD, Wuepper KD: Activation of Hageman factor in solid and liquid phases. A. critical role of kallikrein. J Exp Med 1973; 138: 1564- 1583.

Ringertz B, Palmbald J, Radmark O, et al.: Leukotriene-induced neutrophil aggregation ill vilra. FEBS Letters 1982; 147: 180-182.

Ripley Y, Jackson JR: Role of neutrophils in the deposition of platelets during acute inflammation. Lab. Invest 1983; 49: 716-724.

Robinson DR, Levine L: Prostaglandin concentrations in synovial fluid in rheumatic diseases: action of indomethacin and aspirin. In: Robinson HJ, Vane JR (eds), Prostaglandin synthetase inhibitors. Raven Press. New York 1974; pp. 223-228.

Rocha E, Silva M: Histamine II and anti histamines. Handbook of Experimental Pharmacology, Springer-Verlag, Berlin 1978; vol. 18 (2).

Roth Sh, Polley HF, Code CF: The activity of histamine and related enzyme systems in human synovial membane and fluid. Arthr. Rheum 1964; 7: 749- 750.

Rynes RI, Ruddy S, Schur PH, et al.: Levels of complement component~properdin factors, and kininogen in patients with inflammatory arthritides. J. Rheumatol. 1974; 1: 413-427.

Sacks T, Moldow CF, Craddock PR, et al.: Oxygen radicals mediated endothelial damage by complement-stimulated granulocytes. J Clin Invest 1978; 61: 1161-1167.

Saeki K, Wake K, Yamasaki H: Inhibition of adjuvant arthritis by histamine. Arch. Int. Pharmacodyn. Ther 1976; 222: 132-140.

Saito H, Ratnoff OD, Donaldson VH: Defective activation of clotting, fibrinolytic, and permeability enhancing system in human Fletcher trait plasma. Circ Res 1974; 34: 641 - 651.

Salmon JA, Higgs GA, Vane JR, et al.: Synthesis of arachidonate cyclo-oxygenase products by rheumatoid and nonrheumatoid synovial lining in nonproliferative organ culture. Ann. Rheum Dis 1983; 42: 36-39.

Samuelsson B: Leukotrienes: mediators of immediate hypersensitivity reactions and inflammation. Science 1983; 220: 568-575.

Sawai K, Niwa S, Katori M: The significanl reduction of high molecular weight-kininogen in synovial fluid of patients with active rheumatoid arthritis. Adv. Exp. Med. 1979; 120B: 195-202.

Sawai K: Parameters for indicating the involvement of plasma kallikrein-kinin system in acute inflammation. Agents Actions 1982; 9 (suppl): 645-648.

Schachter M: Kallikrein (kininogenases) a group of serine proteases with biological actions. Pharmac. Rev 1980;31: 1-17.

Scickuma G, Carrereto OA, Hampton A, et al.: Siteofkininogenases secretion in the dog nephron. Am. J Physiol 1976; 230: 533-536.

Scicli AG, Carretero OA: Renal kallikrein-kinin system. Kidney Int. 1986; 29: 120-130.

Scicli AG, Kher V, Carretero OA: Glandular kallikrein in plasma and urine: evaluation of a direct RIA for its determination. Adv Exp Med Biol 1979; 120B: 127-142.

Sharma JN, Brooks OM, Dick WC: Raised plasma kininogen levels in rheumatoid arthritis-response to therapy with non-steroidal anti-inflammatory drugs. Adv Exp Med Biol 1976; 70: 335-343.

Sharma JN: Comparison of the anti-inflammatory activity commiphora mukul (an indigenous drug) with those of phenylbutazone and ibuprofen in experimental arthritis induced by mycobacterial adjuvant. Arzneim. Forsch./ Drug. Res 1977; 27: 1455-1457.

Sharma JN: Studies on plasma kinin-precursors in rheumatoid arthritis. Ph. D. Thesis; The University of Strathclyde, Glasgow, Scotland; United Kingdom, 1976.

Sharon P, Stenson WF: Enhanced synthesis of leukotriene B4 by colonic mucosa in inflammatory bowel disease. Gastroenterology 1984; 86: 453-460.

Silverberg M, Dunn JT, Miller G:: Mechanism for Hageman factor activation and role of HMW kininogen as a coagulation factor. Ann. NY Acad. Sci 1981; 370: 253-260.

Singh YN, Lembeck F, Theiler M: The molecular weights of plasma and inlesiinal kallikreins. Arch Pharmac 1976; 293: 159-161.

Smedly LA, Tonnesen MG, Sandhaus RA, et al.: Neutrophil-mediated injury to endothelial cells. Enhancement by endotoxin and essential role of neutrophil elastase. J Clin Invest 1986; 77: 1233-1243.

Smersam LM, Justen JM, Leach KL, et al.: Human polymorphonuclear neutrophil activation with arachidonic acid. Br. J Pharmac 1987; 91: 641-649.

Smith AN: Mobilization of tissue kallikrein in inflammatory disease of the colon. Gut 1973; 14: 133-138.

Smith H, McGuire MB, Levina L: Prostaglandin synthesis by rheumatoid synovium and its slimulation by colchicine. Prostaglandin 1975; 10: 67-85.

Smith MJH: Leukotriene B_4 Gen. Pharmac. 1981; 12: 211-216.

Snyder F: Chemical and biochemical aspects of platelet activating factor: a novel class of acetylated ether-linked choline phospholipids. Med Res 1985; 5: 107-140.

Soter NA, Lewis RA, Corey EJ, et al.: Local effects of synthetic leukotrienes (LTC_4, LTD_4, LTE_4, LTB_4) in human skin. J Clin Dermatol 1983; 8(): 115-119.

Struge MA, Yates DB, Gordon D, et al.: Prostaglandin production in arthritis. Ann. Rheum Dis 1978; 37: 315-320.

Svensson J, Samuelsson B: Thromboxanes: a new group of biologically active compounds derived from prostaglandin endoperoxides. Proc. Natl. Acad. Sci.. USA. 1975; 72: 2994-2998.

Swerlick RA, Yancey KB, Lawley TJ: A direct in vivo comparison of the inflammatory properties of human C5a and C5a des Arg. in human skin. J Immunol 1988; 140: 2376-2381.

Szpejda M: Evidence that platelet activating factor may mediate some acute inflammatory responses. Studies with the platelet-activating factor antagonist, CV3988. Lab. Invest. 1986: 54: 275-281.

Tanaka K, Harada Y, Ueno A, et al.: Activation of plasma kallikrein-kinin system and its significant role in pleural fluid accumulation of rat carrageenan-induced pleurisy. Inflammation 1983; 7: 121-131.

Tang LE: Prostaglandins and inflammation. Seminar Arth. Rheum 1980; IX: 153-189.

Taylor DJ, Evanson JM, Wooley DE: Comparative effects of interleukin-I and a phobol ester on rheumatoid synovial cell fructose 2, 6-biphosphate content and prostaglandin E production. Biochem. Biophys Res Commun 1988; 150: 349-354.

The kinin system and prostaglandins in the intestine. Pharmacol. ToxicoL 1988a; in press.

The presenc of interleukin-I synovial fluid. Cellul. Immunol. 1986; 103: 54-64.

Thureson-Klein A, Hedqvist P, Ohlen A, et al.: Leukolriene 84, platelet-activating factor and substance P as mediators of acute inflammation Pathol. Immunopathol Res 1987; 6: 190-206.

Tissot M, Pradelles P, Giroud JP: Substance-P-like levels in inflammatory exudates. Inflammation 1988; 12: 25-35.

Uchida Y, Longridge DJ, Labedz T, et al.: New synthetic antagonists of bradykinin. Br. J. Pharmac 1987; 92: 851-855.

Uchida Y, Oh-Oshi S, Tanaka K, et al.: Activation of plasma kallikrein-kinin system and its significant role in the pleural fluid accumulation of rat carrageenin-induced pleurisy. Agents Actions 1982; 9 (suppl): 379-383.

Van Arman CG, Carlson RP: The two distinct phases of inflammatory response in the dog's knee joint. In: Sicuteri F, Rocha E, Silva M, Back N (eds), Bradykinin and related kinins. Plenum Press. New York 1970; pp.525-533.

Vane JR, Hart FD, Mojtulewski JA: Effects af anti-inflammatory drugs on prostaglandin in rheumatoid al1hritis. In: Robinson HJ, Vane JR (eds), Prostaglandin synthetase inhibitors. Raven Press New York 1974; pp 165- 173.

Vane JR: Mode of action of anti-inflammatory agents which are prostaglandin synthetase inhibitors. In : Vane JR, Ferreira SH (eds), Anti-inflammatory drugs, Springer-Verlag, Berlin 1979; pp. 373-389.

Vane JR: Prostaglandins as mediators of inflammation. In: Samuelsson N, Paoletti R (eds), Advances in prostaglandin and thromboxane research. Raven Press, New York. Vol. 2: pp. 791-801.

Vavrek JR, Stewart JM: Competitive antagonists of bradykinin. Peptides 1985; 6: 161-164.

Voelkel NF, Worthen S, Reeves JT, et al.: Nonimmunologieal production of leukotrienes induced by platelet-activating factor. Science 1982; 218: 286-288.

Vogt W: Anaphylatoxins: possible role in disease. Complement 1986; 3: 177-190.

Von euler US, Gaddum JH: An unidentified depressor substance in certain tissue extracts. Physiol (Lond) 1931; 71: 74-87.

Waldmann R, Abraham JP: Fitzgerald trait. Deficiency of a hitherto unrecognized agent, Fitzgerald factor, participating in surface mediated reactions of clotting, fibrinolysis, generation of kinins, and the property of diluted plasma enhancing vascular permeability (PF/dil). J Clin Invest 1975; 55: 1082-1089.

Wallengren J, Ekman JR, Moller H: Substance P and vasoactive intestinal peptide in bullous and inflammatory skin disease. Acta Derrnatol. Venereol 1986; 66: 23-28.

Ward PA, Zvaifler NJ: Complement-derived leukotactic factors in inflammatory synovial fluids of humans. J Clin Invest 1971; 50: 606-616.

Wasi S, Murray RK, Macmorin DRL, et al: The role of PMN-Ieukocytes in tissue injury, inflammation and hypersensitivity. II. Studies on the proteolytic activity of PMN-Ieukocyte Iysosomes of the rabbit. Br. J Exp. Pathol 1966; 47: 411-423.

Watanbe M, Ohuchi K, Sugidachi A, et al.: Platelet-activating factor in the inflammatory exudate in the anaphylactic phase of allergic inflammation in rats. Int. Arch. Allergy Appl Immunol 1987; 84: 396-403.

Webster ME, Goldfinger SE, Seegmiller JE: Presence of a kinin in inflammatory effusion from arthritides of varying etiology. Arthr Rheum 1967; 10: 13-20.

Weiss SJ, Curnutte JT, Regiani S: Neutrophil mediated solubilization of the subendothelial matrix: oxidative and nonoxidative mechanisms of proteolysis used by normal and chronic granulomatous disease phagocytes. J Immunol 1986; 136: 636-641.

Weissmann G: Prostaglandins in acute inflammation. The Upjohn Company. 1980; pp.5-32.

Whaley K, Khong Y, McCartney C, et al.: : Alternative pathway complement activation and its control in gram-negative endotoxin shock. Adv. Inflamm Res 1979; 1: 293-301.

Whalley Et, Cleigg S, Stewart Jm, et al.: The effect of kinin agonists and antagonists on the pain response of the human blister base. Naunyn Schmiedebergs Arch Pharmacol. 1987; 336: 652-655.

Williams Tj, Morely J: Prostaglandins as potentiator of increased vascular pernleability of inflammation. Nature 1973; 246: 215-217.

Willis AL: Release of histamine, kinin and prostaglandin during carrageenan-induced inflammation. In: Monte Gazza P, Horton EW (eds), Prostaglandin, peptides and amines. Academic Press, London 1969; pp.30-39.

Wood DD, Ihrie EJ, Dinarello CA, et al.: Isolation of interleukin-I-like factor from human joint infusions. Arthritis Rheum 1983; 26: 975-983.

Wuepper KD: Prekallikrein deficiency in man. J. Exp. Med. 1973; 138: 1345-1355.

Yaaje K, Pierce JY: Synthesis of kallikrein by rat kidney slices. Br. J. Pharmac 1975; 53: 229-234.

Yancey KB: Review: Biological properties of human C5a: selected in vitro and ill vivo studies: Clin Exp Immunology 1988; 71: 207-210.

Yang HYT, Tague LT, Manning N: Carboxypeptidase in blood and other fluid III. The esterase activity of the enzyme. Biochem Pharmac 1967; 16: 1287-1297.

Zach EP, Werle E: Über den Kininogengehalt von Serum und Plasma nach Gewebeschiidigung bei Ratlen. Arch. Pharmac 1973; 276: 167-180.

Zeitlin IJ, Brooks PM, Buchanan WW, et al.: The action of aspirin on plasma kininogen and other plasma proteins in rheumatoid patients; relationship to disease activity. Clin. Exp. Pharmac Physiol 1980; 7: 347-353.

Zeitlin IJ: Pharmacological characterization of kinin-forrning activity in rat intestinal tissue. Br. J Pharmac 1971; 42: 648-6491p.

Zeitlin IJ: The action of cimetidine hydrochloride and mepyramine maleate in rat adjuvant arthritis. Eur. J Pharmac 1980; 78: 175-185.

Zipser RD, Nast CC, Lee M, et al.: In vivo production of leukotriene B_4 and leukolriene C_4 in rabbit colitis. Relationship to inflammation. Gastroenterology 1987; 92: 33-39.

Chapter 4

Mediation of Kallikrein-Kinin System in the Mechanism of Action of Angiotens in Converting Enzyme Inhibitors

INTRODUCTION

Angiotensin converting enzyme inhibitors (ACEIs): captopril, enalapril, cilazapril, lisinopril, ramipril and spirapril are powerful blood pressure (BP) lowering agents in various forms of hypertensive and normotensive situations (see Sharma, 1988a, b, 1989). These drugs are widely used as most effective anti-hypertensive agents for patients with essential hypertension, as well as for those patients in whom the hypertension is not associated with raised activity of the renin-angiotensin system (RAS) (Oparil et al., 1987). On the one hand, it has been indicated that captopril decreases proteinuria in hypertensive patients with renal disease via the mode of reducing angiotensin II formation (Ikeda et al., 1989). On the other hand, their -BP lowering property in hypertensive patients has been suggested to be due mainly to the blockade of angiotensin II release (Milner, 1988), which has been considered as the prime mode of action of these substances. However, it is postulated that their mode of action may not be due solely to inhibition of ACE production. Since ACE is identical to kininase II, an enzyme that not only inhibits the conversion of angiotensin I into angiotensin II, but also protect the kallikrein-kinin system (KKS) by intervening the biodegradation of the vasodepressor and diuretic polypeptides, kinins (Sharma, 1988b, 1989). It remains, uncertain however, whether kinin participate by local mechanism(s) in the action of ACEIs. Thus, the present review aims to discuss recent data on the significance of kinins in mediating hypotensive effect of ACEIs.

KALLIKREIN-KININ SYSTEM

The kallikrein-kinin system consists of several components which are responsible for its activation and inhibition in regulating the cellular and molecular functions of kinins by stimulating kininoreceptors. Figure 4.1 shows the complex mode of kallikreins-kininogens-kinins releasing, activating and inhibiting pathways. Kinins are produced in the plasma, lymph, heart, smooth muscles and endocrine glands from kininogens by the action of kallikreins. Bradykinin (BK) is a nonapeptide (N-Site: H-Arg-Pro-Pro-Gly-Phen-Ser-Pro-Phe-Arg-OH: C-site) having chemical structure and pharmacological actions similar to other kinins (Sharma 1988a, 1988c). The two forms of kallikreins are plasma and tissue (organ). Plasma kallikrein circulates in an inactive form termed as pre-kallikrein or Fletcher factor, and has been designated to be involved in the haemodynamic processes. Whereas tissue kallikrein is considered as endogenous hormone and occurs in large amounts in various organs and tissues (see Sharma, 1988a). The renal kallikrein contributes to the regulation of renal transport function, blood flow and BP (Guder and Hallbach, 1988; Sharma 1984; 1988a; Carretero and Scicli, 1989). Kininogens are defined as multifunctional proteins derived from $\alpha 2$-globulin and contain kinins sequences in their molecular structures. They are synthesized in the liver and circulate in plasma and other body fluids.

The two forms of human kininogens are low molecular weight and high molecular weight, which are different from each other in molecular weight, sensitivity to plasma and organ kallikreins, and also in physiological responsibilities (for review, see Muller-Esterl et al., 1986). An addition, T-kininogen has been found only in rat plasma and accounts for more than 70% of the total kininogen in plasma that is capable of releasing T-kinin after trypsinazation (Okamoto and Greenbaum, 1983). Their formation in the liver might be increased during various inflammatory stimuli (Sharma et al., 1976, 1988; Borges and Gordon, 1976).

Kinin inactivating enzymes are collectively known as kininases, which are found in circulatory system and in numerous body tissues. Kininase I cleaves the C-terminal arginine, and kininase II (ACE) has been extensively studied that metabolises BK by releasing Phe-Arg-from C-terminal (Erdos, 1979). Des-Arg9- BK formed via kininase I action possesses greater or less activity than BK depending on the preparations used, whereas, des-(Phe^8-Arg^9)-BK released by kininase II is inactive (Marceau et al., 1983). Hence, kininase II does not only inactivate kinins (potent vasodepressors), but also converts angiotensin I into angiotensin II (a powerful vasopressor).

KININ RECEPTORS

The two main kinin receptors such as B_1 and B_2 have been proposed, however, multiple B_2 receptors in the mammalian tissues might also be involved in cellular responses of kinins (Regoli and Barabe, 1980; Vavrek and Stewart, 1985; Plevin and Owen, 1988). Regoli and his co-workers (Marceau et al., 1983) proposed the function for B_1 receptors; vasodilation, hypotension, smooth muscle contraction, and for the B_2; vasodilation, exudation, pain, smooth muscle contraction, inhibition of phagocyte migration and possibly prostaglandins (PGs) release. Thus, it could be concluded that B_2 receptors are mediating and modulating inflammatory reactions, on the other side, B_1 might be responsible for its role in haemostatic regulatory processes. Moreover, kinins act on B_1 and B_2 receptors to release conjointly endothelium-derived relaxing factor and prostacyclin from bovine aortic endothelial cells (Juste et al., 1989). These findings suggest that BK has multifactorial actions in balancing the release of other vasoactive substances. The advancement in the kinin research was hampered mainly because of the unavailability of specific antagonists. Recently, a number of BK analogues have been synthesized which are specific antagonists of BK (Vavrek and Stewart, 1988). These antagonists may provide access to the tools necessary for understanding the kinin functions in various physiopathological conditions. In addition, compound B-3824 is an effective antagonist of BK-induced vascular permeability in rabbit skin (Schachter et al., 1987).

Using specific BK-antagonists, Whalley et al. (1987) confirmed that the kinin receptors mediating pain on human blister base are of the B_2 type which may serve as valuable model substances for developing new anti-inflammatory drugs (Taylor et al., 1989). These antagonists may also be helpful in investigating the role of kinins in the mode of action of various antihypertensive agents, for example ACEIs, beta blockers, calcium channel antagonists and diuretics, since BK is an endogenous vasodilator agent.

KALLIKREIN-KININ AND RENIN-ANGIOTENSIN SYSTEMS INTERATION

The interaction between KKS and RAS is currently of great interest. It is known that kinin and angiotensin I are released from the α2-globulin (synthesized in the liver) termed as kininogens and angiotensinogen respectively (Sharma, 1978; Sharma and Zeitlin, 1982; Murakami et al.) 1980).

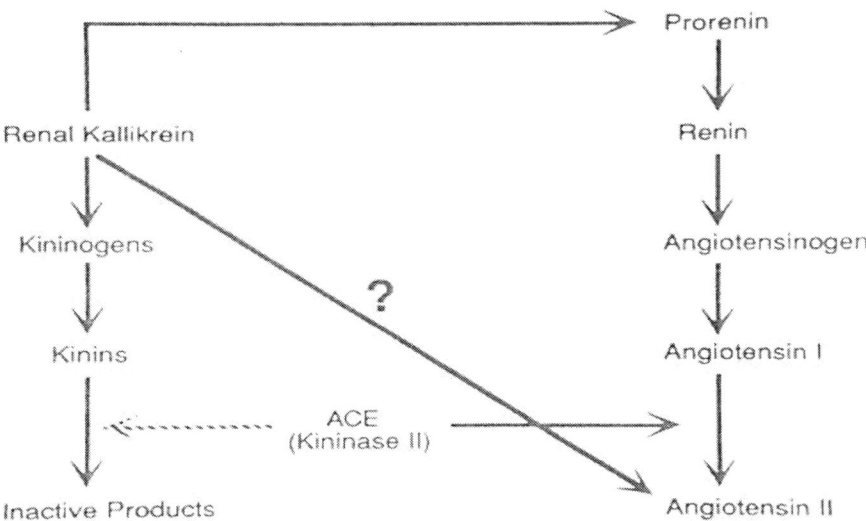

Figure 4.2. Hypothetical presentation of interaction between the kallikrein-kinin and reninangiotensin systems in regulation of physiological responses.

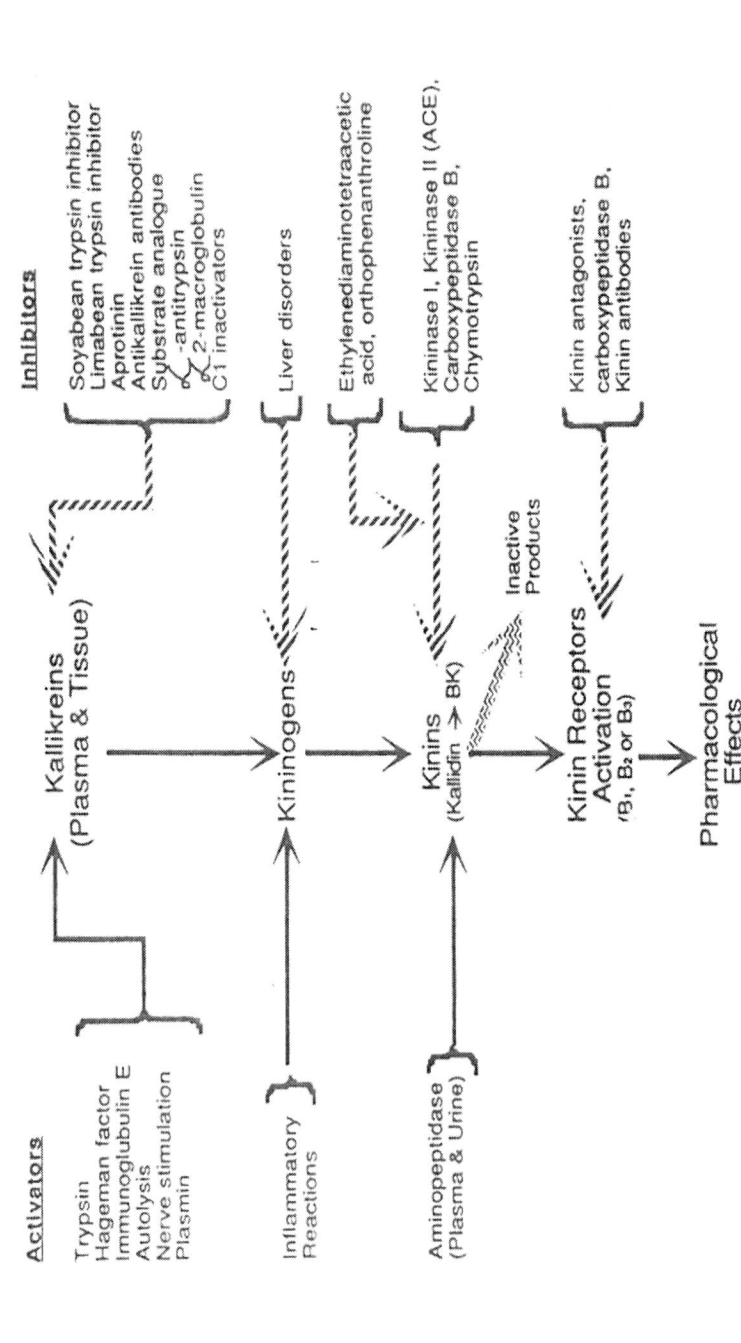

Figure 4.1. Components of the kallikrein-kinin forming system and their activating and inhibiting factors.

ACE (kininase 11, peptidyldipeptidase; E.C. 3.4.15.1) converts angiotensin I to angiotensin II, and hydrolyses BK (see above) Kallikrein has the property to convert inactive plasma renin to active renin (Sealey et al.. 1978). However, work of Hiwada et al. (1983) indicated that tissue kallikrein does not directly activate inactive renin, but participates in the activation process of inactive renin. There is complex evidence to suggest that kallikrein can generate angiotensin II like pressor substance, which has been named as "Kinin—tensin enzyme system" (Arakawa, 1988; Arakawa and Maruta, 1980; Ideishi et al., 1987).

The tissue kallikrein may have an important role in regulation of both kinin and angiotensin II production. It might be therefore assumed that kallikrein is the physiological regulator of these vasoconstrictor (angiotensin II) and vasodilator (BK) in maintaining the normal BP. However, it is a great puzzle; why the renal kallikrein activity reduces and angiotensin II formation raises in essential hypertensive patients? It is conceivable that nature has provided with us a very complex mechanism in researching the biochemical and physiological basis of actions of these autocoids. Figure 4.2 shows an interaction between the KKS and RAS.

KALLIKREIN-KININ SYSTEM DURING HYPERTENSION

It is now widely believed that deficient levels of KKS may lead to alterations in physiological states, such as vasoconstriction, retention of sodium and water, increased peripheral resistance, renovascular constriction, and abnormalities in vascular smooth muscle structure and cell membrane functions (Margolius, 1984; Sharma, 1984; 1988a; Verma et al., 1987). Therefore, the lack of KKS release in systemic circulation may cause the development of hypertension. Berry and coworkers (1989) demonstrated that dominant allele expressed as high urinary kallikrein excretion may be associated with reduced risk of essential hypertension. Hence, population with genetic coding which reduces KKS may have a predisposing factor for the genesis of high BP. Margolius et al. (1971) observed the reduced urinary kallikrein excretion in patients with essential hypertension. It is evident that hypertensive conditions can be treated successfully with kininase II inhibitors (ACEIs) that protect the inactivation of kinins. The role of kallikrein-kinin system in renal function and hypertension has been extensively covered in the proceedings of a symposium held in Sapporo, Japan(limura and Margolius, 1988). Figure4.3 summarises the role of KKS in pathophysiology of essential hypertension.

ANTIHYPERTENSIVE EFFECTS OF KININASE II INHIBITORS (ACEIs)

The discovery of kininase II inhibitors came after the observations made by Ferreira (1965) that various extracts from the venom of Viper Bothrops jaracara potentiated the actions of BK. This property appeared to result from inhibiting the kininases responsible for BK biodegradation. In addition, Bakhle (1968) reported that BK potentiating agent can also inhibit the conversion of angiotensin I to Angiotensin II. Subsequently, it was discovered that the ACE is identical to kininase II, which causes release of angiotensin II on one hand, and on the other hand, it can also cause inactivation of BK (Yang et al., 1971). On this principle, Ondetti et al. (1977) synthesized an orally active agent (SQ, 14,225 or captopril). Since then numerous compounds belonging to this class have been developed which are under vigorous clinical evaluation. These ACE (kininase II) inhibitors have the unique property to cause reduction in BP not only in hypertensive humans and animals, but also in normotensive individuals and animals (Sharma, 1989), whereas other groups of antihypertensive drugs are devoid of these dual properties. Captopril has been shown to be active in lowering BP in various hypertensive models (Ng et al., 1988; Hutchinson and Mendelsohn, 1980; Antonaccio, 1982) and in essential hypertension (Kudo et al., 1988). Administration of captopril (1.5 mg/kg i.v.) to normotensive mongrel dogs was associated with an increased renal blood flow despite a significant fall of 17 mmHg in mean arterial BP (Clappison et al., 1981). These investigators also observed an increased urinary kinin excretion which might be associated in the regulation of renal vasculature. Enalapril is known to possess hypotensive action in experimental and clinical hypertension (Sharma et al., 1983; Gavras, 1986; Cerasola et al., 1987). It has been observed that enalapril can reduce BP in conscious normotensive Dahl-salt resistant (DSR), Dahl salt-sensitive (DSS) rats, and hypertensive DSS rats (Sharma et al., 1984). Cilazapril is a novel ACEI which elicits pronounced antihypertensive effect in spontaneously hypertensive and renal hypertensive rats (Hefti et al., 1986; Ding et al., 1988), as well as causes hypotension in normal dogs (Holck et al., 1986).

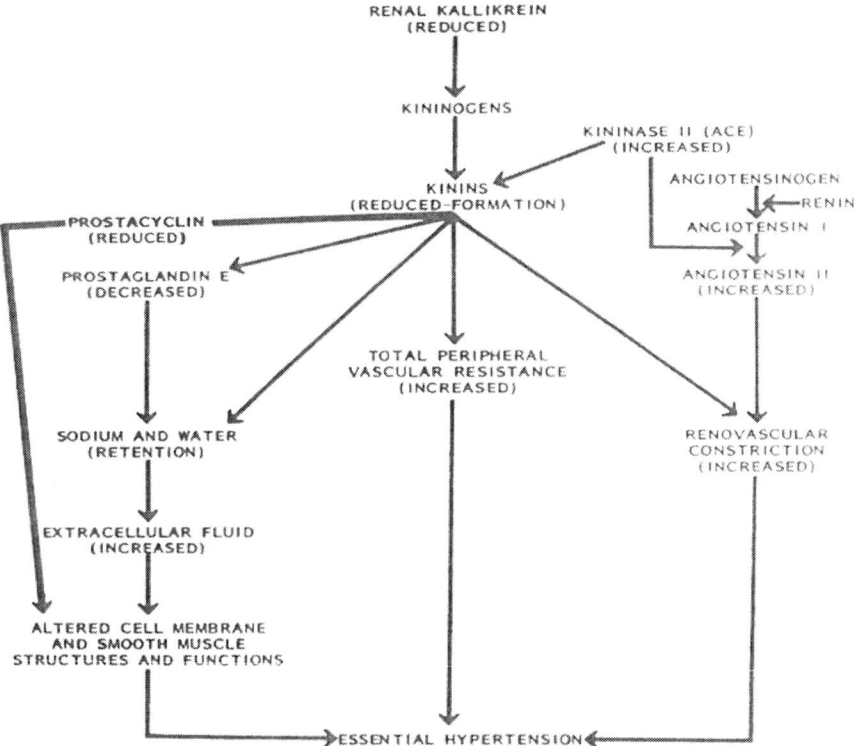

Figure 4.3. Hypothetical role of kallikrein-kinin system in the pathogenesis of essential hypertension.

The hypotensive action of cilazapril in terms of percentage change was greater in hypertensive rats than the normotensive rats (41±6 vs 20±3 mmHg or 25±4% vs 16±2% respectively) (Ding et al., 1988). Following the administration of ramipril in essential hypertensive patients, systolic, diastolic and mean BP decreased significantly without altering the heart rate (Masuda et al., 1988). In conclusion, it seems that these drugs are able to reduce BPin physiological and pathological states. The reduction of physiological BP is suggestive that endogenous mediators of vasodialation might be potentiated in the presence of ACEIs, and the role of RAS in the long term BP regulation may be questionable with reference to the genesis of hypertension (see Figure 4.3).

The modes of actions of ACEIs in normotensive and hypertensive conditions are not clearly described. However, it is documented that BP lowering effects of ACEIs in hypertensive patients is mainly due to the blockade of angiotensin II formation (Winner, 1988), and it is partially due to protection of kinins. Masuda et al. (1988) have proposed both the reduced plasma angiotensin II and the increased plasma kinin may contribute to the hypotensive effect of ramipril in normal renin group, whereas anti-hypertensive action in low renin class should be considered to be mainly based on an increased plasma kinin levels. Aprotinin, a tissue kallikrein inhibitor, blocks the anti-hypertensive effect of captopril in patients with low and normal RAS having essential hypertension (Overlack et al., 1980). In addition, failure of captopril to lower BP in some hypertensive patients might reflect the blunted activity of KKS (Madeddu et al., 1987). Determination of plasma and tissue kinins levels in the presence and in the absence of ACEIs in humans could provide meaningful information concerning the status of KKS in the mode of action of ACEIs. Nevertheless, due to methodological artifacts, the blood concentrations of kinins have been observed to be raised, unchanged or reduced after the administration of ACEIs (Carretero et al., 1981; Johnston et al., 1981; Vinci et al., 1979; Hulthen and Hokfelt, 1978). Thus, it is suggested that kinins participate in the BP regulation of ACEIs. However, other studies contradict this hypothesis, indicating that inhibition of KKS per se will often result in a reduction of stimulated renin activity; therefore, the measurement of kinins in the plasma cannot clarify the role of kinins in ACE inhibition (Winner, 1988). Moreover, reversal of hypotensive action of ACEIs by using specific kinin receptors antagonists may provide the most reliable direct evidence that kinins do play a role in the hypotension-induced by ACEIs.

KININ RECEPTORS ANTAGONISTS AND ANGIOTENSIN COVERTING ENZYME (KININASE II) INHIBITORS

Currently, kinin receptors antagonists are available as valuable tools for the evaluation of the biological functions of kinin with special interest to the mode of action of ACEIs. Stewart and Vavrek (1986) showed that BK antagonists inhibited the BP lowering effect of BK. In the rat, the fall in mean arterial BP induced by i.a. injections of BK was greatly reduced during an i.a. infusion of BK antagonist (B4310) (Griesbacher et al., 1989). A theoretical possibility exists that administration of kinin antagonists should produce a rise in BP if the kinins are indeed, mediators of BP regulations. In this regard, Carbonell and coworkers (1988a) demonstrated that treatment with high doses of a kinin antagonist produced an increase in BP in the rat. Thus, kinins have major role in the controlof BP.To assess the effect of BK antagonist on the acute antihypersive activity of enalapril in hypertensive rats, Carbonell and coinvestigators (1988b) reported reduction in the hypotensive response of ACEIs in the presence of BK antagonist when compared with the saline-infused control group.To obtain additional facts about the pharmacological relationships between the BK, BK antagonists and captopril, a ACEI, we have demonstrated in acute experiments in spontaneously hypertensive rats that (1) BK induced hypotension was greatly potentiated after captopril treatment, (2) hypotensive responses produced by BK and captopril were significantly antagonized in the presence of BK antagonist (B5630) and (3) heart rate did not change during administration of these agents (Sharma et al., 1989) Figure 4.4 represents the tracing of the hypotensive effect of BK and captopril in the absence and in the presence of kinin antagonist in hypertensive rats.Although, there is indication that circulating BK does not actively participate in normotensive BP control, endogenous BK might play an important role in cardiovascular regulation by blunting the BP effect of pressure amines and hormones (Waeber et al., 1988).

Nevertheless, the critical analysis of present data suggests that kinin is directly responsible for the mode of action of ACE (kininase II) inhibitors and in the pathogenesis of hypertension.

SUMMARY

The kallikrein-kinin system has a most significant role in the regulation of both normotensive and hypertensive BP. Hence, reduced activity of kinin receptors mediated via decreased circulating endogenous kinin might explain the cause of high BP. This system also governs the activation of RAS at various axis in control of the physiological state of BP. The kinin receptor antagonists can block the hypotensive action of captopril-like drugs in hypertensive and normotensive animals. The hypotensive action of BK is greatly increased after ACE (kininase II) inhibitors treatment. On the basis of these two pharmacological properties, it is probable to conclude that these drugs do not only protect inactivation of kinins, but also possess most significant action as kinin receptors agonists, since hypotensive action induced by ACEIs is antagonized by specific BK receptors antagonist. Hence, I propose here that the mode of action of ACEIs are due to protection of kinin system, and these drugs act like kinin receptor activators (Figure4.5). The discovery of specific BK antagonists offers a new dimension concerning the experimental approach for examining the role of kinins in hypertension and other pathological situations, and potential therapeutic agents were the kinin system is abnormally raised.

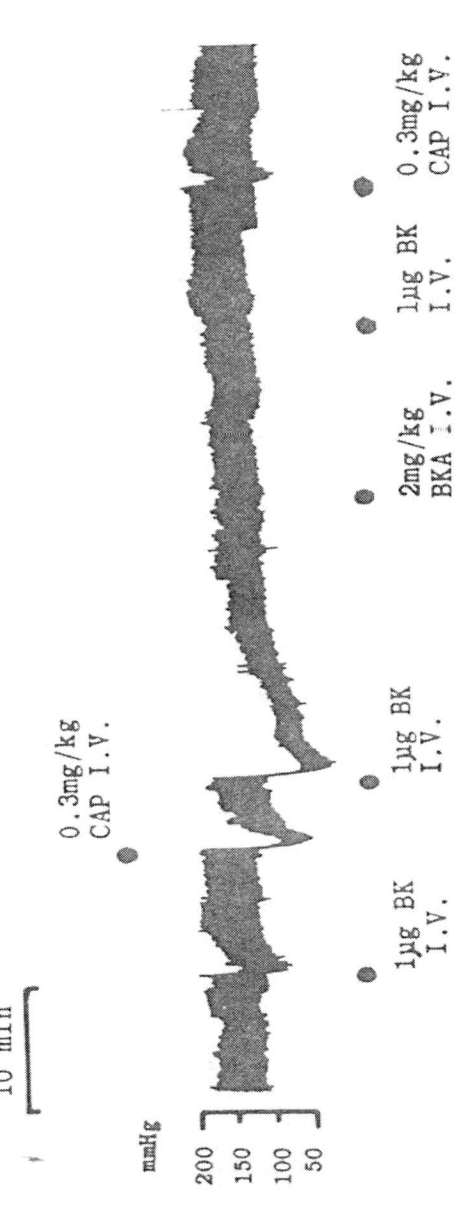

Figure 4.4. Effects of bradykinin(BK: 1μg i.v.),captopril (CAP; 0.3mg/kg i.v.) and BK antagonist (BKA; 2 mg/kg i.v.) on the systolic and diastolic blood pressure of a spontaneously hypertensive rat aneathetized with pentobarbitone sodium (50mg/kg i.p.). Bradykinin induced a fall in blood pressure and duration of hypotension were increased by CAP treatment. Bradykinin antagonist (B5630) and caused blockade of hypotensive effects of BK and CAP (This is an unpublished work of Sharma J. N.. Mohsin S.S.J..Stewart J.M. and Vavrek R.J).

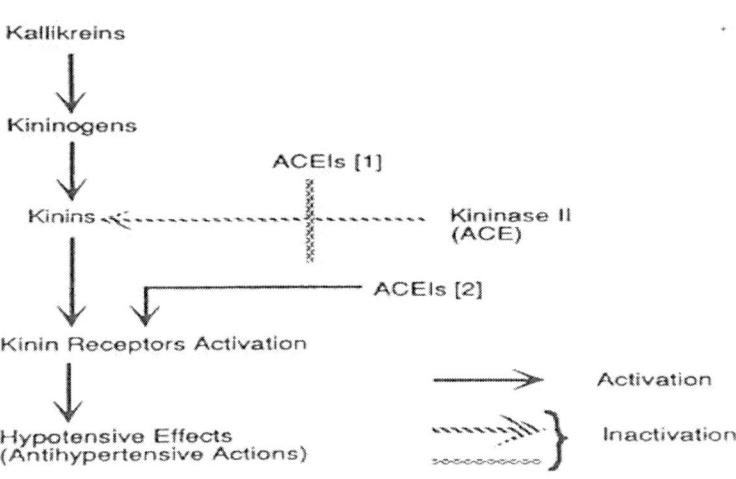

Figure 4.5. Kinin receptor activator.

REFERENCES

Antonaccio MJ: Angiotensin converting enzyme (ACE) inhibitors. A. Rev. Pharmacol. Toxicol 1982; 22: 57-87.

Arakawa K: Alternative pathways of angiotensin II and kinin formation by kallikreinIn Renal function, Hypertension and Killikrein-Kinin System (Edited by Iimura O. and Margolius H. S.) University of Tokyo Press, Tokyo 1988; pp: 61-66..

Arakawa K, Maruta H: Ability of kallikrein to generate angiotensin II-like pressor substance and a proposed 'kinin-tensin enzyme system'. Nature 1980; 288: 705-706.

Bakhle YS: Conversion of angiotensin I to angiotensin II by cell free extract of dog lung. Nature 1968; 220: 919-921.

Berry TD, Hasstedt SJ, Hunt SC, et al: A gene for high urinary kallikrein may protect against hypertension in utah kindreds. Hypertension 1989; 13: 3-8.

Bonner G: Haben die Kinine eine Bedeutung fur die antihypertensive Wirkung der ACE-Hemmer? Z. Kardiol. 1988; 7 (Suppl. 3): 23-27.

Borges DR, Gordon AH: Kininogen and kininogenase synthesis by the liver of normal and injured rats. J Pharm. Pharmacol 1976; 28: 44-48.

Carbonell LF, Carretero OA, Madeddu P et al : Effect of a kinin antagonist on mean blood pressure. Hypertension 1988a; 11 (Suppl. I): 1-84-1-88.

Carbonell LF, Carreterro OA, Stewart JM et al : Effect of a kinin antagonist on the acute antihypertensive activity of enalaprilat in severe hypertension. Hypertension 1988b; 11: 239-243.

Carretero OA, Scicli AG: Kinins, paracrine hormones, in the regulation of blood flow, renal function, and blood pressure. In Endocrine Mechanisms in Hypertension (Edited by Laragh J. H., Brenner B. M. and Kaplan N. M.) Raven Press, New York.1989; pp: 219-239.

Carretero OA, Scicli AG, Maitra SR: Roles of kinins in the pharmacological effects of converting enzyme inhibitors. In Angiotensin Converting Enzyme Inhibitors (Edited by Horovitz Z. P.), Urban and Schwarzenberg, Baltimore 1981; pp: 105-121..

Cerasola G, Cottone S, D'Ignoto G, et al : Effect of enalapril maleate on blood pressure, renin-angiotensinaldosterone system, and peripheral sympathetic activity in essential hypertension. Clin Ther 1987; 9: 390-399.

Clappison BH, Anderson WP, Johnston Cl: Role of the kallikrein-kinin system in the renal effects of angiotensin converting enzyme inhibition in anaesthetized dogs. Clin Exp Pharmac Physiol 1981; 8: 509-513.

Ding YN, Chang ST, Shieh SM, et al : Antihypertensive and renal effect if cilazapril and their reversal by angiotensin in renovascular hypertensive rats.
Clin Sci 1988; 74: 365-372.

ErdOs EG: Kininases. Handbook Exp Pharmac 1979; 25: 427-448.

Ferreira SH: A bradykinin-potentiating factor (BPF) present in the venom of Bothropsjararaca. Br. J Pharmac 1965; 24: 163-169.

Gavras H: A multicenter trial of enalapril in the treatment of hypertension. Clin Ther 1986; 9: 15-29.

Griesbacher T, Lembeck F, Saria A: Effect of the bradykinin antagonist B4310 on smooth muscle and blood pressure in the rat, and its enzymatic degradation. Br JPharmac 1989; 96: 531-538.

Guder WG, Hallbach J: Localization and regulation of the renal kallikreinkinin system: possible relations to renal transport functions. Klin Wochenschr 1988; 66: 849-856.

Hefti F, Fischli W, Gerald M: Cilazapril prevent hypertension in spontaneously hypertensive rats. J Cardiovas Pharmac 1986; 8: 641-648.

Hiwada K, Matsumoto C, Kokubu T: Role of glandular kallikrein in the activation process of human plasma inactive renin. Hypertension 1983; 5: 191-197.

Holck M, Fischli W, Hefti F et al: Cardiovascular effects of the new angiotension-converting enzyme inhibitor, cilazapril, in anesthetized and conscious dogs.J Cardiovas Pharmac 1986; 8: 99-108.

Hulthen UL, Hdkfelt B: The effect of the converting enzyme inhibitor SQ 20,881 on kinins, reninangiotensin-aldosterone and catecholamine in relation to blood pressure in hypertensive patients. ActaMed Scand 1986; 204: 497-502.

Hutchinson JS, Mendelsohn FAO: Hypotensive effects of captopril administered centrally in intact conscious spontaneously hypertensive rats and peripherally in anephric anaesthetized spontaneously hypertensive rats. Clin Exp Pharmac Physiol 1980; 7: 555-558.

Ideishi M, Ikeda M, Arakawa K: Direct angiotensin II formation by rat submandibular gland kallikrein. J Biochem 1987; 102: 859-868.

Iimura O, Margolius HS (Eds): Renal Function, Hypertension and KallikreinKinin System, Tokyo University Press, Tokyo 1988.

Ikeda T, Nakayama D, Gomi T, et al : Captopril, an angiotensin I--converting enzyme inhibitors, decreases proteinuria in hypertensive patients with renal diseases. Nephron 1989; 52: 72-75.

Johnston Cl, Yasujima M, Clappison BH: The kallikrein-kinin system and angiotensin converting enzyme inhibition in hypertension. In Angiotensin Coverting Enzyme

Inhibitors (Edited by Horovitz Z. P.) Urban and Schwarzenberg, Baltimore.1981; pp: 123-139.

Juste PD, de Nucci G, Vane JR: Kinins act on B, and E, receptors to release conjointly endothelium-derived relaxing factor and prostaglandin from bovine aortic endothelial cells. Br J Pharmac 1989; 96: 920-926.

Kudo K, Abe K, Chiba S, et al : Role of thromboxine A, in the hypertensive effect of captopril in essential hypertension. Hypertension 1988; 11: 147-152.

Madeddu P, Oppes M, Rubattu S, et al: Role of renal kallikrein in medulating the antihypertensive effect of a single oral dose of captopril in normal and low-renin essential hypertensives. J Hyperten 1987; 5: 645 648.

Marceau F, Lussier A, Regoli D, et al: Pharmacology of kinins: their relevance to tissue injury and inflammation. Gen Pharmac 1983; 14: 209-229.

Margolius HS: The kallikrein-kinin system and the kidney. A Rev Physiol 1984; 46: 309-326.

Margolius HS, Geller R, Pisano JJ, et al: Altered urinary kallikrein excretion in human hypertension Lancet 1971; 2: 1063-1065.

Masuda A, Shimamoto K, Ando T, et al: The mechanism of the hypotensive effect of ramipril (Hoe 498) in patients with essential hypertension. In Renal Function, Hypertension and Kallikrein Kinin System (Edited by Iimura o. and Margolius H. S.)University of Tokyo Press, Tokyo 1988; pp: 189-194..

Muller-Esterl WS, Iwanga S, Nakani-Shi S: Kininogens revişited. Trends Biochem Sci 1986; 11: 336-339.

Murakami E, Hiwada K, Kokubu T: Effect of prostaglandins on renin substrate production by the liver.Clin Sci 1980; 59: 137-139.

Ng CF, Gautieri RF, Lember PM: The effect of chronic administration of indomethacin in captopriltreated renal hypertensive rats. Res. Commun. Chem. Path.Pharmac 1988; 59: 321-338.

Okamoto H, Greenbaum 1M: Kininogen substrate for trypsin and cathepsin D in human, rabbit and rat plasmas. Life Sci 1983; 32: 207-213.

Ondetti MA, Rubin B, Cushman DW: Design of specific inhibitors of angiotensin-converting enzyme: new class of orally active antihypertensive agents.Science 1977; 196: 441-444.

Oparil S, Horton R, Wilkins 1H, et al: Antihypertensive effect of enalapril in essential hypertension: role of prostacyclin. Am J Med Sci 1987; 294: 395402.

Overlack O, Stumpe KO, Kuhnert M, et al: Altered blood pressure and renin responses to converting enzyme inhibition after aprotinin-induced kallikrein-kinin system blockade. Clin Sci 1980; 59: (Suppl1.), 129-132.

Plevin R, Owen PJ: Multiple B, kinin receptors in mannnalian tissues. Trends Pharmac Sci 1988; 9: 387-389.

Regoli D, Barabe J: Pharmacology of bradykinin and related kinins. Pharmac.Rev 1980; 32: 1-46.

Schachter M, Uchida Y, Longridge DJ,et al: New synthetic antagonists of bradykinin. Br J Pharmac 1987; 92: 851855.

Sealey JE, Atlas SA, Laragh JH, et al: Human urinary kallikrein converts inactive to active renin and is a possible physiological activator of renin. Nature 1978; 275: 144-145.

Sharma JN: The effect of prostaglandins (PGE, and PGF,,) on plasma kininogen levels in the rat. Biomedicine 1978; 29: 292-293.

Sharma JN: Kinin-forming system in the genesis of hypertension. Agents Actions 1984; 14: 200-205.

Sharma JN: Interrelationship between the kallikrein-kinin system and hypertension: a review. Gen Pharmac 1988a; 19: 177-187.

Sharma JN: The kallikrein-kinin system in hypertension. In Renal Function, Hypertension and KallikreinKinin System (Edited by Iimura O. and Margolius H. S.),. University of Tokyo Press, Tokyo.1988b; pp: 147-154

Sharma JN: The kinin system and prostaglandins in the intestine. Pharmac Toxic 1988c; 63: 310-316.

Sharma JN: Contribution of kinin system to the antihypertensive action of angiotensin converting enzyme inhibitors. Adv Exp Med Biol 1989; 247 A: 179-205.

Sharma JN, Zeitlin IJ: Reduced plasma kininogen concentrations by prostaglandin E, in rats.. Eur J Pharmac 1982; 83: 119-121.

Sharma JN, Zeitlin IJ, Brooks PM, et al: A novel relationship between plasma kininogen and rheumatoid disease. Agents Actions 1976; 6: 148-153.

Sharma JN, Fernandez PG, Kim BK, et al: Cardiac regression and blood pressure control in the Dahl rat treated with anlapril maleate (MK-421), and angiotensin converting enzyme inhibitor and hydrochlorothiazide. J Hyperten 1983; 1: 251-256.

Sharma JN, Fernandez PG, Kim BK, et al: Systolic blood pressure responses to enalapril maleate (MK-421) (an angiotensin converting enzyme inhibitor) and hydrochlorothiazide in conscious Dahl sensitive(s) and resistant (R) rats. Can J Physiol. Pharmac 1984; 62: 486-489.

Sharma JN, Zeitlin IJ, Mackenzie JF, et al: Plasma kinin precursor levels in clinical intestinal inflammation. Fund Clin. Pharmac 1988; 2: 399-403.

Sharma JN, Stewart JM, Mohsin SSJ, et al: Influence of a kinin antagonist on acute hypotensive responses induced by bradykinin and captopril in spontaneously hypertensive rats. Agents Actions 1992; 38: (suppl III) 258-269.

Stewart JM, Vavrek RJ: Bradykinin competitive antagonists of bradykinin.
Adv Exp Med Biol 1986; 198: 537-542.

Taylor JE, DeFeudis FV, Moreau JP: Bradykinin-antagonists: therapeutic perspectives. Drug Dev Res 1989; 16: 1-11.

Vavrek RJ, Stewart JM: Competitive antagonists of bradykinin. Peptides 1985; 6: 161-164.

Vavrek RJ, Stewart JM: New bradykinin antagonist peptides as tools for the study of the kallikreinkinin system. In Renal Function, Hypertension and Kallikrein Kinin System (Edited by Iimura O. and Margolius H. S.),. University of Tokyo Press, Tokyo. 1988; pp: 85-90

Verma PS, Gagnon JA, Miller RL: Intrarenal kallikrein-kinin activity in acute renovascular hypertension in dogs. Renal Physiol 1987; 10: 311-317.

Vinci JM, Horwitz D, Zusman RM, et al: The effect of converting enzyme inhibition with SQ 20, 881 on plasma and urinary kinins, prostaglandin E, and angiotensin II in hypertensive man. Hypertension 1979; 1: 416-426.

Waeber B, Aubert JF, Fluckiger JP, et al: Role of endogenous bradykinin in blood pressure control of conscious rats. Kidney Intern 1988; 34 (Suppl. 26.): S63-S68.

Whalley ET, Clegg S, Stewart JM, et al: The effect of kinin agonists and antagonists on the pain response of human blister base. Naunyn-Schmiedeb. Arch Pharmac 1987; 336: 652-655.

Yang HYT, Erdos EG, Levin Y: Characterization of a dipeptide hydrolase (kininase II; angiotensin I converting enzyme). J Pharmac Exp Ther 1971; 177: 29-300.

Chapter 5

The Kinin System and Prostaglandins in the Intestine

The tissues of the intestinal tract constitute a large number of biologically active endogenous mediators such as kallikrein-kinin system (KKS) and prostaglandins (PGs). There is a growing conviction that these agents interact with each other in the regulation of motility, blood supply, secretion of electrolyte and protection of gastroduodenal mucosa in normal physiological concentrations. Pharmacologists, neuroscientists, endocrinologists and gastroenterologists have led other groups in recognizing the likely pathophysiological and clinical significance of these vasoactive substances, which are released in the intestine. The prime aim of this brief review is to identify the role of KKS and PGs in the gut.

THE KALLIKREIN-KININ SYSTEM

Kinins are generated in plasma, lymph, smooth muscle and endocrine organs from precursor kininogens by the enzymatic actions of a group of proteases called kallikreins (Figure5.1). Bradykinin is a nonapeptide (H-Arg-Pro-Pro-Gly-Phen-Ser-Pro-Phe-Arg-OH) which has chemical structure and pharmacological properties like other kinins (for review see Sharma 1988). Kinins are quickly inactivated by enzymestermed kininases. These kininases are localized in the endothelial cells, kidney, intestine and lung (Erdos 1977). Kininase I (carboxypeptidase N) cleaves the C-terminal arginine. Kininase II (angiotensin-converting enzyme) has been extensively studied and metabolises kinins by releasing the C-terminal Phc-Arg (Erdos 1979).

KALLIKREINS

Kallikreins are divided into two groups(plasma and tissue or glandular). These enzymes differ in molecular weight, biological functions, physicochemical, immunological properties, and in their localization in the body. Plasma kallikrein is present in the circulation in an inactive form called prekallikrein or Fletcher factor. Plasma lacking prekallikrein (designated

Fletcher trait deficiency) possesses a reduced rate of surface-mediated coagulation which reaches normal when the incubation time is increased in the presence of kaolin (Hathway & Alsever 1970). Prekallikrein is activated by Hageman factor (HF) (Kaplan & Austen 1971). Active plasma kallikrein has been shown to convert inactive HF into active HF in the fluid phase (Cochrane et al. 1973).

Tissue kallikreins are found in the kidney, pancreas, intestine, salivary gland and synovial tissue (Nustad et al. 1975; Zeitlin 1971; Amundsen & Nustad 1965; Sharma et al. 1983). The renal kallikrein has been suggested to regulate blood pressure and is possibly involved in the physiopathology of hypertension (Sharma 1984 & 1988). Amundsen & Nustad (1965) observed the presence of tissue kallikrein-like activity in the rabbit and rat intestine. Schachter and his co-workers (Schachter et al. 1983) demonstrated tissue kallikrein in the goblet cells of the intestine in the rat and cat by using immunohistochemical techniques. In the small intestine of the rat, two kallikreins of varying molecular weights (33,000-35,000) have been reported (Moriwaki et al. 1980), while in the whole length of intestine, a tissue kallikrein of 33,000 molecular weight was observed (Zeitlin et al. 1976). Furthermore; it has been proposed that activation of intestinal kallikrein via bile acids may be responsible for the biological effects of bile acids (Zeitlin et al. 1986). A high rate of tissue kallikrein synthesis in the rat colon has also been observed (Miller et al. 1984). The kinin forming enzyme in the rat stomach has been found to be of a higher rate when compared with that in various regions of the intestine (Kobayashi & Ohata 1981). These investigators suggest that this enzyme is similar to cathepsin D, and the enzyme is involved in the function of the stomach. This latter kallikrein differed from plasma kallikrein and had the inhibitor and substrate specificities of a glandular kallikrein (Zeitlin 1971).

KININOGENS

Two kinin-forming substrates, low molecular weight (LMW) and high molecular weight kininogens (HMWK)have been isolated from bovine plasma (Komiya et al. 1974). They differ in molecular weights (HMW - 76,000; LMW -48,000), and in their susceptibility to plasma and tissue kallikreins. HMW kininogen is the main substrate for plasma kallikrein, and LMW kininogen is the most suitable substrate for tissue kallikrein. Two kininogens with different molecular weights (HMW - 120,000, LMW - 78,000) have also beenisolated from human plasma (Jacobsen 1966; Nagayasu and Nagasawa 1979). The presence of a third form of human kininogen of about 200,000 daltons has been demonstrated (Pierce & Guimaraes 1975). Deficiency of HMW kininogen appears to be the source of the multiple defects such as impaired clotting, kinin-release, and surface-activated fibrinolysis in plasma. HMW kininogen is also known as "Fitzgerald factor", because its absence was found first in the Fitzgerald family (Donaldson et al. 1977; Lutcher 1976). Moreover, an immunochemical evidence has been shown for the presence of HMW Kininogen in human platelets and its secretion after platelet activation with a divalent cationophore A23I87, collagen, and thrombin (Schmaier et al. 1983).

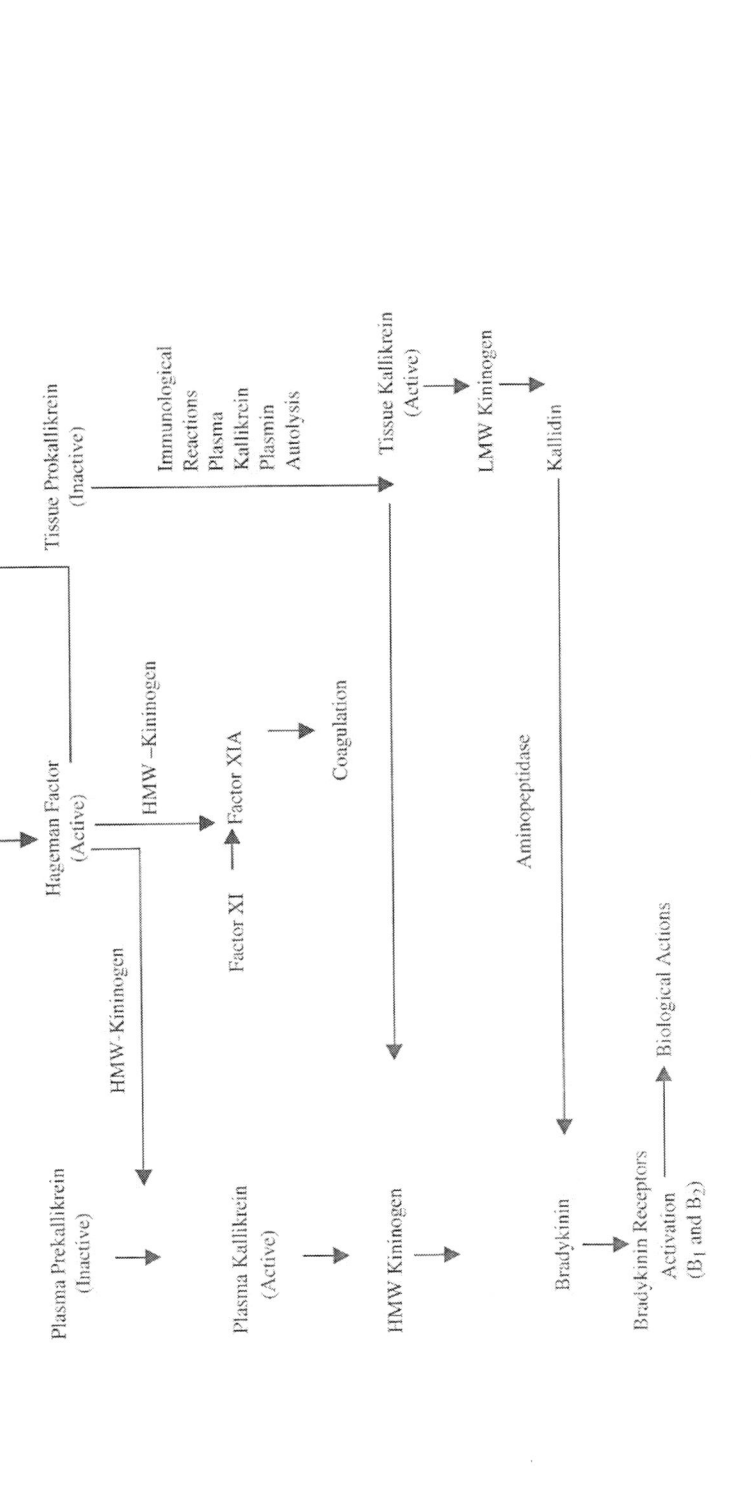

Figure 5.1. A scheme showing the mode of kinin-formation and its inhibition in the circulatory system.

In rat plasma, three types of kininogens (HMW kininogen, LMW kininogen and T-kininogen) have been reported (Okamoto & Greenbaum 1983a & b). T-kininogen accounts for more than 70% of the total kininogen in the plasma which is able to release kinin upon trypsinazation. A major part of rat urinary T-kininogen originates from the circulation (Okamoto et al. 1987). Principally, all kininogens are synthesized in the liver and secreted into the blood plasma and various organs where they serve a variety of physiological functions (for review see Muller-Esterl et al. 1986) such as kinin-production. Nevertheless, kinins can cause increased vascular permeability, vasodilation and pain (Sharma & Buchanan 1979).

KININ SYSTEM AND THE INTESTINE

The main physiological functions of the kinins are vasodilation, increased vascular permeability and hyperaemia of the mucosa of the gastrointestinal tract (GIT) (Gautvik et al. 1972; Hilton & Jones 1968; Hilton & Lewis 1956). On the other side, pharmacological evidence shows that kinins alter the GIT motility and the transepithelial transport of water, electrolytes, aminoacid, glucose, macromolecules and vitamin B_{12} (Fasth & Hulten 1973; Rohen & Peterhoff 1972; Dennhardt & Haberich 1972; Moriwaki et al. 1972; Rumpeltes et al. 1975). Further, Moriwaki and coworkers (Moriwaki et al. 1977) suggested that kinin stimulates Na + transport in the membrane. The influence of KKS on the intestinal transport of amino acids and sugar might be the result of acceleration of Na + flow. Similar phenomenon has been found in the kidney, where an infusion of kinin into the renal artery causes high renal sodium excretion (MarinGrez et al. 1982).

Tissue kallikrein and its inactive precursor have been reported in every segment of the GIT (Zeitlin 1971; Amundsen & Nustad 1965; Frankish & Zeitlin 1977). Using immunohistochemical techniques, kallikrein has been localized in the goblet cells of the colon of rats (Schachter et al. 1983; Miller et al. 1984). Excessive kinin-formation in human colon may account for inflammation of the gut wall (Zeitlin & Smith 1973). Moreover, it has been suggested that infiltration into the intestinal fluid of increased levels of plasma kallikrein and plasma proteins (possibly kininogen) could take place in ulcerative colitis and Crohn's disease (Fasth et al. 1978), indeed, it seems that most of the components present in the inflamed gut may have originated from the systemic circulation. Therefore, raised amounts of plasma kininogen observed by Sharma et al. (1988) in clinical intestinal inflammatory diseases might be due to an increased synthesis resulting from high utilization to kininproduction at the site of intestinal inflammation. In this regard, it has been reported that during allergic reaction, there is an increase in vascular permeability and a trasudation of kininogens from plasma into nasal fluids, where they provide substrate for kinin-release (Baumgarten et al. 1985).

High amounts of kinin-forming enzyme has been noted in the tissue taken from carcinoid tumours that arise from argentaffin cells of the intestinal glands (Oates et al. 1964; Zeitlin & Smith 1966), Thus, it is possible that the kallikrein in the GIT may be formed in the exocrine glands of the mucosa. It has also been known that adrenergic stimulation of submandibular gland releases tissue kallikrein into vascular compartment, which has vasodilator action in the peripheral circulation (Ørstravik et al. 1982). Recently, it has been shown that the biological actions of bile acids are also mediated via activation of a serine proteinase possibly intestinal tissue kallikrein (Zeitlin et al. 1986). It is of interest to note that kinin acts independently of the intramural cholinergic and adrenergic neurones, since it causes the guinea-pig terminal ileum to contract after blocking both cholinergic and adnergic transmissions (Matusak & Bauer 1986). It clearly appears that the physiological and pathological functions of kinins in the intestinal system are not yet known. It would be possible to understand distinctly the actions of kinins in the pathophysiology of intestinal tract when systemic, digestive, renal, autonomic and vascular smooth muscle pharmacological activities of KKS are investigated. Furthermore, BK is involved in the mediation and modulation of the biological actions of PGs in the bowel.

RELEASE OF PROSTAGLANDIN BY BRADYKININ

Kinin-induced PG biosynthesis in various tissues, irrespective of whether it contracts or relaxes intestinal smooth muscle, indicates that a common pathway underlies in the physiopathological processes of the gut. BK mediated release of PGs has been demonstrated in a variety of tissue such as the kidney (McGiff et al. 1972), spleen (Ferreira et al. 1971), lungs (Palmer et al. 1973), and intestine (Musch et al. 1983). Further, BK stimulates the synthesis of PGE_2 in the rabbit ileal and colonic mucosa, this action is abolished by PGs synthetase inhibitor such as indomethacin (Musch et al. 1983). In addition, Cuthbert & Margolius (1982) suggested that kinins stimulate net cloride secretion in the rat colon via PGs mediated pathway. It is well known that an enzyme, phospholipase A_2, can be activated by kinin in the process of PGs production. In this connection, it has been observed that pharmacological effects of BK on the ileumand colon might be due to PGs release which can be antagonized by the phospholipase inhibitor, mepacrine (Musch et al. 1983). Phospholipase A_2 activity is localized in the rat jejunal brush-border membranes (Pind & Kuksis 1988). Thus, it is possible that BK releases PGs in the gut by the process of activating intestinal phospholipase A_2. PGE_2 may also cause kinins release by positive feedback mechanism as suggested by Sharma & Zeitlin (1982). The pharmacological interactions between the KKS and PGE_2 in the intestinal system are presented in Figure5.2.

PROSTAGLANDINS IN THE INTESTINE

Arachidonic acid (AA) can be metabolized into a spectrum of biologically active eicosanoids via three major pathways; the lipooxygenase, cyclooxygenase and cytochrome P450-dependent monooxygenase. PGs constitute a family of 20-carbon polyunsaturated acids whose initial synthesis involves the release of the precursor from phospholipids of the cell membrane due to the action of an enzyme known as phospholipase A_2 (Flower & Blackwell 1976). The cyclooxygenase pathway converts AA into transient endoperoxides e.g. PGG_2 and PGH_2. PGH_2 is converted by enzymatically-catalyzed to form several biologically active products. These products are PGE_2, PGD_2, PGA_2, $PGF_{2\alpha}$ thromboxane A_2 (TXA_2) and prostacyclin (PGI_2) (Hamburg et al. 1975; Hamberg & Samuelsson 1973). The lipoxygenase pathway can convert AA into 5 hydroperoxyeicosatetraenoic acid (5- HPETE) and 5- monohydroxyeicosatetraenoic acid (5- HETE). They are produced along with the leukotrienes

(LTs) (Murphy et al. 1979). The most recently known pathway is cytochrome P450-dependent epoxygenase which metabolizes AA into pharmacologically active agents e.g. expoxides and diols (Carroll et al. 1987). The biologically active products of AA metabolites are summarized in Figure5.3.

Prostaglandins are produced in the intestinal smooth muscle, and have been implicated in the control of intestinal motility, and water and electrolyte transport in the gut (Field et al. 1981; Knapp et al. 1978). Exogenously administered PGs have considerable variations in their actions on the gastrointestinal smooth muscle. PGE_2 and PGI_2 types cause inhibition, whereas F types produce stimulation of intestinal contractility (Konturek et al. 1982; Thor et al. 1985). PGE2, AA and PGI_2 administration into the mesenteric artery elicit a significant vasodilation in the intestine, whereas inhibition of cyclooxygenase shows opposite effects (Pawlik et al. 1975; Tepperman & Jacobson 1981). Furthermore, the same series can increase 02 consumption by the intestine, probably due to stimulation of intestinal transport (Gallavan & Jacobson 1982), however, $PGF_{2\alpha}$ causes the intestinal vascular smooth muscle to constrict and reduces 02 consumption. These actions have been suggested to indicate that PGs have an important role in the blood flow regulation of the gut (Konturek & Pawlik 1986). Also, there is evidence that PGE_2 stimulates intestinal epithelial cell adenylate cyclase by the receptor-mediated mechanism (Smith et al. 1987). These receptors may be responsible for the control of mucosal transport through PGs in the gut. Moreover, in physiological concentrations, PGs have protective actions on the gastroduodenal mucosa by mobilizing mucosal defence factors (Johanson & Bergstrom 1982). In addition, PGs are capable of producing most of the signs of inflammation; their raised concentrations have been found in the inflammatory exudate from various tissues (Kaley & Weiner 1971). Raised PGE_2 levels have been detected consistently in the inflamed rectal mucosa and colonic venous plasma of patients with ulcerative colitis (Harris et al. 1978; Gould et a!. 1977) as well as in the tissue in a guinea-pig model of immune colitis (Norris et al. 1982). In male Wistar rats, PGE_2, and $PGF_{2\alpha}$ treatment (400 µg/kg in 4 divided doses given with 15 min. intervals intraperitoneally) produced severe diarrhoea, passage of blood and significant loss of body weight (Sharma 1983). In these rats, macroscopic evaluation of GIT showed induration with marked haemorrhage, and PGE_2 was found to be more active than $PGF_{2\alpha}$. These differences could be only explained on the assumption that PGE_2 may be able to release plasma kinins which may potentiate the inflammatory actions of PGE_2 (Sharma 1983). This observation demonstrates that diarrhoea may result from excess of PGs production by the inflamed gut. Intestinal tissue of man, rat, mouse, guinea-pig and rabbit can convert (14C) AA into both cyclooxygenase and lipoxygenase products (Capasso et al. 1987). These investigators also suggested that these products are likely to play an important part in the effects of some laxatives and a substantial primary contribution to the cathartic effect. Recently, Lauritsen et al. (1987) failed to reduce the raised levels of the mucosal release of PGE_2 and LTB_4 in ulcerative colitis patients after treatment with oral vitamin E.

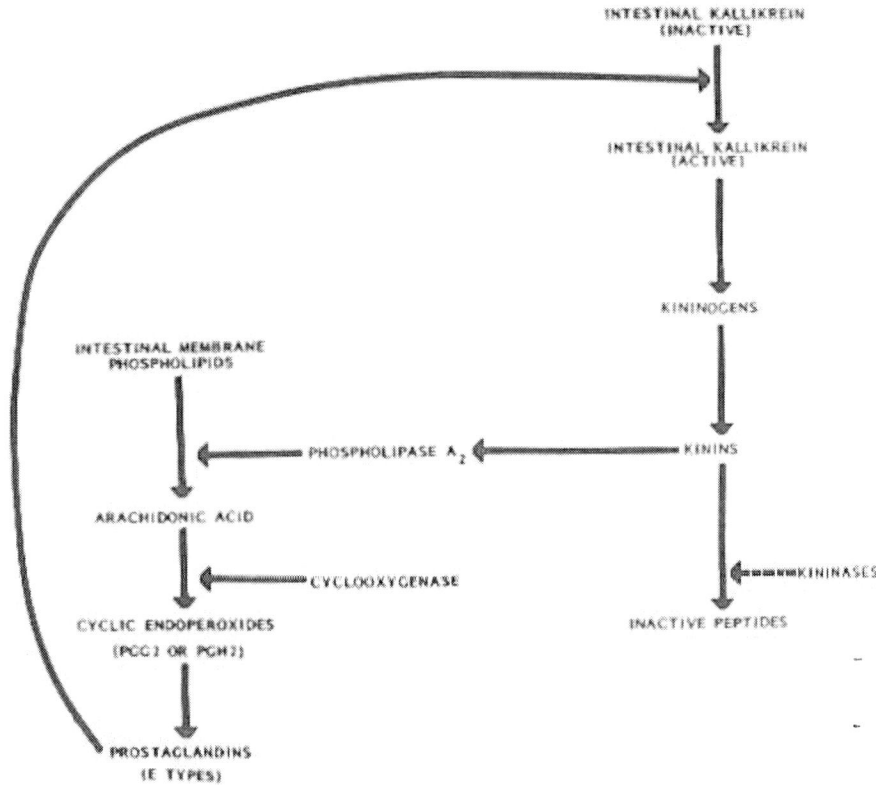

Figur e5.2. A possible interaction of the kallikrein-kinin system and prostaglandin in the intestinal mucosa. Activation (); inactivation (.) ⟶

GASTROPROTECTION

The term "gastroprotection (e.g. organoprotection)" has been introduced into GIT pharmacology and physiopathology by Szabo & Szelenyi in 1987 (Szabo & Szelenyi 1987) instead of "cytoprotection" until true cell preservation can be demonstrated. According to Robert (1979) cytoprotection refers to protection against chemically (concentrated ethanol, acid or base) or physically (heat) induced haemorrhagic acute gastric erosions and ulcers by PGs in doses much smaller than those needed to reduce gastric acid secretion in the rat. However, the mechanisms and primary targets of cytoprotection are not known and the term has lapsed into a state of confusion due to misuse and excessive use (Szabo & Szelenyi 1987). Hence, it is intended here to use the terminology "gastroprotection" in place of "cytoprotection". Several prostaglandins at normal physiological concentrations have been shown to act as gastroprotective agents. This is evident from the fact that non-steroidal anti-inflammatory drugs (NSAIDs) can produce lesions in the GIT within a short period in the fasted rat and guinea-pig (Whittle 1976; Garner 1978). These toxic effects of NSAIDs are associated with the inhibition of PGs biosynthesis, and PGs treatment prevented the GIT lesions without interfering with drug absorption (Lippman 1974; Guth & Paulsen 1979).

PGE$_2$ can prevent intestinal blood loss during indomethacin therapy in patients with rheumatoid arthritis (Johansson et al 1980). In addition, PGE$_2$, and methylated PGE analogues in clinical trials have been shown to have protective actions on gastric and duodenal ulcers (Johansson & Kollberg 1981; Vantrappen et al. 1980). Also, indomethacin-induced gastric lesions were closely associated with the inhibition of PGI$_2$ in the rat (Whittle 1981). Peskar et al. (1984) have suggested that inhibition of cycleoxygenase by NSAIDs could be the mechanism underlying the anti-inflammatory and ulcerogenic actions of these agents. It has been indicated that high levels of LTB$_4$ may potentiate mucosal damage by aspirin, however, in low concentrations; LTB$_4$ may have modest gastroprotective activity against aspirin in rats (Rainsford 1984). Further studies on LTs in the GIT may help us to understand the mechanism of GIT physiopathology. The mechanism of gastroprotection is not yet known. However, some workers (Flemstrom & Garner 1982; Takeuchi et al. 1986; Konturek et al. 1981) have suggested that PGs stimulate HCO$_3$ secretion (non-mediated by carbonic anhydrase) which could be involved in the mechanisms of gastroprotection. In addition PGEs, PGI$_2$, PG precursors and the endoperoxides all inhibit acid secretion (Robert 1979). Prostraglandins increase mucus secretion (Johansen & Kollberg 1978) and the thickness of the mucosal mucus layer (Bickel & Kauffman 1981). On the other hand, it has been observed that intravenous or oral pre-treatment with 16, 16-dimethyl PGE$_2$ (10. 20 µg/kg) or PGE$_2$ (10, 100 µg/kg) significantly augmented platelet activating factor (PAF)-induced gastric mucosal damage (Steel et al. 1987). The reason for the failure of the PGs to protect against PAF - induced gastric mucosal damage is not clear and emphasizes our lack of understanding of the mechanism underlying the gastric damage produced by this agent. Furthermore, relationship between inhibition of PG production and gastric mucosal damage induced by anti-inflammatory drugs may depend on type of drugs and species (Rainsford et al. 1981). Therefore, pharmacogenetics of gastroprotection by PGs and their intestinal toxic effects may be important in the physiology and pathology of the gut. Inhibitors of 5-lipoxygenase and some LT antagonists have been shown to protect the gastric mucosa in mice against lesions induced by oral or parenteral administration of aspirin - like drugs (Rainsford 1987). It has been suggested that high production of LTs and other products of 5-lipooxygenase may play a role in the development of acute gastric mocosal damage induced by NSAIDs.

REFERENCES

Amundsen E, Nustad K: Kinin-forming and destroying activities of cell homogenates. J Physiol. (Lond.) 1965; 179: 479-488.

Baumgarten CR, Togias AG, Naclario RM, et al: Influx of kininogens into nasal secretion after antigen challenge of allergic individuals. J Clin Invest 1985; 76: 191-197.

Bickel M, Kauffman GL: Gastric gel mucus thickness: effect of distension, 16, 16-dimethyl prostaglandin E$_2$ and carbenoxolone.Gastroenterology 1981; 80: 770-775.

Capasso F, Tavares IA, Tsang R, et al.: Eicosanoid formation by mammalian intestine. Effect of some intestinal secretagogues. Eur J Pharmacol 1987; 138: 107-113.

Carroll M, Schwartzman AM, Capdevila J, et al: Vasoactivity of arachidonic acid epoxides. Eur J Pharmacol 1987;138: 281-283.

Cochrane CG, Revak SD, Wuepper KD : Activation of Hageman factor in solid and liquid phases. A critical role of kallikrein. J Exp Med 1973; 138: 1564-1583.

Cuthbert AW, Margolius HS: Kinins stimulate net chloride secretion by the rat colon. Brit. J Pharmacol 1982; 75: 587-598.

Dennhardt R, Haberick FJ: Effect of kallikrein on the absorption of water, electrolytes and hexoses in the intestine of rats. In: Kininogenases. (edited by: Haberland GL, Rohen JW) Schattauer Verlag, Stuttgart. 1972; pp. 81-88.

Donaldson VH, Kleniewski J, Saito H, et al.: Prekallikrein deficiency in a kindred with kininogen deficiency and Fitzgerald trait clotting defect. Evidence that high molecular weight kininogen and prekallikrein exist as a complex in normal human plasma. J Clin Invest 1977; 60: 571-583.

Erdos EG: The angeotensin converting enzyme. Fed Proc 1977; 36: 1760-1765.

Erdos EG: Kininases. In: Handbook of experimental pharmacology. Ed: Erdos EG Heidelberg, Springer-Verlag. 1979; 25: pp. 427-448.

Fasth S, Hulten L: The effect of bradykinin on intestinal motility and blood flow. Acta chir scand 1973; 139: 699-705.

Fasth S, Hulten L, Johnson BJ, et al.: Mobilization of colonic kallikrein following pelvic nerve stimulation in the atropinized cat. J Physiol (Lond) 1978; 285: 471-478.

Ferreira SH, Moncada S, Vane JR: Indomethacin and aspirin abolish prostaglandin release from the spleen. Nature 1971; 231: 237-239.

Field M, Musch MW, Stoff JS: Role of prostaglandin in the regulation of intestinal electrolyte transport. Prostaglandins 1981; 21: (Suppl) 73-79.

Flemstrom G, Garner A: Gastroduodenal HCO_3 transport: characteristics and mucosal protection. Amer. J Physiol 1982; 242: G 183-G 193.

Flower RJ, Blackwell GJ: The importance of phospholipase A_2 in prostaglandin biosynthesis. Biochem. Pharmacol 1976; 25: 285-291.

Frankish NH, Zeitlin IJ: The assay of tissue kallikrein in rat intestine. Brit. J Pharmacol 1977; 59: 517P.

Gallavan RH Jr, Jacobson ED: Prostaglandins and the splanchnic circulation. Proc. Soc Exp Biol Med 1982; 170: 391-397.

Garner A.: Mechanisms of action of aspirin on the gastric mucosa of the guinea-pig. Acta physiol scand 1978; Suppl. 101-110.

Gautvik KM, Kriz M, Lund-Larsen K: Plasma kinins and adrenergic vasodilatation in submandibular salivary gland of the cat. Acta physiol scand 1972; 86: 419-426.

Gould SR, Brash AR, Connolly ME: Increased prostaglandin production in ulcerative colitis. Lancet 1977; 2: 98.

Guth PH, Paulsen G: Prostaglandin cytoprotection does not involve interference with aspirin absorption. Proc. Soc Exp Biol Med 1979;162: 128-130.

Hamberg M, Samuelsson B: Detection and isolation of an endoperoxide intermediate in prostaglandin biosynthesis. Proc Natl A cad. Sci USA. 1973; 70: 899-903.

Hamberg M, Svensson J, Samuelsson B: Thromboxanes: A new group of biologically active compounds derived from prostaglandin endoperoxides. Proc. Natl Acad Sci USA. 1975; 72: 2994-2998.

Harris DW, Smith PR, Swan CHJ: Venous prostaglandinlike activity in diarrhoeal states. Gut 1978; 19: 1057-1058.

Hathway WE, Alsever J: The relation of "Fletcher factor" to factor XI and XII. Brit. J Haematol 1970;18: 161-169.

Hilton SM, Lewis GP: The relationship between glandular activity, bradykinin formation and functional vasodilatation in the submandibular salivary gland. J Physiol (Lond) 1956; 134: 471-483.

Hilton SM, Jones M: The role of plasma kinin in functional vasodilatation in the pancreas. J Physiol (Lond) 1968; 195: 521-533:

Jacobsen S: Substrate for plasma kinin-forming enzymes in human, dog and rabbit plasma. Brit. J Pharmacol 1966; 26: 403-411.

Johansson C, Bergstrom S: Prostaglandins and protection of the gastroduodenal mucosa. Scand. J Gastroentrol 1982; Suppl 21-46.

Johansson C, Kollberg B: Stimulation by intragastrically administered E_2 prostaglandin on human gastric mucus output. Eur. J Clin Invest 1978; 9: 229-232.

Johansson C, Kollberg B: Clinical trails with prostaglandin E_2 in the gastrointestinal tract during indomethacin treatment in rheumatic diseases. Gastroenterology 1981; 78: 479-483.

Johansson C, Kollberg B, Nordemer B, et al.: Protective effect of prostaglandin E, in the gastrointestinal tract during indomethacin treatment of rheumatic diseases. Gastroenterology 1980; 78: 479-484.

Kaley G, Weiner R: Prostaglandin E_1 - a potential mediator of the inflammatory response. Ann. NY Acad. Sci 1971; 180: 338-350.

Kaplan AP, Austen KF: A prealbumin activator of prekallikrein II. Derivation of activators of prekallikrein from active Hageman factor by digestion with plasmin. J Exp Med 1971; 133: 696-712.

Knapp HR, Oelz O, Sweet BJ, et al.: Synthesis and metabolism of prostaglandins E_2, $F_{2\alpha}$ and D_2 by the rat gastrointestinal tract: stimulation by a hypertonic environment in vitro. Prostaglandins 1978; 15: 751-757.

Kobayashi M, Ohata K: Properties of kinin-forming enzyme in rat stomach. Japan. J Pharmacol 1981; 31: 369-373.

Komiya M, Kato H, Suzuki T: Structural comparison of high molecular weight and low molecular weight kininogens. J Biochem 1974; 76: 833-845.

Konturek SJ, Pawlik W: Physiology and pharmacology of prostaglandins. Dig. Dis. Sci 1986; 31: 6S-19S.

Konturek SJ, Piastucki I, Brzozowski T: Role of prostaglandins in the formation of aspirin-induced ulcers. Gastroenterology 1981; 80: 4-9.

Konturek SJ, Thor P, PawlikW, et al.: Role of prostaglandins in the myoelectric, motor, and metabolic activity of the small intestine in the dog. In: Motility of the digestive tract. Ed.: M. Wienbeck. Raven Press, New York, 1982; pp. 437-443.

Lauritsen K, Laursen LS, Bukhave K, et al.: Does vitamin E supplementation modulate in vivo arachidonate metabolism in human inflammation? Pharmacology Toxicology 1987; 61: 246-249.

Lippman W: Inhibition of indomethacin-induced gastric ulceration in the rat by perorally administered synthetic and natural prostaglandin analogues. Prostaglandins 1974; 7: 1-10.

Lutcher CL.: Reit trait: a new expression of high molecular weight kininogen deficiency. Clin Res 1976; 24: 440A (Abst.).

Marin-Grez M, Schaechtelin G, Bonner G, et al.: Renal kallikrein activity and urinary kallikrein excretion in rats with experimental renal hypertension. Clin Sci 1982; 63: 349-354.

Matusak O, Bauer V: Effect of desensitization induced by adenosine 5'-triphosphate, substance p, bradykinin, serotonin, γ-amino-butyric acid andendogenous noncholinergic-nonadrenergic transmission in the guinea-pig ileum. Eur. J Pharmacol 1986; 126: 199-209.

McGiff JC, Terrango NA, Malik Ku, et al.: Release of a prostaglandin E-likesubstance from canin kidney by bradykinin: Comparison with elediosin. Circulation Res 1972; 31: 36-43.

Miller DH, Chao J, Margolius HS: Tissue Kallikrein synthesis and its modification by testosterone or low dietary sodium. Biochem. J 1984; 218: 37-43.

Moriwaki C, Fujimori H, Toyono Y, et al.: Studies on kallikrein V. Purification and Characterization of rats intestinal kallikrein. Chem. Pharm Bull 1980; 28: 3612-3620.

Moriwaki C, Fujimori H, Toyno Y: Intestinal kallikrein and the influence of kinin on the intestinal transport. In: Kininogenase 4. Ed.: Haberland GL, Rohen RW, Suzuki T Schattauer Verlag, Stuttgart, New York. 1977; pp. 283-290.

Moriwaki C, Moriya H, Yamaguchi K, et al.: Intestinal absorption of pancreatic kallikrein and some aspects of its physiological role. In: Kininogenases. Ed.: Haberland GL and Rohen JW. Schattauer Verlag, Stuttgart, New York. 1972; pp. 57-66.

Murphy RC, Hammerstrom S, Samuelsson B: Leukotriene C: A slow reacting substance from murine mastocytoma cells. Proc. Natl. Acad. Sci USA 1979; 76: 4275-4279.

Musch MW, Kachur JF, Miller RJ, et al.: Bradykininstimulated electrolyte secretion in rabbit and guinea-pig intestine. Involvement of arachidonic acid metabolites. J Clin Invest 1983; 71: 1073-1083.

Muller-Esterl W, Iwanaga S, Nakani-Shi S: Kininogens revisited. Trends Biochemical Sci 1986; 11: 336-339.

Nagayasu T, Nagasawa S: Studies of human kininogen: Isolation, characterization, and cleavage by plasma kallikrein of high molecular weight (HMW) kininogen. J Biochem 1979; 85: 249-258.

Norris AA, Lewis AJ, Zeitlin IJ: Changes in colonic tissue levels of inflammatory mediators in guinea-pig model of immune colitis. Agents Actions 1982; 12: 243-246.

Nustad K, Vaaje K, Pierce JV: Synthesis of kallikrein by rat kidney slices. Br. J Pharmac 1975; 53: 229-234.

Oates JA, Melmon KL, Sjordsma A, et al.: The release of a kinin peptide in carcinoid Syndrom. Lancet 1964; 1: 514-518.

Okamoto H, Greenbaum LM: Kininogen substrate for trypsin and cahtepsin D in human rabbit and rat plasmas. Life Sci 1983a; 32: 2007-2013.

Okamoto H, Greenbaum LM: Isolation and structure of Tkinin. Biochem. Biophys Res Commun 1983b; 112: 701-708.

Okamoto H, Itoh N, Uwani M: Identification of T-kininogen in rat urine. Biochem Pharmac 1987; 36: 2979-2984.

Palmer MA, Piper PJ, Vane JR: Release of rabbit aorta contracting substance (RCS) and prostaglandins induced by chemical or mechanical stimulation of guinea-pig lungs. Brit JPharmacol 1973; 49: 226-246.

Pawlik W, Shpherd AP, Jacobson ED: Effect of vasoactive agents on intestinal oxygen consumption and blood flow in dogs. J Clin Invest 1975; 56: 484-490.

Peskar BM, Weiler H, Meyer CH: Inhibition of prostaglandin production in gastrointestinal tract by anti-inflammatory drugs. Adv Inflam Res 1984; 6: 39-50.

Pierce JV, Guimaraes JA: Further characterization of highly purified human kininogen. Life Sci 1975;16: 790-791.

Pind S, Kuksis A: Solubilization and assay of phospholipase A, activity from rat jejunal brush-border membrane. Biochem Biophys Acta 1988; 939: 211-221.

Rainsford KD: The effects of 5-lipoxygenase inhibitors and leukotrienes antagonists on the development of gastric lesions induced by non-steroidal anti-inflammatory drugs in mice. Agents Actions 1987; 21: 316-319.

Rainsford KD: Mechanisms of gastrointestinal ulceration by nonsteroidal anti-inflammatory/analgesic drugs. Adv. Inflamm Res 1984; 6: 51-64.

Rainsford KD, Peskar BM, Brune K: Relationship between inhibition of prostaglandin production and gastric mucosal damage induced by antiinflammatory drugs may depend on type of drugs and species. J Pharm Pharmacol 1981; 33: 127-128.

Robert A.: Cytoprotection by prostaglandins. Gastorenterology 1979; 77: 761-767.

Rohen JW, Peterhoff I: Stimulation of mitotic activity by kallikrein in the gastrointestinal tract of rats. In: Kininogenases. Ed.: Haberland GL, Rohen JW, Schattauer Verlag, Stuttgart, New York, 1972, pp. 148-157.

Rumpeltes H, Koeppe P, Pribilla W: Influence of a kallikrein preparation (BAY d 7687) on the intestinal absorption of vitamin B_{14} in man. In: Kininogenases 3. Ed.: Haberland GL, Rohen JW, Blumer G, Huber P. Schattauer Verlag, Stuttgart, New York, 1975; pp. 63-72.

Schachter M, Peret MW, Billing AG, et al.: Immunolocalization of the protease kallikrein in the colon. J. Histochem. Cytochem 1983; 31: 1255-1260.

Schmaier AH, Zuckerberg A, Silverman C, et al.: High molecular weight kininogen.A secreted platelet protein. J Clin Invest 1983; 71: 1477-1489.

Sharma JN: Ability of prostaglandins to induce acute inflammatory bowel disease in the rat: a preliminary report. J Med 1983; 14: 157-160.

Sharma JN: Kinin-forming system in the genesis of hypertension. Agents Actions 1984; 14: 200-205.

Sharma JN: Interrelationship between the Kallikrein-kinin system and hypertension. A review. Gen. Pharmac 1988; 19: 177-187.

Sharma JN, Buchanan WW: Kinin system in clinical and experimental rheumatoid arthritis: a short review. Curro Med Res Opin 1979; 6: 314-321.

Sharma JN, Zeitlin IJ: Reduced plasma kininogen concentration by prostaglandin E2 in rats. Eur. J Pharmacol 1982; 83: 119-121.

Sharma JN, Zeitlin IJ, Deodhar SD, et al.: Detection of kallikrein-like activity in inflamed synovial tissue. Arch. Int Pharmacodyn Therap 1983; 262: 279-286.

Sharma JN, Zeitlin IJ, Mackenzie JF, et al.: Plasma kinin-precursor levels in clinical intestinal inflammation. Fundamental Clin Pharmacol 1988; In Press.

Smith G, Warhurst JL, Lee M, et al.: Evidence that PGE_2 stimulates intestinal epithelial cell adenylate cyclase by a receptormediated mechanism. Dig. Dis Sci 1987; 32: 71-75.

Steel G, Wallace JL, Whittle BJR: Failure of prostaglandin E_2 and its 16, 16-dimethyl analogue to prevent the gastric mucosal damage induced by Paf. Brit. J Pharmacol 1987; 90: 365-371.

Szabo S, Szelenyi I: 'Cytoprotection' in gastrointestinal pharmacology. Trends Pharmacol Sci 1987; 8: 149-154.

Takeuchi K, Ohtsuki H, Okabe S: Mechanisms of protective activity of 16, 16-dimethyl PGE2 and acetazolamide on gastric and duodenal lesions in rats. Dig. Dis Sci 1986; 31: 406-411.

Tepperman BL, Jacobson ED: Mesenteric circulation. In: Physiology of the gastrointestinal tract. Ed: Johnson LR. Raven Press, New York, 1981; pp. 1317-1336.

Thor P, Konturek JW, Konturek SJ, et al.: Role of prostaglandins in control of intestinal motility. Amer. J Physiol 1985; 248: G353-G359.

Vantrappen G, Popiela T, Tytgat DNJ, et al.: A multicenter trail of 15 (R)-15-methyl prostaglandin E_2 in duodenal ulcer. Gastroenterology 1980; 78: 1283.

Whittle BJR: Relationship between the prevention ofrat gastric erosions and the inhibition of acid secretion by prostaglandins. Eur. J Pharmacol 1976; 40: 233-239.

Whittle BJR: Temporal relationship between cyclooxygenase inhibition, as measured by prostacyclin biosynthesis, and the gastrointestinal damage induced by indomethacin in the rat. Gastroenterology 1981; 80: 94-98.

Zeitlin IJ: Pharmacological characterization of kinin-forming activity in rat intestinal tissue. Brit. J Pharmacol 1971; 42: 648-649P.

Zeitlin IJ, Al\l-Dhahir AHR, Cook S, et al.: Bile acids and the intestinal kallikrein-kinin system. Adv. Exp Med Biol 1986; 198B: 47-53.

Zeitlin IJ, Singh YN, Lembeck F, et al.: The molecular weights of plasma and intestinal kallikreins in rats. Arch. Pharmacol 1976; 293: 159-161.

Zeitlin IJ, Smith AN: 5-Hydroxyindoles and kinins in the carcinoid and dumping syndromes. Lancet 1966; 2: 986-991.

Zeitlin IJ, Smith AN: Mobilization of tissue kallikrein in inflammatory disease of the colon. Gut 1973; 14: 133-138.

Ørstravik TB, Carretero OA, Scicli AG: The kallikreinkinin system in the regulation of submandibular gland blood flow. Amer. J Physiol 1982; 242: H1010-H1014.

Chapter 6

Pro-inflammatory Actions of the Platelet Activating Factor: Relevance to Rheumatoid Arthritis

The mechanisms causing inflammation in rheumatoid arthritis (RA) are not yet clearly known. They may be associated with different types of inflammatory cells and probably numerous mediators (Sharma and Mohsin 1990). Nowadays, the platelet activating factor (PAF) is discussed as an important mediator in RA.

BIOCHEMISTRY OF PAF

The platelet activating factor has been characterized as a phospholipid (1-alkyl-2-acetyl-sn-glycero-3 phosphocholine) (Benveniste et al. 1979; Demopoulos et al. 1979). This lipid mediator can be generated by various tissues and cells such as macrophages, mast cells, platelets, neutrophils, basophils, eosinophils, endothelial cells and monocytes (Braquest et al.. 1987; Sipka et al. 1989; Doebber and Wu 1988). The PAF is also known as acetylglyceryl ether phosphocholine, PAF-acether (a concentration of acetate and ether) and alkylacetylglycerophosphocholine. The mechanisms of the production of the molecular PAF species under various conditions by different cells are not clearly known (for review see Snyder 1989). PAF having an 18:0 alkyl chain at the sn-I position is less active than the PAF with a 16:0 alkyl strain, and unsaturated alkyl moieties have been found to be biologically more active on human leukocytes and rat erythrocytes than saturated forms (Satouchi et al. 1981; Surley et al. 1985; Czarnetzki and Muramatsu 1981 Kaya et al. 1984). Basophil degranulation and the release of PAF are involved in the pathogenesis of various immune diseases, allergic reactions and inflammatory processes (Ninio and Benveniste 1987).

PRO-INFLAMMATORY ACTIONS OF PAF

After systemic administration of PAF severe hypotension and shock are to be found (PAGE et al. 1984; Pretolani et al. 1987; Snyder 1985; Issekutz and Szpeda 1986; Watanabe et al. 1987). After 30 min the intrapleural injection of PAF leads to a marked exudation accompanied by a reduction in the pleural leukocyte counts in rats (Tarayre et al. 1987;Martins et al. 1989).

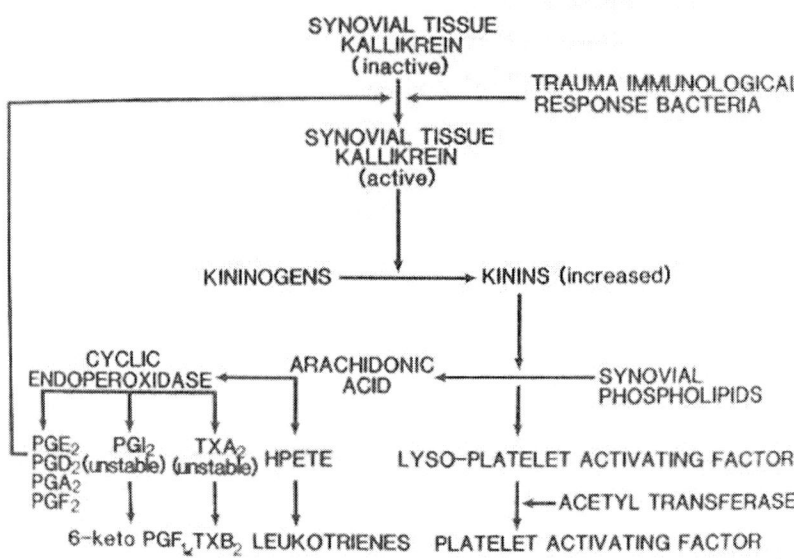

Figure 6.1. A hypothetical presentation indicating the mode of the release of platelet-activating factor (PAF) in inflammed rheumatoid joints. The kallikrein-kinin system may mediate and modulate the release of PAF, prostaglandins (POs) and leukotrienes (LTs) within the synovial joints to induce chronic synovitis leading spontaneously to cartilage and bone damage.

Furthermore, these authors report that the pretreatment of animals with the PAF antagonist WEB2086 inhibited pleurisy induced by zymosan. On the other hand, this pretreatment failed to modify pleurisy induced by carrageenin. This suggests that PAF plays an important role in inflammatory reaction caused by zymosen, but not by carrageenin. Nonetheless, the intradermal injection of PAF is followed by increased vascular permeability, oedema, vascular lesion, and thrombosis in rats (Martins et al. 1987; Pirotzyky et al. 1984). Similar proinflammatory actions of PAF were known in the rabbit (Humphrey et al. 1982, 1984).

Intradermal administration of PAF to humans can induce a biphasic inflammatory response characterised by acute and late-onset components (Archer et al. 1984). PAF causes PMNL chemotaxis and degranulation in vitro (Goetzi. et al. 1980), and when injected into human skin it produces accumulation of PMNL and mononuclear cells (Archer et al. 1985).

High concentrations of PAF are present in the synovial fluid of adjuvant-induced arthritis in the rabbit (Pettifer et al. 1987). To my knowledge there are no data available on the presence of PAF in RA synovial fluid. Hence, the experimental model of antigen-induced arthritis in the rabbit is an appropriate model to search for the role of PAF in the pathogenesis of rheumatoid arthritis (Sharma 1977; Sharma and Sharma 1977; Dumonde and Glynn, 1962). The involvement of PAF has also been suggested in the genesis of inflammatory skin disorders, such as psoriasis. PAF has been detected in psoriatic scales (Ramesha et al. 1987; Mallet and Cunningham .1985) and is responsible for the perseverance of the disease.

Furthermore, the synthesis of PAF initially involves the activation of phospholipase A_2 resulting in the formation of lyso-PAF from membrane phospholipids (Albert and Snyder 1983). This enzyme is also responsible for the release of prostaglandins (PGs) and leukotrienes (LTs) which are powerful inflammatory mediators. It is possible that the release of PAF is accompanied by PGs, LTs and kinin production at the inflammatory site. In the anaphylactic phase of allergic air pouch inflammation in rats, lyso-PAF concentrations in the pouch fluid were significantly raised as compared to normal rats (Watanabe et al. 1987). ThissuggeststhatPAFmight play arelevantrolein causing allergic inflammation. Furthermore, topical application of PAF, LTB_4, or substance P cause leukocyte migration and leukocyte dependent extravasation of macromolecules in rabbit and hamster (Thureson-Klein et al. 1987). Also a noteworthy observation is that the simultaneous presence of PAF and other inflammatory mediators like LTB_4, $PGF_{1\alpha}$, and $PGF_{2\alpha}$, in the supernatant of human neutrophils treated with phospholipase A2 obtained from human monocytes (Sipka et al. 1989). These findings strongly suggest the pathogenic role of PAF in joint inflammatory disease. Figure6.1 summarizes the possible mode of PAF release and interactions with other mediators in the pathogenesis of RA. Numerous PAF antagonists have been recently described (Braquet et al. 1987). These antagonists have been classified into 3 groups. Firstly, the nonspecific inhibitors of PAF effects, which include drugs interfering with intracellular calcium activities, modulation of cyclic nucleotides and phosphocolinesterase inhibitors (Issekutz, and Szpejda 1986; Coeffier et al. 1986). Secondly, the specific inhibitors of PAF which are compounds derived from chemical modification of the PAF structure (Braquet et al. 1987). Thirdly, synthetic compounds such as derivatives of the hetrazepines (Weber and Heuer 1989). The clinical significance of these PAF antagonists have yet to be evaluated in chronic inflammatory diseases, such as RA. Future clinical investi gations may provide evidence for their usefulness as antirheumatic agents.

REFERENCES

Albert DH, Snyder F: Biosynthesis of l-alkyl-2-acetyl-sn-glycero-3 phospho choline (platelet-activating factor) from l-alkyl-2-acyl-sn-glycero-3 phosphocholine by rate alveolar macrophages. Phospholipase Az and inophore stimulation. J Biol Chem1983; 258: 97-102.

Archer CB, Page CP, Paul W, et al.: Inflammatory characteristics of platelet activating factor (PAF-acether) in human skin. Br. J Dermatol 1984; 110: 45-50.

Morely J, MacDonald DM: Accumulation of inflammatory cells in response to intracutaneous platelet activating factor (PAF-acether) in man. Br. J Dermatol 1985; 112: 285-290.

Benveniste J, Camussi J, Polonsky I: Platelet activating factor. Monogr. Allergy 1977; 12: 138-142.

Tence M, Varenne P, Bidault J, et al.: Semi-synthese et structure proposee du facteur activant les plaquettes (P.A.F.): PAF-acether, un alkyl ether analogue de la lysophos-phatidyecholine. CR. Acad. Sci Paris 1979; 289: 1037-1040.

Braquet P, Touqui L, Shen TY, et al.: Perspectives in platelet-activating factor research. Pharmac Rev 1987; 39: 97-145.

Coefier E, Borrel MC, Lefort J, et al.: Effects of PAF-acether and structural analogues on platelet activation and bronchoconstriction in guinea pigs. Eur. J Pharmacol 1986; 131: 179-188.

Czarnetzki BM, Muramatsu T: Saturated and nonsaturated 1-0-alkyl-2-0-acetoyl-sn-glycero-3-phosphocholines derived from ratfish liver oil: effect of human leukocyte migration. Chem Phys Lipids 1891; 29: 309-315.

Demopoulos CA, Pinckard RN, Hanahan DJ: Platelet-activating factor: Evidence for 1-0-alkyl-2acetyl-sn-glycerol-3-phosphorylcholine as the active component (A new class of lipid chemical mediators). J Biol Chem 1979; 254: 9355-9358.

Doebber TW, Wu MS: Platelet-activating factor-induced cellular and pathophysiological responses in the cardiovascular system. Drug Develop. Res. 1988; U: 151-161.

Dumonde DC, Cylnn LE: The production of arthritis in rabbits by an immunological reaction to fibrin. Br. J Exp. Pathol 1962; 43: 373-383.

Goetzl E, Derian CK, Tauber AI, et al.: Novel effect of 1-0-hexadecyl-2-Acylsn-glycero-3phosphorylcholine mediators of human leukocyte function: delineation of the specific roles of the acyl substituents. Biochem Biophys Res Commun 1980; 94: 881-888.

Humphrey DM, Hanahan DJ, Pinckard RN: Induction ofleukocytic infiltrates in rabbit skin by acetyl ether phosphorylcholine. Lab. Invest. 1982; 47: 227-234.

McManus LM, Hanahan DJ, Pinckard RN: Morphologic basis of increased vascular permeability induced by acetylglyceryl ether phosphorylcholine. Lab Invest 1984; 50: 16-25.

Issekutz AC, Szpejda M: Evidence that platelet activating factor may mediate some acute inflammatory responses. Studies with the platelet-activating factor antagonist, CV3988. Lab Invest 1986; 54: 275-281.

Kaya K, Miura T, Kubota K: Different incorporation rates of arachidonic acid into kalenylacyl-, alkylacyl-, and diacylphosphatidylethanolamine ohat erythrocytes. Biochem Biophys Acta 1984; 796: 304-311.

Mallet AI, Cunningham FM: Structural identification of platelet activating factor psoriatic scale.Biochem Biophys Res Commun 1985; 126: 192-198.

Martina MA, Silva PMR, Neto HCCF, et al.: PharmacologicalmodulationofPaf-induceratpleurisy and its role in inflammation by zymosan. Br. J Pharmacol 1989; 96: 363-371.

Ninio E, Benveniste J: Relationship between PAF-acether and arachidonic acid. Biol Eicosanoids 1987; 152: 51-60.

Page CP, Paul W, Dewar A, et al.: PAF-acether: a putative mediator of asthma and inflammation. Agents Actions 1983; 13: 177-183.

Pettipher ER, Higgs GA, Henderson B: PAF-acether in chronic arthritis. Agents Actions 1987; 21: 98-103.

Pirotzyky E, Page CP, Roubin R, et al.: PAF-acetherinduced plasma exudation in rat skin is independent of platelets and neutrophils. Microcirc Endothel Lymphatics 1984; 1: 107-122.

Pretolani M, Lefort J, Malanchere E: Interference by the novel PAF-acether antagonist WEB2086 with the bronchopulmonary responses to P AF-acether and to active and passive anaphylactic shock in guinea-pigs. Eur. J Pharmacol 1987; 140: 311-321.

Ramesha CS, Soter N, Pickett WC: Identification and quantitation of P AF from psoriatic scales. Agents Action 1987; 21: 382-383.

Satouchi K, Pinckard RN, Hanahan DJ: Influence of alkyl ether chain length of acetyl glyceryl ether phosphorylcholine and its ethanolamine analog on biological activity toward rabbit platelets. Arch. Biochem Biophys 1981; 211: 683-688.

Sharma JN: Changes in biochemical parameters associated with experimental arthritis in rabbits. Biomedicine 1977; 27: 252-255.

Mohsin SSJ: The role of chemical mediators in the pathogenesis of inflammation with emphasis on the kinin system. Exp Pathol 1990; 38: 73-96.

Sharma JN: Comparison of the antiinflammatory activity of cornrniphoramukul (an indigenous drug) with those of phenylbutazone and ibuprofen in experimental arthritis induced by mycobacterial adjuvant. Arzneim. Forsch./Drug Res 1977; 27: 1455-1457.

Sipka S, Dinya Z, Gergely P, et al.: Simultaneous presence of platelet activating factor, leukotriene B4, prostaglandin $F_{1\alpha}$ and $F_2\alpha$ in the supernatant of human neurophils treated with phospholipase A2 of human monocytes. Klin. Wochenschr 1989; 67: 123-125.

Snyder F: Chemical and biochemical aspects of platelet-activating factor, a class of acetylated ether-linked choline phospholipids. Med. Res Rev 1985; 5: 107-140.

- Biochemistry of platelet-activating factor: a unique class of biologically active phospholipids, P.S. Exp Biol Med. 1989; 190: 125-135.

Surles JR, Wykle RL, O'flaherty JT, et al.:Facile Synthesis of platelet-activating factor and racemic analogues containing unsaturation in the sn-l-alkyl chain. J Med Chem 1985; 28: 73-78.

Tarayre JP, Delhon A, Aliaga M, et al.: Pharmacological modulation of P AF-acether-induced pleurisy in rats. Pharmacol Res Commun 1987; 19: 859-876.

Thureson-Klein A, Hedqvist P, Ohlen A, et al.: Leukotriene B_4, platelet-activating factor and substance P as mediators of acute inflammation. Pathol Immunopathol Res 1987; 6: 190 - 206.

Watanbe M, Ohuchi K, Sugidachi A, et al.: Platelet-activating factor in the inflammatory exudate in the anaphylactic phase of allergic inflammation in rats. Int. Arch. Allergy Appl Immunol 1987; 84: 396-403.

Weber KH, Heuer HO: Hetrazepines as antagonists of platelet activating factor. Med Res Rev1989; 9: 181-218.

Chapter 7

Role of Tissue Kallikrein-Kininogen-Kinin Pathways in the Cardiovascular System

INTRODUCTION

A number of observations focus on the kinins as potential mediators in endogenous cardiovascular protective mechanisms. This is due to the fact that kallikrein–kinin system (KKS) components are localized in the heart and in the vascular tissues (Nolly et al.1981., Sharma and Uma.1996., Sharma et al.1998., Sharma et al.1999., Oza and Goud.1992., Nolly et al.1993). Kinins are released during ischemia (Vegh et al.1991) and cause beneficial cardiac effects (Linz et al 1993). Bradykinin (BK) antagonists worsen ischemia-induced effects (Vegh et al 1994), and BK can contribute to the cardioprotective effects of preconditioning (walls et al 1994). On the other hand, the reduction in cardiac infarct size by BK after preconditioning in rabbits was prevented by a BK antagonist (Hoe 140) treatment (walls et al 1994). BK at a dose that has no effect on blood pressure (BP) can prevent left ventricular hypertrophy (LVH) in rats with hypertension caused by aortic banding (Linz et al 1993). Reduction in peripheral and cardiac KKS components may also be the cause of developing high BP in human and experimental animals (Sharma JN.1984., Sharma JN.1988., Sharma JN. 1989, Sharma et al.1996). In the present review, the current concept on the role of kinins in the cardiovascular system is presented.

THE KININ SYSTEM

The kinins are pharmacologically active polypeptides released in the tissues and body fluids as a result of the enzymatic action of kallikrein on kininogens. The kinin family includes BK (Arg-Pro-Pro-gly-Phe-Ser-Pro-Phe-Arg), kallidin (Lys-Arg-Pro-Pro-Gly-Phe-Ser-Pro-Phe-Arg) and methionyl-lysyl-BK (Met-Lys-Arg-Pro-Pro-Gly-Phe-Arg). Kallidin and methionyl-lysyl-BK are converted into BK by aminopeptidases present in plasma and urine (Sharma JN 1990). Kinins are rapidly (<15 sec) inactivated by circulating kininases (Sharma JN 1992).

Kininogens are multifunctional proteins derived mainly from α2-globulin. In humans, the two forms of kininogens are high molecular weight kininogen (HMWK) and low molecular weight kininogen (LMWK) (Nagayasa and Nagasawa 1979).

These kininogens differ from each other in molecular weight, susceptibility to plasma and tissue kallikreins and in their physiological properties (Muller et al 1986). They are synthesized in the liver and circulate in the plasma and other body fluids. In addition, there is a T-kininogen in the rat plasma considered to be an acute phase reactant of inflammation (Greenbaum LM 1982). This kininogen releases T-kinin by the enzymatic action of T-kallikrein in rats (Okamoto and greenbaum 1983). Tissue kallikrein is found in various organs such as the kidney, heart and synovial tissue (Nolly et al.1981., Sharma and Uma1996, Sharma et al.1998). These kallikreins differ from one another in molecular weight, biological function, and physicochemical and immunological properties (Bhoola et al 1992). The tissue kallikrein is synthesized in the cells as a precursor and converted into active form by the cleavage of an amino terminal peptide (Takada et al 1985). Active tissue kallikrein acts on LMWK to release kallidin. The plasma kallikrein is found in circulation in an inactive form, which is known as prekallikrein or Fletcher factor. (Weiss et al. 1974). This inactive prekallikrein is converted to active kallikrein by activated Hageman factor (XIIa) (Cochrane et al 1973). In addition, plasma kallikrein is able to convert inactive factor XII to XIIa by positive feedback reaction. The plasma prekallikrein and HMWK are present together in a complex form (Griffin et al 1976). Factor XIIa and factor XI circulate with HMWK in bound form (Mandle et al 1976). In this way, factor XI can be converted into XIa for the participation in the intrinsic coagulation cascade . In immunological reactions, the tissue proteoglycan and mast cell heparin might act as an initiating surface for initial activation of the Hageman factor (Silverberg et al 1987). It seems that the kinins may be generated in parallel with the formation of thrombin at inflammatory sites, because inactive plasma kallikrein can be activated by coagulant Hageman factor. The tissue kallikrein multigene family comprises a closely related cluster of genes that vary in number among the different mammalian species: 24 genes have been identified in the mouse, 20 in the rat, 3 in humans and 3 in the hamster (Bhoola et al 1992).

Several restriction fragment length polymorphisms (RFLP) have been mapped in tissue kallikrein gene and their regulatory regions in spontaneously hypertensive rats (SHR) (Wooley-Miller et al 1989). These findings may reflect a possible difference in the tissue kallikrein gene locus between SHR and normotensive Wistar-Kyoto rats (WKYR). A tissue kallikrein RFLP has been indicated to co-segregate with high BP in the F2 offspring of SHR and normotensive Brown Norway rat crosses (Pravene et al 1991). This finding strongly suggests a possibility of SHR The kininases, kinin-inactivating enzymes, are present in the plasma, endothelial cells and in the tissues to regulate the physiological functions of the kinins in the body. These are known as kininase I, kininase II or angiotensin-converting enzyme (ACE) and enkaphalinase. In plasma, kininase I cleaves the C-terminal arginine of BK to form des-Arg^9-BK. Kininase II causes inactivation of BK by releasing pentapeptide (Arg-Pro-Pro-Gly-Pheo and tripeptide (Ser-Pro-Phe) fragments. Figure7.1 shows the kinin formation, activation and inhibition pathways.

Role of Tissue Kallikrein-Kininogen-Kinin Pathways in the Cardiovascular System

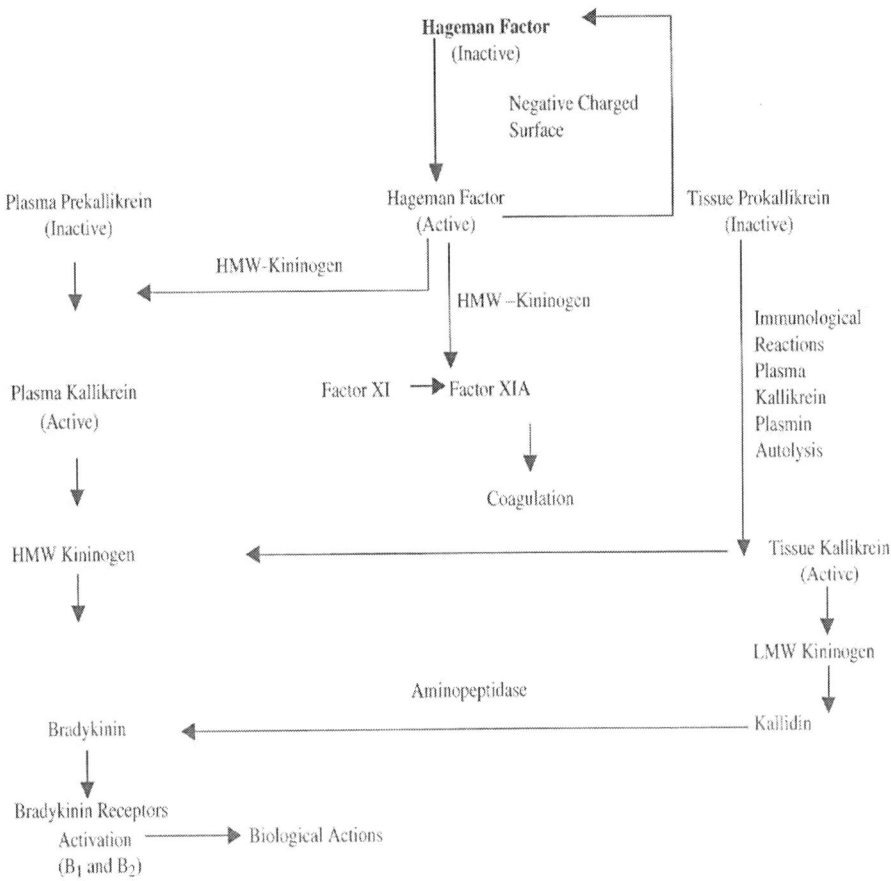

Figure 7.1. The mode of kinin formation.

KININ RECEPTORS AND ANTAGONISTS

Kinins exert their pharmacological actions through the activation of two receptor types, B_1 and B_2, which have been cloned and belong to the seven-transmembrane G-protein coupled receptor family (Marceau et al 1998). The kinin B_1 receptor displays high affinity and selectivity for kinin metabolites lacking the C-terminal arginine residue, such as des-Arg^9-BK. The B_1 receptor is rarely expressed in normal tissue, but seems to be upregulated in pathological states associated with inflammation and tissue injury(Marceau et al 1998). This may indicate an important area of research within the study of KKS. B_1 receptor activation may produce stimulation of smooth muscle, increased cell proliferation and collagen synthesis (Regoli et al 1984). In addition, it may also cause release of nitric oxide (NO) and prostacyclin (PGI_2) from bovine endothelial cells (D'Orleans-Juste et al 1989). Kinins stimulate the release of tumor necrosis factor and interleukin from macrophages through activating B_1 receptors (Tiffany et al 1989). The kinin B_2 receptors may participate in pathological conditions such as pain, inflammation (Sharma JN and Yusof APM 1998; Sharma JN and Yusof APM 1988), bronchoconstriction (Jin et al 1989), hypertension (Sharma et al 1992) and cardiac arrhythmias induced in rats (Abbas et al 1999). The B_2 receptor is thought to mediate contractions of rat uterus, guinea pig ileum and tracheal smooth muscles (Barabe et al 1977). Kinins act on kinin B_2 receptors to release conjointly NO and PGI_2 from the endothelial cells in vitro (D'Orleans-Juste 1989). B_2 receptors exhibit higher affinity for BK and kallidin. Farmer et al. (Farmer et al 1989) suggested that the large airways contain a novel B_3 receptor that may produce BK-induced bronchoconstriction. These investigators noted that several B_2 receptor antagonists such as D-Arg(Hyp^3,D-Phe^7)-BK and DArg(Hyp^3,$Thi^{5,8}$,D-Phe^7)-BK as well as B_1 antagonist (des-Arg^9(Leu^8)-BK) did not block the BK-induced contraction of guinea pig tracheal smooth muscle preparations. The presence of a kinin B_3 receptor has also been proposed in the opossum esophageal longitudinal smooth muscle. This receptor has been characterized by rapid desensitization, causes contraction of longitudinal smooth muscle via PG release and is activated by kinin B_2 receptor antagonists (PheS-D-Phe^7-BK and D-Phe^7-hyp^8-BK). Furthermore, Saha et al.proposed the presence of a B_4 receptor in the opossum esophageal longitudinal smooth muscle. This receptor shows no tachyphylaxis; its action does not involve PG, and is activated by kinin B_2 receptor antagonists. The development of kinin receptor antagonists has been pursued for more than two decades (Regoli D. and Barabe J. 1980; Wirth et al 1991). The kinin B_1 receptor antagonist was first introduced as des-Arg^9-(leu8)-BK by Regoli and Barabe (Regoli D. and Barabe J. 1980). The 'second generation' of B2 receptor antagonists came with the introduction of hoe-140(D-Arg-Arg-Pro-Hyp-Gly-Thi-Ser-D-Tic-Ag; Icatibant) (Cheronis et al 1992) and CP-0127 (D-Arg-Arg-Pro-Hyp-Gly-Thi-Cys-D-Phe-Leu-Arg; bradycor) (Henson et al 1996). The 'third generation' of BK antagonist, B9430 (D-Arg-Arg-pro-Hyp-Gly-Igl-Ser-Digl-Oic-Arg) is known to be extremely potent and long lasting at both B_1 and B_2 receptors (Burgess et al 2000). The development of this compound not only demonstrates that a polypharmaceutic approach covering both receptor types is possible, but also that the structures of the B_1 andB_2 receptors are sufficiently similar to be antagonized by a single drug. This fact was not appreciated until recently. Most recently, bradyzide, a potent non-peptide B_2 BK receptor with long-lasting oral activity in animal models of inflammatory hyperalgesia has been described (Farmer SG and Burch RM 1992). These BK receptor antagonists may prove to be therapeutically applicable in pathological states, which are caused by hyperactivity of kinins.

MODE OF ACTION OF KININS

Interaction between the kinins and their specific receptors can lead to activation of several second-messenger systems. The kinin receptor stimulation in the intact cells or in tissues appears to initiate the second-messenger pathways such as arachidonic acid products and the activation of calcium-sensitive systems (Burch RM 1990). The elevation of cellular inositol phosphates by BK involves G-protein-coupled activation of phospholipase A_2 and C that are used in the synthesis of eicosanoids (Sharma JN and Zeitlin IJ 1977). It is of interest that indomethacin, a cyclooxygenase inhibitor, was able to cause potentiation of BKinduced contractions of both isolated estrous rat uterus and guinea pig tracheal smooth muscle preparations (Akbar et al 1998; Ransom et al 1992). These findings may suggest that there could be non-eicosanoid pathways for the cellular and molecular actions of BK. Furthermore, it is known that BK significantly stimulates phosphoinositide hydrolysis in guinea pig ileum longitudinal muscle that may result in elevation of cytosolic calcium ion levels to induce contractile responses (Schini et al 1990). Schini et al. (Adetuyibi A and Mills IH 1972) demonstrated that the kinin B_2 receptor stimulation causes production of cyclic guanosine monophosphate (cyclic GMP) in cultured porcine aortic endothelial cells. The formation of cyclic GMP may be an important step for the biological actions as well as release of NO evoked by BK in the endothelial cells and in the vascular smooth muscles.

THE KININ SYSTEM IN CARDIOVASCULAR DISORDERS
HYPERTENSION

Hypertension is a major risk factor for the development of cardiovascular diseases, such as coronary heart disease, congestive heart failure and peripheral vascular and renal diseases (Sharma JN 1988). There is ample evidence documenting the role of KKS in pathogenesis of hypertension (Sharma et al 1996). The pharmacological action of BK in the regulation of systemic BP was vasodilatation in most areas of the circulation, a reduction of total peripheral vascular resistance and a regulation of sodium excretion from the kidney (De Freitas et al 1964; Webster ME and Gilmore JP 1964). When BK is injected into the renal artery, it causes diuresis and natriuresis by increasing renal blood flow(McGiff et al 1975). These actions of BK have been attributed to PG release in the renal circulation (Margolius et al 1971). The role of KKS in hypertension was established by Margolius et al. (Margolius et al 1972; Sharma JN and Zeitlin IJ 1981) with the observations that urinary kallikrein excretion is significantly reduced in hypertensive patients and hypertensive rats. This led to the suggestion that reduced urinary kallikrein excretion might result from a defect in kinin generation in hypertensive situations. Research on the systemic changes in the KKS has provided further insight regarding the mechanisms of various hypertensive conditions. In this connection, it is known that kininogen levels and a kinin-potentiating factor are reduced in essential and malignant hypertension (Sharma JN 1988; James FW and Donaldson VH). It may be possible that the deficiency in plasma HMWK is due to decrease in liver synthesis in individuals who develop hypertension after mild exercise (Mohsin et al 1992). It can be proposed that a deficient KKS might be a significant factor in the pathophysiology of hypertension. In this connection, it is suggested that the role of renal KM is to excrete excess of sodium. Therefore, a reduction in the generation of renal KKS may cause development of hypertension as a result of sodium accumulation in the body (Katori M and Majima M 1997; Wang et al 1994). Thus, the development of a compound having renal kallkrein-like activity may serve the purpose of excreting excessive sodium from the kidney. This action may be useful for the treatment of hypertension. Also, it has been demonstrated that transgenic mice overexpressing renal tissue kallikrein were hypotensive and that the administration of aprotinin, a tissue kallikrein inhibitor, restored the BP in the transgenic mice (Sharma et al 1995). The suppression of the hypotensive responses of ACE inhibitors by aprotinin in SHR has been documented (Chao J and Chao L 1998). These findings highlight a role of tissue kallikrein in the regulation of BP. Recently it has been proposed that tissue kallikrein gene delivery into various hypertensive models exhibits protection, such as a reduction in high BP, attenuation of cardiac hypertrophy, inhibition of renal damage and stenosis (Silberbauer et al 1982). These findings may indicate the prospect of this kallikrein gene therapy for cardiovascular and renal pathology. Kininase II (ACE) inhibitors are currently used in the treatment of both clinical and experimental hypertension (Antonaccio M 1982; Edery et al 1981). Kininase II inhibitors could lower BP by inhibiting the biodegradation of kinin as well as blocking the formation of angiotension (Ang II) at the renal site. A calcium-channel blocker, nifedipine, used to treat patients with essential hypertension, can normalize the reduced urinary kallikrein excretion (Smith et al 1980). Our previous investigations demonstrated differential sensitivity for the genetically Dahl-salt-sensitive (DSS) hypertensive and genetically Dahl-salt-resistant (DSR) normotensive rats to the hypotensive action on nifedipine (Edery et al 1981). This might reflect a significantly more important function of diminished renal KKS activity in DSS hypertensive rats as compared with the DSR normotensive rats. It is unknown whether a similar situation may exist in genetically predisposed humans with hypertension. Furthermore, Smith et al. (Sharma JN 1993) have proposed that women with reduced activity of the renal KKS combined with increased sympathetic drive may be at increased risk of developing pregnancy-induced hypertension. It is a generally accepted view that the BK-induced BP-lowering effect is mediated by the kinin B_2 receptor, but B_1 might also be involved under special situations (Regoli D 1984). It has been demonstrated that the B_2 receptor antagonist (B5630) can abolish the hypotensive effects of BK as well as captopril, an ACE inhibitor (Sharma JN 1992). This led to the proposal that the hypotensive action of ACE inhibitors might be due to the activation of the kinin B_2 receptor (Braunwald E. 1997). The accumulation of BK after treatment with ACE inhibitors with subsequent release of NO, PGs and PGI_2 could account for the additional mediators released by these drugs in hypertensive patients. However, the use of BK antagonist can abolish the effectiveness of anti-hypertensive drugs; therefore, these drugs must be contraindicated in patients with hypertension.

CARDIAC FAILURE AND ISCHEMIA

Cardiac failure and ischemia are the leading causes of death in developed and many developing countries (Lochner W. and Parratt JR 1966). These conditions are considered as the new emerging epidemic of the third millennium ((Lochner W. and Parratt JR 1966). The role of kinins in the heart has not received much attention, despite the fact that it was shown earlierthat local and systemic administration of BK can increase coronary blood flow and improve myocardial metabolism. It is well known that ACE inhibitors limit ventricular dilatation, delay the progression of clinical symptoms, and improve mortality rate. This beneficial action appears to be related to the reduced formation of Ang II, which results in a decreased growth response and attenuated pressure load (Linz et al 1995). In addition, the ability of ACE inhibitors to prevent kinins from enzymatic breakdown represents a relevant mechanism contributing to cardioprotection (Zhu et al. 1995). This concept fueled a series of studies demonstrating the presence of a local KKS in the heart (Nolly HL and Brotis J. 1981; Sharma JN and Uma K. 1996; Sharma et al. 19991). The binding of kinins to endothelial B2 receptors leads to the release of NO and PGI_2, exerting vasodilator, ischemic, and anti-proliferative effects and preserving myocardial stores of energy-rich phosphates and glycogen

(Madeddu et al. 1998). Kinins contribute to the maintenance of cardiovascular homeostasis by opposing the vasoconstrictor activity of Ang II (Kichuck et al. 1996). Circumstantial evidence also suggests that a dysfunctional KKS may contribute to the pathogenesis of heart failure. In fact, reduced local kinin generation and blunted NO formation have been reported in microvessels of failing human hearts (Whalley et al. 1992). Furthermore, in dogs with pacing-induced congestive heart failure, selective blockade of B2 receptors by Hoe 140 reduces coronary blood flow and contractility and increases left ventricular end diastolic pressure (Koide et al. 1993). Thus, the reduced activity of the cardiac KKS may facilitate the development of cardiac failure. On the other hand, kinins are continuously released during cardiac hypoxia and ischemia (Linz et al. 1993; Scholkens BA 1996). They act as cardioprotective agents in perfusion and participate in the process of ischemic preconditioning (Vegh et al. 1991; Walls et al. 1994). There is evidence to suggest that BK infusion into coronary artery reduces significantly the severity of ischemia-induced arrhythmia in anesthetized dogs (Scholkens BA 1996). Studies undertaken in rats, dogs, and humans revealed that kinins are released under the conditions of ischemia and myocardial infarction (Rubin LE and Levi R. 1995; Dela et al. 1993). This process may be indicative of the role of kinins in protecting the heart at the time of myocardial infarction. This raised local kinin release might be able to exert a protective effect on the heart by activating signal transduction pathways generating NO and PGI_2. Coronary artery ligation for shorter and longer duration in SHR and WKY rats showed that administration of BK could increase the survival time of these rats (Abbas et al. 1999). This effect of BK was reverted by pretreatment with a specific B_2 receptor antagonist (Abbas et al. 1999). In conclusion, these results support the hypothesis that KKS might be regarded as a prime mediator in protecting the heart in ischemic conditions. However, extensive investigations on the molecular biology and gene mapping of KKS in the heart during health and cardiovascular diseases can provide many questions to be answered regarding the significance of KKS in cardiovascular pathophysiology. This may allow us to develop KKS-based therapeutics for cardiovascular diseases.

LEFT VENTRICULAR HYPERTROPHY

Left ventricular hypertrophy (LVH) is regarded as an independent risk factor in hypertensive patients (Sharma et al. 1998). BK can counter the development of LVH in rats with hypertension produced by aortic banding (Linz et al. 1993). This anti-hypertrophic effect of BK was abolished by treatment with B_2 receptor antagonist and NO synthetase inhibitor. Thus, BK has a role in protecting the heart against developing LVH by releasing NO in this model of hypertension induced by aortic banding. In this regard, we have for the first time demonstrated that a lack of cardiac KKS could be responsible for the induction of LVH in SHR and SHR with diabetes 4). Therefore, it is suggested that reduced cardiac tissue kallikrein and cardiac kininogen may be responsible for reduced BK generation in the heart. Therefore, deficient components of KKS in the heart may be the cause of myocardial dysfunction in maintaining high BP and cardiac LVH. It is highly desirable to develop the stable compounds of KKS to evaluate their efficacy and potency in cardiac failure and cardiac ischemia, as well as myocardial infarction. Recently, we have shown that, in hypertensive rats, BP reduction and regression of LVH with captopril treatment might be due to enhanced renal tissue kallikrein activity (Nies et al. 1993). This may further support the view that tissue kallikrein may act as a cardioprotective agent. It has recently been proposed that kinins have modulatory effects in preventing myocardial ischemia (Marcondes S. and Antunes E. 2005). It is of interest to note that Madeddu and co-workers (Maestri et al. 2003) described the cardiac hypertrophy and microvascular deficit in kinin B_2 receptor knockout mice.

REFERENCES

Abbas SA, Sharma IN, Yusof APM: The effect of bradykinin and its antagonist on survival time after coronary artery occlusion in hypertensive rats. Immunopharmacology 1999; 44: 93-98.

Abbas SA, Sharma JN, Yusof APM: Effect of bradykinin and its antagonist on survival time after coronary artery occlusion in rats. Gen Pharmacol 1999; 33: 243-247.

Adetuyibi A, Mills IH: Relationship between urinary kallikrein and renal function, hypertension, and excretion of sodium and water in man Lancet 1972; 2: 203-207.

Akbar A, Sharma IN, Yusof APM, Gan EK: Potentiation of bradykinin-induced responses in the intact and denuded epithelium of guinea pig tracheal preparations. Tissue Reactions 1998; 20: 95-100.

Almeida FA, Stella RCR, Voos A, et al: Malignant hypertension: a syndrome associated with low plasma kininogen and kinin potentiating factor. Hypertension 1981 ; 3: 46-50.

Antonaccio M: Angiotensin converting enzyme (ACE) inhibitors Annu RevPharmacol Toxicol1982; 22: 57-87.

Barabe J, Droulin JN, Regoli D, et al: Receptors for bradykinin in intestine and uterine smooth muscle. Can J Physiol Pharmacol 1977; 96: 920-926.

Bhoola KD, Figueroa CD, Worth K: Bioregulation of kinin, kallikrein, kininogen and kininases. Pharmacal Rev 1992; 44:1-80.

Braunwald E: Cardiovascular medicine at turn of the millennium:triumphs, concern and opportunities. N Engl J Med 1997; 337: 1360-1369.

Burch RM. Kinin signal transduction: role of phosphoinositides and eicosanoids. J Cardiovasc Pharmacol 1990; 15(Suppl 6): S44-46.

Burgess GM, Perkins MN, Rang PR, et al: Bradyzide, a potent non-peptide B_2 bradykinin receptor antagonist with long-lasting oral activity in animal models of inflammatory hyperalgesia. Br J Pharmacol 2000; 129: 77-86.

Chao J, Chao L: Kallikrein gene therapy in hypertension, cardiovascular and renal diseases. Gen Ther Mol Biol 1998; 1: 301-308.

Cheronis JC, Whally ET, Nguyen KT: A new class of bradykinin antagonist: synthesis and in vitro activity of bissuccinimidoalkane peptide dimers. J Med Chem 1992; 35: 1563-1572.

Cochrane CG, Revak SD, Wuepper D: Activation of Hageman factor in solid and fluid phase. A critical role of kallikrein. J Exp Med 1973; 138: 1564-1583.

De Freitas FM, Farraco EZ, de Azevedo DE General circulatory alterations induced by intravenous infusion of synthetic bradykinin in man.Circulation 1964; 29: 66-70.

Dela CR, Suffredini A, Page JD, et al: Activation of kallikrein-kinin system after endotoxin administration to normal human volunteers. Blood 1993; 81: 3313-3317.

D'Orleans-Juste P, de Nussi G, Vane JR: Kinins act on B_1 or B_2 receptors to release conjointly endothelium-derived relaxing factor and prostacyclin from bovine aortic endothelial cells. Br J Pharmacol 1989; 96: 920-926.

Edery H, Rosenthal T, Amitzur G, et al: The influence of SQ 20881 on the blood kinin system of renal hypertensive patients. Drug Exp Clin Res 1981; VII: 749-756.

Erdos EG: Some old and some new ideas on kinin metabolism. J Cardiovasc Pharmacal 1990; 15(Suppl 6): S20-24.

Farmer SG, Burch RM, Meeker SA, et al: Evidence for a pulmonary B_3 bradykinin receptor. Mol Pharmacol 1989; 36: 1-8.

Farmer SG, Burch RM: Biochemical and molecular pharmacology of kinin receptors. Annu Rev Pharmacol Toxicol 1992; 32: 511-536.

Greenbaum LM: T-kinin and T-kininogen. Children of technology. Biochem Pharmacal 1982; 33: 2943-2944.

Griffin JH, Cochrane CG: Mechanism for the involvement of high molecular weight kininogen in surface-dependent reactions of Hageman factor. Proc Natl Acad Sci 1976; 73: 2554-2558.

Hanson L, McCullough RG, Selig WM: In vivo pharmacological profile of novel, potent, stable BK antagonist at B_1 and B_2 receptors. Immunopharmacology 1996; 33: 191-193.

James FW, Donaldson VH. Decrease exercise tolerance and hypertension in serve hereditary deficiency of plasma kininogen. Lancet 1981; 1: 889.

Jin LS, Seeds E, Page C, et al.: Inhibition of bradykinininduced bronchoconstriction in guinea-pig by a synthetic B_2 receptor antagonist. Br J Pharmacol 1989; 97: 598-602.

Katori M, Majima M: Role of the renal kallikrien-kinin system in the development of hypertension. Immunopharmacology 1997; 36: 237-242.

Kichuck MR, Seyedi N, Zhang X, et al: Regulation of nitric acid production in human coronary microvessels and the contribution of local kinin formation. Circulation 1996; 94: 44-51.

Koide A, Zeitlin IJ, Parratt JR: Kinin formation in ischaemic heart and aorta of anaesthetized rats. J Physiol (Lond) 1993; 467: 125P.

Linz W, Wiemer G, Gohlke P. Contribution of kinin to the cardiovascular action of converting-enzyme inhibitors. Pharmacol Rev 1995; 47: 25-50.

Linz W, Wiemer G, Scholkens BA: Bradykinin prevents left ventricular hypertrophy in rats. J Hypertens 1993; 11(Suppl 5): S96-97.

Linz WW, Wiemer G, Scholkens BA: Contribution of bradykinin to the cardiovascular effects of ramipril. J Cardiovasc Pharmacol 1993; 22(Supp19): SI-8.

Lochner W, Parratt JR: A comparison of the effects of locally and systemically administered kinin on coronary blood flow and myocardial metabolism. Br J Pharmacol Chemother 1966; 26: 17-26.

Madeddu P, Milia AF, Salis ME, et al: Renovascular hypertension in bradykinin B_2-receptor knockout mice. Hypertension 1998; 23: 305-509.

Maestri R, Milia AF, Salis MB, et al: Cardiac hypertrophy and microvascular deficit in Kinin B_2 receptor knock-out mice. Hypertension 2003; 41: 1151-1155.

Mandle R, Colman RW, Kaplan A: Identification of prekallikrein and HMW- kininogen as a complex in human plasma. Froc Natl Acad Sci 1976; 73: 4176-4183.

Marceau F, Hess JF, Bachvarov DR: The B_1 receptors for kinin. Pharmacal Rev 1998; 50: 357-386.

Marcondes S, Antunes E: The plasma and tissue kininogen-kallikrein-kinin system: role in cardiovascular system. Curr Med Chern 2005; 3: 33-44.

Margolius HS, Geller R, deJong W, et al: Altered urinary kallikrein excretion in rats with hypertension. Circ Res 1972; 30: 358-362.

Margolius HS, Geller R, Pisano JJ, et al: Altered urinary kallikrein excretion in human hypertension. Lancet 1971; 2: 1063-1065.

McGiff JC, Itskovitz HD, Terrango NA: The action of bradykinin and eledoicin in the canine isolated kidney: relationship to prostaglandins Clin Sci Mol Med 1975; 49: 125-131.

Mohsin SSJ, Majima M, Katori M, et al: Important suppressive roles of the kallikrein-kinin system during the developmental stage of hypertension in spontaneously hypertensive rats. Asia Pacific J Pharmacol 1992 ;71: 73-82.

Muller-Esterl W, Iwanaga S, Nakanishi S: Kininogens revisited. TIBS 1986; 11: 336-339.

Nagayasa T, Nagasawa S: Studies of human kininogen. Isolation, characterization, and cleavage by plasma kallikrein of high molecular weight (HMW) kininogen. J Biochem 1979; 85: 249-258.

Nally HL, Brotis J: Kinin-forming enzyme in rat cardiac tissue. Am J Physiol1981; 265: H1209-1214.

Nally HL, Carretero OA, Sclicli AJ: Kallikrein release by vascular tissue. Am J Physiol 1993; 265: H1209-1214.

Nies AS, Forsyth RP, Williams HE, et al: Contribution of kinins to endotoxin volunteers. Blood 1993; 81: 3313-3317.

Nustad KK, Vaaje K, Pierce JY: Synthesis of kallikrein by rat kidney slices. Br J Pharmacol 1975; 53: 229-234.

Okamoto H, Greenbaum LM: Pharmacological properties of T-kinin. Biochem Pharmacol 1983; 32: 2637-2638.

Oza NB, Gaud HD: Kininogenase of the aortic wall in spontaneously hypertensive rats. J Cardiovasc Pharmacol 1992; 20(Suppl 9): 1-3.

Pravenc M, Ken V, Kunes J: Cosegregation of blood pressure with a kallikrein gene family polymorphism. Hypertension 1991; 17: 242-246.

Ransom W, Young GS, Schneck K, Goodman CB: Characterization of solubilized bradykinin B_2 receptors from smooth muscle and mucosa of guinea-pig ileum. Biochem Pharmacol 1992; 43: 1823-1827.

Regoli D, Barabe J: Pharmacology of bradykinin and related kinins. Pharmacol Rev 1980; 32: 1-46.

Regoli D: Neurohumoral regulation of precapillary vessels: the kallikrein-kinin system. J Cardiovasc Pharmacol 1984; 6(Suppl 3): S401-412.

Rubin LE, Levi R: Protective role of bradykinin in cardiac anaphylaxis. Circ Res 1995; 79: 434-440.

Saha JK, Sengupta JN, Goyal RK: Effect of bradykinin and bradykinin analogs on the opossum lower esophageal sphincter: characterization of an inhibitory bradykinin receptor. J Pharmacol Exp Ther 1991; 259: 265-273.

Saha JK, Sengupta JN, Goyal RK: Effect of bradykinin on opossum longitudinal smooth muscle: evidence for novel bradykinin receptors. J Pharmacol Exp Ther 1990; 252: 1012-1020.

Schini VB, Boulanger C, Regoli D, et al: Bradykinin stimulates the production of cyclic GMP via activation of B_2 receptors in cultured porcine aortic endothelial cells. J Pharmacol Exp Ther 1990; 252: 581-585.

Scholkens BA: Kinins in the cardiovascular system. Immunopharmacology 1996; 33: 209-217.

Sharma IN, Uma K, Yusaf APM: Left ventricular hypertrophy and its relation to the cardiac kinin-forming system in hypertensive and diabetic rats. lnt J Cardiol 1998; 63: 229-235.

Sharma IN, Uma K, Yusof APM: Altered cardiac tissue and plasma kininogen levels in hypertensive and diabetic rats. Immunopharmacology 1999; 34: 129-132.

Sharma IN, Uma K. Cardiac kallikrein in hypertensive and diabetic rats with and without diabetes. Immunapharmacology 1996; 33: 341-343.

Sharma IN, Zeitlin IJ: Indomethacin in low concentrations potentiates the action of some spasmogens on the isolated oestrous rat uterus J Pharm Pharmacol 1977; 29: 316-317.

Sharma JN, Amrah SS, Noor AR; Suppression of hypotensive responses of captopril and enalapril by kallikrein inhibitors aprotinin in spontaneously hypertensive rats. Pharmacology 1995; 50: 363-369.

Sharma JN, Ferandez PG, Kim BK, et al: Systolic blood pressure responses to enalapril maleate (MK 421), an angiotensin converting enzyme inhibitor and hydrochlorothiazide in conscious Dahl salt-sensitive (S) and salt-resistant (R) rats. Can J Physiol Pharmacol 1984; 62: 241-243.

Sharma JN, Kesavarao U: Effect of captopril on urinary kallikrein, blood pressure and myocardial hypertrophy in diabetic spontaneously hypertensive rats. Pharmacology 2002; 64: 196-200.

Sharma JN, Stewart JM, Mohsin SSJ: Influence of a kinin antagonist on acute hypotensive responses induced by bradykinin and captopril in spontaneously hypertensive rats. Agents Actions 1992; 38(III): 258-269.

Sharma JN, Vma KK, Noor AR: Blood pressure regulation by the kallikrein-kinin system. Gen Pharmacol 1996; 27: 55-63.

Sharma JN, Yusof APM, Wirth KJ: The kinin antagonist Hoe 140 reduceacute paw oedema in rats caused by carrageenan, bradykinin and kaolin. Inflammopharmacology 1988; 6: 9-17.

Sharma JN, Yusof APM: Pro-inflammatory properties of the kallikreinkinin system: potential for new drug therapy. Inflammopharmacology 1998; 6: 289-296.

Sharma JN, Zeitlin IJ, Deodhar SD, et al.: Detection of tissue kallikrein-like activity in inflamed synovial tissue. Arch Int Pharmacody Ther 1983; 262: 279-286.

Sharma JN, Zeitlin IJ: Altered plasma kininogen in clinical hypertension. Lancet 1981; 1: 125-126.

Sharma JN. Contribution of kinin system to the antihypertensive action of angiotensin converting enzyme inhibitors. Adv Exp Med Biol 1989; 247A: 197-205.

Sharma JN. Interrelationship between the kallikrein-kinin system and hypertension: a review. Gen Pharmacal 1988; 19:177-187.

Sharma JN: Does kinin mediate the hypotensive action of angiotensin converting enzyme (ACE) inhibitors. Gen Pharmacal 1990; 21: 451-457.

Sharma JN: Involvement of the kinin-forming system in physiopathology of rheumatoid inflammation. Agents Actions 1992; 38(III): 343-361.

Sharma JN: Kinin system and prostaglandins in the intestine. Pharmacol Toxicol 1988; 63: 310-316.

Sharma JN: Kinin-forming system in the genesis of hypertension. Agents Actions 1984; 14: 200-205.

Sharma JN: Therapeutic prospects of bradykinin antagonists. Gen Pharmacol 1993; 24: 267-274.

Silberbauer K, Stanek B, Temple H: Acute hypotensive effect of captopril in man modified by prostaglandian synthesis inhibition. Br J Clin Pharmacol 1982; 14: 87S-93S.

Silverberg M, Diehl S: The auto activation of factor XII (Hageman factor) induced by low-heparin and dextran sulfate. Biochem J 1987; 248: 715-720.

Smith C, Campbell S, Albano J: Urinary kallikrein excretion in normotensive and hypertensive pregnancies: 8 years later. Immunopharmacology 1990; 44: 177-182.

Takada Y, Skidgel RA, Erdos EG: Purification of human urinary prokallikrein: identification of the site of activation by the metalloproteinase thermolysin. Biochem J 1985; 232: 851-856.

Thampson RE, Mandle R, Kaplan AP: Association of factor XI and high molecular weight kininogen in human plasma. J Clin Invest 1977; 60: 1376-1380.

Tiffany CW, Burch M: Bradykinin stimulates tumor necrosis factor and interleukin-1 release from macrophages. FEBS Lett 1989; 247: 189-192.

Vegh A, Rapp JG, Parratt JR: Attenuation of the antiarrhythmic effects of ischaemia preconditioning by blocked of bradykinin B_2 receptors. Br J Pharmacol 1994; 107: 1167-1172.

Vegh A, Szekeres L, Parratt JR: Local intracoronary infusions of bradykinin profoundly reduce the severity of ischaemia-induced arrhythmia in anaesthetized dogs. Br J Pharmacal 1991; 104: 294-295.

Walls TM, Sheehy R, Hartman JC: Role of bradykinin in myocardial preconditioning. J Pharmacal Exp Ther 1994; 270: 681-689.

Wang C, Chao L, Chao J: Human tissue kallikrein induces hypotension in transgenic mice. Hypertension 1994; 23: 236-243.

Webster ME, Gilmore JP. Influence of kallidin-10 on renal function. Am J Physiol 1964; 206: 714-718.

Weiss AS, Gallin JL, Kaplan AP: Fletcher factor deficiency: a diminished rate of Hageman factor activation caused by absence of prekallikrein with abnormalities of coagulation, fibrinolysis, chemotactic activity and kinin generation. J Clin Invest 1974; 53: 622-633.

Whalley ET, Clegg S, Stewart JM: The effect of kinin agonists and antagonists on the pain response of human blister base. Naunyn-Schmiedeberg's Arch Pharmacol 1987; 336: 652-655.

Whalley ET, Solomon JA, Modafferi DM: CP-0127, a novel potent bradykinin antagonist increases survival in rat and rabbit model of endotoxin shock. Agents Actions 1992; 38(Suppl): 413-420.

Wirth KJ, Hock FJ, Albus U, et al: Hoe 140 a new potent and long acting bradykinin antagonist-in vitro studies. Br J Pharmacol 1991; 102: 774-777.

Woolly-Miller C, Chao J, Chao L: Restriction fragment length polymorphism's mapped in spontaneously hypertensive rats using kallikrein probes. J Hypertens 1989;7:865-871.

Yoshida H, Zhang N, Chao L, et al: Kallikrein gene delivery attenuates myocardial infarction and apoptosis after myocardial ischemia and perfusion. Hypertension 2000; 35: 25-31.

Zhu P, Zugga CE, Simper D, et al: Bradykinin improves post ischemic recovery in the rat heart: role of high energy phosphates, nitric oxide and prostacyclin. Cardiovasc Res 1995; 29: 658-663.

Chapter 8

Role of Nitric Oxide in Inflammatory Diseases

Abstract

Nitric oxide (NO) is a signaling molecule that plays a key role in the pathogenesis of inflammation. It gives an anti-inflammatory effect under normal physiological conditions. On the other hand, NO is considered as a pro-inflammatory mediator that induces inflammation due to over production in abnormal situations. NO is synthesized and released into the endothelial cells by the help of NOSs that convert arginine into citrulline producing NO in the process. Oxygen and NADPH are necessary co-factors in such conversion. NO is believed to induce vasodilatation in cardiovascular system and furthermore, it involves in immune responses by cytokine-activated macrophages, which release NO in high concentrations. In addition, NO is a potent neurotransmitter at the neuronal synapses and contributes to the regulation of apoptosis. NO is involved in the pathogenesis of inflammatory disorders of the joint, gut and lungs. Therefore, NO inhibitors represent important therapeutic advance in the management of inflammatory diseases. Selective NO biosynthesis inhibitors and synthetic arginine analogues are proved to be used for the treatment of NO-induced inflammation. Finally, the undesired effects of NO are due to its impaired production, including vasoconstriction, inflammation and tissue damage.

Key words: Nitric oxide; Asthma; Rheumatoid arthritis; Inflammatory bowel diseases

Introduction

Nitric oxide (NO) is a member of the labile radical entities known as reactive oxygen species (ROS) and contains one nitrogen atom covalently bonded to an oxygen atom with one unpaired electron. It is particularly reactive with oxygen and heme-iron containing groups which reduce NO to more stable nitrate compounds (Ignarro, 1989) For this reason, the bioavailability of NO in certain tissues (notably blood-rich in haemoglobin and muscle rich in myoglobin) is extremely low and the biological actions are restricted temporally and spatially close to its site of synthesis (Ignarro et al., 1993). Paradoxically, NO is also lipid soluble, making it highly membrane permeant (Subczynski et al., 1996). Therefore, many of its most well described actions involve its diffusion between cells to act as a paracrine-signaling molecule.

The NO's role was first discovered by several groups of scientists who were attempting to identify the agent responsible for promoting blood vessel relaxation and regulating vascular tone. This agent was termed endothelium-derived relaxing factor (EDRF), and was initially assumed to be a protein like most other signaling molecules. The discovery that EDRF was in fact nitric oxide has led to explosion of interest in this field and resulted in many thousands of publications over the last few years.

NO has now been demonstrated to be a versatile molecule that plays its actions in a variety of biological processes including immune defenses, inflammation and neurotransmission.

NO is a fairly short-lived molecule (with a half life of 6s) produced from enzymes known as nitric oxide synthases (NOSs) and provides its actions through the L- arginine substrate that is transported into the cells (Moncada et al., 1991).

Since it is a small molecule, NO is able to penetrate rapidly across cell membranes and diffuse through distances of more than several microns. This means that NO can be formed or synthesized in a variety of tissues and as a consequence it is capable of affecting a number of important biological processes and has been implicated in several diseases (Gonon et al., 2004).

This paper is going to concern more on specific disease conditions related to joint, gut and asthmatic inflammatory disorders.

FORMATION OF NO

To begin with, nitric oxide (NO) is a paracrine mediator that is released by endothelial cells and by certain neurons. Because NO is rapidly oxidized, its biological lifetime is only several seconds. For this reason, NO affects only cells in the immediate vicinity of the cell that produces it.

The formation of NO is catalyzed by nitric oxide synthases (NOS), which are dimeric flavoproteins, contain tetrahydrobioprotein and have homology with cytochrome P450 and is most likely to be in the cardiovascular and central nervous systems. These enzymes convert arginine into citrulline, producing NO in the process. Oxygen and NADPH (nicotinamide adenine dinucleotide Phosphate with extra hydrogen) are necessary co-factors. There are three isoforms of NOS named according to their activity or the tissue type in which they were first described. The isoforms of NOS are neuronal NOS (or nNOS), constitutive endothelial NOS (or eNOS) and inducible NOS (or iNOS). These enzymes are also sometimes referred to by number, so that nNOS is known as NOS 1, iNOS is known as NOS 2 and eNOS is NOS 3. Despite the names of these enzymes, all three isoforms can be found in a variety of tissues and cell types (Kolb-Bachofen et al., 2006).

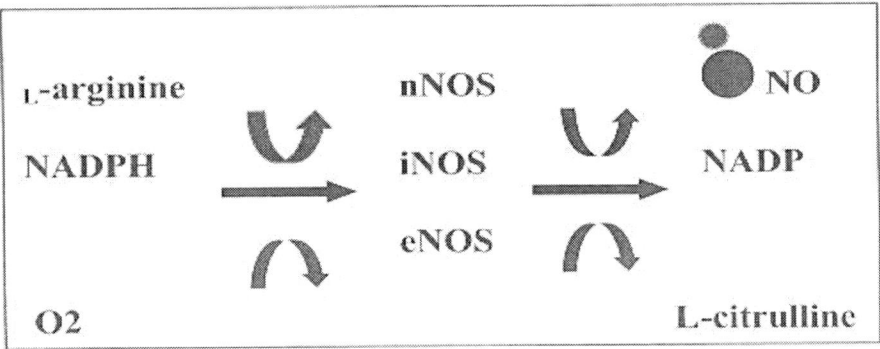

Figure 8.1. General mechanism of NO formation by NOSs.

Figure8.1 shows the nitrogen atom of NO is derived from the terminal guanido group of L-arginine. Details of the reaction mechanism are controversial, but it is known that NOS enzymes are functionally 'bimodal' in that they combine oxygenase and reductase activities associated with distinct structural domains. The oxygenase domain contains haem, while the reductase domain binds calcium-calmodulin, FMN (flavin mono-nucleotide), FAD (Flavin adenine di-nucleotide) and NADPH By analogy with cytochrome P450, it is believed that the flavins accept electrons from NADPH and transfer them to the haem iron, which binds to oxygen and catalyses the stepwise oxidation of L,-arginine (essential alpha-amino acid) to NO and citrulline (alpha-amino acid).

GENERAL STRUCTURE OF THE NOS

The functional NOS protein is a dimer formed of two identical sub-units. There are three distinct domains in each NOS sub-unit: a reductase domain, a calmodulin-binding domain and an oxygenase domain (Liu and Gross, 1996).

1. The reductase domain: This domain contains the calcium calmodulin, FMN, FAD moieties and NADPH. It acts to transfer electrons from NADPH to the oxygenase domain. It should be noted that the reductase domain transfers electrons to the oxygenase domain of the opposite sub-unit of the dimer, and not to the domain on the same sub-unit (Liu and Gross, 1996).
2. Calmodulin binding: The binding of calmodulin is required for the activity of all the NOS isoforms. It detects changes in intracellular calcium levels, although its precise function is slightly different in each of the three isoforms (Phil Dash, 2001).
3. The oxygenase domain: This domain contains the binding sites for tetrahydrobiopterin, haem (heme) and arginine. The oxygenase domain catalyses the conversion of arginine into citrulline and NO (Knowles and Moncada, 1994).

Two of the enzymes (nNOS and eNOS) are constitutively expressed in mammalian cells and synthesize NO in response to increases in intracellular calcium levels. In some cases, however, they are able to increase NO release indirectly, in response to stimuli such as shear stress. The shearing forces act on the luminal surface of the vascular endothelium and increase the flow velocity of the calcium atoms, which in turn, increase the activity of nNOS and eNOS (Suschek et al., 2004)..

iNOS activity is independent of the level of calcium in the cell; however its activity – like all of the NOS isoforms – is dependent on the binding of calmodulin. Increases in cellular calcium leads to increases in levels of calmodulin and the increased binding of calmodulin to eNOS and nNOS leads to a transient increase in NO production by these enzymes. By contrast iNOS is able to bind tightly to calmodulin even at very low cellular concentration of calcium. Consequently, iNOS activity isn't able to respond to changes in calcium levels in the cell. As a result the production of NO by iNOS lasts much longer than from the other isoforms of NOS, and tends to produce much higher concentrations of NO in the cell (Koppenol and Traynham, 1996).

PHYSIOLOGICAL ROLES OF NO

Since the discovery that nitric oxide is able to induce vasodilation in the cardiovascular system, a large number of other roles have been described for NO. It is also known to play a role in the immune system, the nervous system and in programmed cell death (apoptosis) (Kolb and Kolb-Bachofen, 1998).

In the Cardiovascular system (CVS)

NO formed in the endothelium from the amino acid precursor L-arginine by the activity of the constitutive endothelial NOS isoenzymes has been shown to play an important role in the regulation of local vasomotor tone and other vascular roles and is thought, on the other hand to be due to transcriptional diversity (Ignarro et al., 1993). Based on such mechanisms, NO roles in the CVS are vasodilatation (ligand mediated and flow dependent), inhibition of vasoconstrictor influences (e. g., inhibits angiotensin II and sympathetic vasoconstriction), inhibition of platelet adhesion to the vascular endothelium (anti-thrombotic), inhibition of leukocyte adhesion to vascular endothelium (anti-inflammatory), anti-proliferative (e. g., inhibits smooth muscle hyperplasia following vascular injury) (Hocher et al., 2004). COX-inhibiting NO donors (CINODs) have been suggested as potentially beneficial drugs on cardiovascular and renal abnormalities ((Muscara and Wallace. 2006).

Release of NO as an important inflammatory mediator

In inflammatory reactions, pro-inflammatory cytokines lead to expression of the inducible NO synthase in monocyte/ macrophages, neutrophil granulocytes and many other cells; in the case of bacterial infection, endotoxin is another strong inducer of expression. In consequence, large amounts of NO are synthesized, exceeding the physiological NO production by up to 1000-fold (Forstermann et al., 1994; Knowles and Moncada, 1994; Weinberg et al., 1995; Cook and Cattell, 1996).

NO is secreted by neutrophils and macrophages in the following sequence:

With the onset of inflammation, circulating neutrophils begin to move out of the blood across the endothelium of venules to enter the inflamed area. This multistage process is known as chemotaxis. It involves a variety of protein and carbohydrate adhesion molecules on both endothelial cell and the neutrophil, and is regulated by messenger molecules released by cells in the injured area, including the endothelial cells. These messengers are collectively termed chemoattractants (also termed chemotaxins or chemotactic factors) (Scales et al., 1988).

In the first stage, the neutrophil is loosely tethered to the endothelial cells via a particular class of adhesion molecules; this event is associated with rolling of the neutrophil along the vessel surface. In essence, this initial reversible event permits the neutrophil to be exposed to chemoattractants being released in the injured area. These chemoattractants act on the neutrophil to induce the rapid appearance of another class of adhesion molecules in its plasma membrane-molecules that bind tightly to their matching molecules in the endothelial cells. In the next stage, via still other adhesion molecules, a narrow projection of the neutrophil is inserted into the space between two endothelial cells, and the entire neutrophil squeezes through the endothelial wall and into the interstitial fluid. In this way, huge numbers of neutrophils migrate into the inflamed area and move toward the microbes (Scales et al., 1988).

Movement of leukocytes from the blood cells into the damaged area is not limited to neutrophils. Monocytes follow later, and once in the tissue they undergo anatomical and functional changes that transform them to macrophages (Scales et al., 1988)

Killing by Phagocytes

The initial step in phagocytosis is contact between the surfaces of the phagocyte and microbe. One of the major triggers for phagocytosis during this contact is the interaction of phagocyte receptors with certain carbohydrates or lipids in the microbial cell walls. Contact is not itself always sufficient to trigger engulfment, however, particularly with those bacteria that are surrounded by a thick, gelatinous capsule. Chemical factors produced by the body can bind the phagocyte tightly to the microbe and markedly enhance phagocytosis. Any substance that does this is known as an opsonin, from the Greek word that means 'to prepare for eating' (Scales et al., 1988). As the phagocyte engulfs the microbe, the internal, microbe-containing sac formed in this step is called a phagosome. A layer of plasma membrane separates the microbe from the phagocyte's cytosol. The phagosome membrane then makes contact with one of the phagocyte's lysosomes, which is filled with a variety of hydrolytic enzymes. The membranes of the phagosome and lysosome fuse, and the combined vesicles are now called the phagolysosome. Inside the phagolysosome, the microbe's macromolecules are broken down by the lysosomal enzymes. In addition, other enzymes in the phagolysosome membrane produce NO as well as hydrogen peroxide and other oxygen derivatives, all of which are extremely destructive to the microbe's macromolecules (Scales et al., 1988).

Such intercellular destruction is not the only way phagocytes can kill microbes. The phagocytes also release anti-microbial substances into the extracellular fluid, where these chemicals fight and destroy the microbes without prior phagocytosis. These chemicals can also damage normal tissue (Scales et al., 1988).

Some of these substances such as NO secreted into the extracellular fluid also function as inflammatory mediators. Thus, positive feedback occurs such that when phagocytes enter the area and encounter microbes, inflammatory mediators, including chemokines, are released that brings in more phagocytes.

The overproduction of NO as an inflammatory mediator can lead to tissue destruction such as in inflammatory autoimmune diseases. Thus, depending on the concentration of NO, it can process pro- or anti-inflammatory effects. As a result NO is called 'double-edged sword' or `Jekll and Hide' (Pfeilsehifter et al., 1996).

ROLE OF NO IN INFLAMMATION-MEDIATED NEURODEGENERATION

Several studies provided evidences of the close association between inflammation in the brain and the pathogenesis of several degenerative neurologic disorders, including Parkinson's disease, Alzheimer's diseases, multiple sclerosis, amyotrophic lateral sclerosis, AIDS and dementia. The brain inflammation is mainly caused by activation of glial cells, especially in microglia that in turn produce a variety of pro-inflammatory and neurotoxic factors, including cytokines, fatty acid metabolites, free radicals-such as NO and superoxide. Excessive production of NO, as a consequence of NOS induction in activated glia, has been attributed to be involved in neurodegeneration and neuroprotection (Moncada and Higgs, 2006a).

Possible pro-inflammatory pharmacological effects of NOS NO are to be produced by specific mechanisms (as mentioned earlier) with the help of NOSs. The two isoforms (iNOS and eNOS) involved in inflammation produce NO that acts as an inflammatory mediator. On the other hand, the neuronal enzyme contributes only in the production of NO in the central nervous system to act as a neurotransmitter. Thus, our focus will be on iNOS and eNOS, which have pro-inflammatory effects (Moncada and Higgs, 2006b).

Once there is a bacterial invasion (for example), the bacteria will release endotoxins (part of the bacterial cell wall). And when the immune cells are exposed to these bacterial endotoxins or pro-inflammatory cytokines, they (immune cells) start to produce iNOS, which in turn results in an increase in cellular NO that contributes to inflammation and host defenses. Furthermore, the scientists suggested that the endotoxins activate the eNOS in macrophages that is essential in triggering the induction of iNOS (Corraliza and Moncada, 2002).

NO aids host defenses by killing the invading organism through inhibition of metabolic enzymes and destruction of DNA. However, overproduction of NO by iNOS can lead to septic shock (sepsis, a systemic bacterial infection) that causes host-damage. In sepsis, this is manifested predominantly as a profound hypotension, inadequate tissue perfusion and organ failure, which often result in death. Sepsis and other forms of host-damage (due to overproduction of NO) can be managed by many drugs that can inhibit NO synthesis or action by several mechanisms (Kolb-Bachofen et al., 2006).

INVOLVEMENT OF NO IN JOINT, GUT AND LUNG INFLAMMATORY DISORDERS

It is mainly the inducible form of NO synthase (iNOS) that is involved in inflammatory reactions. Virtually, all inflammatory cells express the inducible form of the enzyme in response to cytokine stimulation. NOS is also present in the bronchial epithelium of asthmatic subjects, in mucosa of the colon in patients with ulcerative colitis and in synoviocytes in inflammatory joint diseases. Inhibitors of iNOS are under investigation for treatment of inflammatory conditions (Hocher et al, 2000).

NO in joint inflammatory disorders

NO is not only a marker, but also a pro-inflammatory mediator of arthritis.

Increased serum concentration of nitrate, indicating enhanced NO production in serum and synovial fluid of the inflamed joints in patients with rheumatoid arthritis (RA), osteoarthritis (OA) and ankylosing spondylitis (Farrell et al., 1992; Kanno et al., 1992; Bode-Boger et al., 1996). Urinary nitrate (NO present in the kidney as nitrate) and c-GMP excretion are influenced in parallelwhen the constitutive NO synthase is activated (Stichtenoth et al., 1995; Van der Vliet et al., 1994).The urinary nitrate excretion was decreased significantly by therapy with prednisolone or non-steroidal anti-inflammatory drugs (NSAIDs) (Stichtenoth et al., 1995).

Further evidence is given by the measurement of elevated nitrotyrosine concentrations in serum and synovial fluid from patients with RA. Nitrotyrosine is formed by reaction of peroxynitrate with tyrosine and is an index of NO-dependent oxidative damage (Van der Vliet et al., 1994). Statins have been reported to possess a number of so-called pleiotropic (vasculoprotective actions that include improvement of endothelial function, increased nitric oxide (NO) bioavailability, antioxidant properties, stabilization of atherosclerotic plaques, regulation of progenitor cells, inhibition of inflammatory responses and immunomodulatory actions) actions. The anti-inflammatory effects of statins may have clinical impact in a number of non-vascular conditions including multiple sclerosis and rheumatoid arthritis (Matthias Endres., 2006).

CELLULAR ORIGIN AND ACTIONS OF NO IN ARTHRITIS

Nearly, all mammalian cells can express the inducible NO synthase after stimulation by cytokines, which are enhanced in inflammatory joint diseases as mentioned above. In humans, the following extra- and intra-articular sources of inflammatory NO production were identified: synovial fibroblasts, synoviocytes, endothelial cells, monocytes/macrophages in blood stream and synovial membrane, osteoblasts and chondrocytes. In patients with active RA, blood mononuclear cells had increased NO synthase activity due to expression of the inducible isoenzymes; the NO synthase activity correlated with the tender and swollen joint count (Weinberg et al., 1994).

Physiological NO production inhibits bone resorption by osteoclasts and it may have some acute protective effects in cartilage breakdown. On the other hand, the high amounts of NO produced by inflamed synovium lead to enhanced bone resorption, diminished bone proliferation and may induce chondrocyte apoptosis (Ralston et al., 1993).

All of these effects contribute to joint damage, thus NO must be considered as an important effector molecule of disease progression.

NO in gut inflammatory disorders

The role of NO as a pro-inflammatory mediator is proven for other chronic inflammatory diseases, such as chronic inflammatory bowel diseases. An increased NO production by the inducible NO synthase was found. Cellular sources of this NO production were mucosal neutrophils in the acute phase, and monocytes/macrophages and lymphocytes in the chronic phase (Miller and Clark, 1994).

In a study of patients with ulcerative colitis or Crohn's disease, there is a demonstration of enhanced activity of NO synthase in the inflamed mucosa. This activity was calcium independent, suggesting expression of the iNOS. As in RA, in ulcerative colitis there will be an increased urinary nitrate excretion as compared to healthy individuals. And after treatment with hydrocortisone by which the disease was inactivated, urinary nitrate excretion was normalized (Weinberg et al., 1994; Ralston et al., 1993; Miller and Clark, 1994). Since the iNOS is the most important isoenzyme in the production of NO in gut inflammatory disorders, the majority of studies have shown improvement in experimental bowel diseases with iNOS inhibition.

CELLULAR EFFECTS OF NO

NO can have potent effects on leukocyte adherence and chemotaxis. NO production leads to decreased expression of adhesion molecules on neutrophils and endothelial cells. These effects can result in changes in leukocyte adhesion and recruitment of postcapillary venules in vivo (Banick et al., 1997; Crisham et al., 1998).

NO can down-regulate macrophage cytokine production. However, it is important to consider that iNOS-derived NO from macrophages is also critical component of mucosal defense against luminal pathogens, such as Helicobacter pylori. Furthermore, NO can modulate neutrophil and monocyte chemotaxis induced by a variety of factors (Gobert et al., 2002; Sato et al., 2000).

Under conditions of oxidative stress, NO can scavenge free radicals and thus prevent cellular injury. However, iNOS activity is associated with inhibition of proliferation, increased apoptosis and cytotoxicity. High levels of NO are associated with mutagenesis and other forms of DNA damage (Liu and Hotchkiss, 1995). NO can also act to alter the function of iron-sulfur-containing enzymes and disrupt mitochondrial respiration (Kurose et al., 1995).

Tissue Effects of NO: NO role in Gastrointestinal Secretion, Permeability and Mucosal Blood Flow

In Gastro-intestinal Secretion: Mucus and epithelial cell fluid secretion are important in host defense in the intestine against microbes, toxins and irritants such as bile salts. NO has been shown to play an important role in both of these epithelial cell functions. NO induces gastric mucus and electrolyte secretion via activation of soluble guanylate cyclase, and this NO production appears to be due to activation of cholinergic receptors. However, prolonged over-expression of iNOS has been linked to decreased intestinal electrolyte transport (Weinberg et al., 1995; Cook and Cattell, 1996).

In permeability: In addition to effects on transcellular transport, NO has also been linked to alterations in paracellular permeability and barrier function. Interferon (INF) gamma has been well shown to cause alterations in permeability and several reports have linked this effect to induction of NO production (Sugi et al., 2001). The exact mechanism of how NO may alter the tight junctional complex or have other effects remains to be determined.

In Mucosal Blood Flow: NO is a potent vasodilator, an effect that is well documented in sepsis. This effect is also of great importance in the gastrointestinal mucosa. The increase in mucosal blood flow that can occur in response to injury from a variety of causative factors can have obvious effects in that there is resulting buffering of acid, dilution of toxins and stimulation of angiogenesis, all of which are critical in mucosal protection (Lippe and Holzer, 1992).

NO in Lung Inflammatory Disorders

Introduction

Inflammatory diseases of the respiratory tract are commonly associated with elevated production of NO and increased indices of NO-dependent oxidative stress. Although NO is known to have anti-microbial, anti-inflammatory and antioxidant properties, various studies support its involvement to lung injuries in several diseases. Such studies are also often presumed that NO dependent oxidations are clue to the formation of the oxidant peroxynitrate, although alternative mechanisms involving the phagocyte-derived heme proteins myeloperoxidase and eosinophil peroxidase might be operative during conditions of inflammation (Moncada et al., 1991).

Roles, cellular origin and generation of NO in the respiratory tract

Since its discovery as a biological messenger molecule more than 10 years ago, NO is now well recognized for its roles and actions in diverse biological processes, including vasodilation, bronchodilation, neurotransmission, tumor surveillance, anti-microbial defenses and regulation of inflammatory-immune process (Moncada et al., 1991; Weinberger et al., 1999).

In the respiratory tract, NO is generated by the three distinct isoforms of NO synthase (nNOS, iNOS and eNOS) that are present to different extents in numerous cell types, including airway and alveolar epithelial cells, neuronal cells, macrophages, neutrophils, mast cells, and endothelial and smooth muscle cells (Gaston et al., 1994).

In contrast with the other two NOS isoforms (nNOS and eNOS), which are expressed constitutively and activated by mediator-induced or stress-induced cell activation, iNOS activity is primarily regulated transcriptionally and is commonly induced by bacterial products and pro-inflammatory cytokines. As such, inflammatory diseases of the respiratory tract, such as asthma, acute respiratory distress syndrome (ARDS) and bronchiectasis, are commonly characterized by an increased expression of iNOS within respiratory epithelial and inflammatory-immune cells, and a markedly elevated local production of NO, as an additional host defense mechanism against bacterial or viral infection. The drawback of such excessive NO production is its accelerated metabolism to a family of potentially harmful reactive nitrogen species (RNS), including peroxynitrate and nitrogen dioxide, especially in the presence of phagocyte-generated oxidants. The formation of such RNS is thought to be the prime reason why NO can be considered as a pro-inflammatory mediator (contribute to the etiology of inflammatory lung diseases) (Gaston et al., 1994; Grisham et al., 1999).

Reynaert et al. in 2005 discussed the presence of high levels of nitric oxide in the expired breath of asthmatic patients and proposed the possible therapeutic benefits of NO inhibitors in the treatment of these patients. NO containing steroid moiety in its structure may provide useful anti-inflammatory drugs along with bronchodilating property.(Tallet et al., 2002).

POSSIBLE FUTURE PROSPECTS OF NO-RELATED THERAPY FOR INFLAMMATORY CONDITIONS

NO has a double-edged role endogenously. It is an essential physiological signaling molecule mediating various cell functions, but on the other hand, it induces cytotoxic and mutagenic effects when present in excess (under oxidative stress condition). Thus, in this objective the concern will be on suppressing the overproduction of NO in which it causes inflammatory tissue damage.

Such suppression will occur through inhibition of the L-arginine/nitric oxide pathway by different mechanisms using several agents including:

1. Selective NO biosynthesis inhibitors which inhibit the inducible (but not constitutive) NOS.
2. Synthetic arginine analogues, which compete with arginine and are useful experimental tools.

Selective NO biosynthesis inhibitors

The selective inhibition of enhanced NO synthesis is a new, so far exclusively experimental therapeutic strategy in the treatment of chronic inflammatory, non-infectious diseases (Di Rosa et al., 1990; Radomski et al., 1990).

Some established drugs for the therapy of these diseases inhibit activity or expression of the inducible NO synthase, which may contribute to their anti-inflammatory effects (Radomski et al., 1990).

Glucocorticoids inhibit expression of the inducible NO synthase, but have no effects on the activity of both inducible and constitutive NO synthases (Di Rosa et al., 1990; Radom-ski et al., 1990). The mechanism of action is complex and includes inhibition of transcription and translation, as well as reduced enzyme stability (Kunz et al., 1994).

Cyclosporin derivatives inhibit NO synthase expression. This could be explained by their actions on IL secretion and by direct effects on gene transcription (Muhl et al., 1993). Similar effects on the expression of inducible NO synthase are described for non-steroidal anti-inflammatory drugs (Kepka-Lenhart et al., 1996). However, the mechanism and clinical implications of these findings remain unclear.

In addition, salicylates are scavengers of NO. 5-Aminosalicylic acid was found to reduce both NO production and disease activity in inflammatory diseases especially in adjuvant arthritis (Grisham and Miles, 1994; Stichtenoth et al., 1997).

Specific and selective inhibition of the inducible NOS is so far possible only in animal experiments to some extent. For use in humans, only highly selective and non-toxic substances are suitable, since the pro-inflammatory NO production by the inducible NO synthesis, but not the homeostatic NO synthesis by the constitutive enzymes, must be inhibited. The latter inhibition can lead to vasoconstriction and platelet aggregation, both of which would augment the inflammatory tissue damage (Miller and Clark, 1994).

A number of substances for selective inhibition of pathological NO over production are now under development.

Synthetic arginine analogues

Drugs can inhibit NO synthesis or action by several mechanisms. Currently, the most useful drugs are arginine analogues, which compete with arginine for NOS and in some cases, also compete with the carrier that transports arginine into endothelial cells. Several such compounds, e.g. NG- monomethyl-L-arginine (L-NMMA) and NG-nitro-L-arginine methyl ester (L-NAME), have proved to be of great value as experimental tools. The use of L-NMMA is being investigated in disorders where there is overproduction of NO (e.g. inflammation and neurodegenerative diseases). Disappointingly, L-NMMA increases mortality in one such condition (sepsis) (Grisham and Miles, 1994; Stichtenoth and Frölich, 1998).

Besides selective inhibitors of the inducible NOS activity and synthetic arginine analogues, several other targets of pharmacological intervention have emerged: inhibition of enzyme transcription and translation, cofactor and substrate supply (Miller and Clark, 1994).

UNDESIRED EFFECTS OF NO

The undesired effects of NO are due to over or impaired production of such mediator and the affected endothelium becomes, as a result, damaged or dysfunctional. The following effects can result in vasoconstriction (e.g., coronary vasospasm, elevated systemic vascular resistance, hypertension), platelet aggregation and adhesion, which can lead to thrombosis, up-regulation of leukocyte and endothelial adhesion molecules leading to enhanced inflammation, vascular stenosis or restenosis as occurs following balloon angioplasty and stent placement and increased inflammation and tissue damage mediated by reactive oxygen species such as superoxide anion and hydroxyl radical (MalmstrOm and Weitzberg, 2004).

REFERENCES

Banick PD, Chen Q, XU YA, et al: Nitric oxide inhibits neutrophil beta 2 integrin function by inhibiting membrane-associated cyclic GMP synthesis J. Cell Physiol 1997; 172: 12-24.

Bode-Boger SM, Boger RR, Alike R, et al: L-arginine induces nitric oxide-dependent vasodilation in patients with critical limb ischemia Circulation 1996; 93: 85-90.

Brzozowski T, Konturek PC, Konturek SJ, et al: Gastroprotective and ulcer healing effects of nitric oxide-releasing non-steroidal anti-inflammatory drugs. Dig liver dis 2000; 32: 583-594.

Cook RT, Cattell V: Role of nitric oxide in immune-mediated diseases. Clin Sci 1996; 91: 375-384.

Corraliza I, Moncada S: Increased expression of arginase II in patients with different from of atrhtritis. Inplications of the regulatuion of nitric oxide. J Rheumatol 2002; 29: 2261-2265.

Crisham MB, Granger DN, Lefer DJ: Modulation of leukocyte-endothelial interaction by reactive metabolites of oxygen and nitrogen: relevance to ischemic heart disease. Free Radic Biol Med 1998: 25: 404-433.

Di Rosa M, Radomski M, Carnuccio R, et al: Glucocorticoids inhibit the induction of nitric oxide synthase in macrophages. Biochem Biophys Res Commun 1990; 172: 1246-1252.

Ellis JL, Augustyniak ME, Cochran ED, et al: NMI-1182, a gastroprotective cyclo-oxygenase-inhibiting nitric oxide donor Inflammopharmacology 2005; 12: 521-534.

Farrell AJ, Blake DR, Palmer RMJ, et al: Increased concentrations of nitrite in synovial fluid and serum samples suggest increased nitric oxide synthesis in rheumatic diseases. Ann Rheum Dis 1992; 51: 219-222.

Fiorucci S, Di Lorenzo A, Renga B, et al: Nitric oxide (NO) releasing naproxen (HCT-3012[(s)-6-methoxy-alpha-methyl-2-naphthalene acetic acid4-(nitrooxyObutyl ester]) interactions with aspirin in gastric mucosa of arthritic rats reveal a role for aspirin triggered lipoxin, prostaglandins, and NO in gastric protection J Pharmacol Exp Ther 2004; 311: 1264-1271.

Forstermann U, Closs El, Pollock JS, et al: Nitric oxide isozymes, Characterization, purification, molecular cloning, and functions. Hypertension 1994; 23: 112-131.

Gaston B, Drazen JM, Loscalzo 1, et al: The biology of nitrogen oxides in the airways. Am J Respir Crit Care Med 1994; 149: 538-551.

Gonon AT, Erbas D, Broijerswen A, et al: Nitric oxide mediates protective effect of endothelin receptors antagonism during myocardial ischemia and perfusion Am J. Physiol Heart Circ Physiol 2004; 286: Hl767-Hl774.

Gobert AP, Mersey BD, Cheng Y, et al: Cutting edge: urease release by Helicobacter pylori stimulates macrophage inducible nitric oxide synthase Immunol 2002; 168: 6002-6006.

Grisham MB, Miles AM: Effects of aminosalicylates and immunosuppressive agents on nitric oxide-dependent N-nitrosation reactions. Biochem. Pharmacol 1994; 47: 1897-1902.

Grisham MB, Jourd'Heuil D, Wink DA: Nitric oxide. 1 Physiological chemistry of nitric oxide and its metabolites: implications in inflammation. Am J Physiol 1999; 275: G315-G321.

Hocher B, Schwarz A, Slowinski T, et al: In-vitro interaction of nitric oxide and endothelin J Hypertens 2004; 22: 111-119.

Hocher B, Schwarz A, Fagan KA, et al; Pulmonary fibrosis and chronic lung inflammation in ET-l transgenic mice Am J Respir Cell Mol Biol 2000; 23: 19-26.

Hoogstraate J, Andersson LI, Berge OG, et al: COX-inhibiting nitric oxide donators (CINODs) - a new paradigm in the treatment of pain and inflammation. Infiammopharmacology 2003; 11: 423--428.

Ignarro LJ: Biological actions and properties of endothelium derived nitric oxide formed and released from artery and vein. Circ Res 1989; 65(1): 1-12.

Ignarro LJ, Fukuto JM, Griscavage, et al: Oxidation of nitric oxide in aqueous solution to nitrite but not nitrate: Comparison with enzymatically formed nitricoxide from L-arginine. Proc Nalt Acad Sci USA 1993; 90(17): 8130-8107.

Kanno K, Hirata Y, Emori T, et al: L-arginine infusion induces hypotension and diuresis/natriuresis with concomitant increased urinary excretion of nitrite/nitrate and cyclic GMP in humans. Clin Exp Pharmacol Physiol 1992; 19: 619-625.

Kepka-Lenhart D, Chen LC, Morris SM. Jr: Novel actions of aspirin and sodium salicylate: discordant effects on nitric oxide synthesis and induction of nitric oxide synthase m RNA in a murine macrophage cell line J Leukocyte Biol 1996; 59: 840-846.

Knowles RG, Moncada S: Nitric oxide synthases in mammals. Biochem J 1994; 298: 249-258.

Kolb-BuchofenV, Kuhhn A, Suschek CV: The role of nitric oxide. Rheumatol 2006; 45 (Suppl 3): iii17-iii19.

Kolb H, Kolb-Bachofen V: Nitric oxide in autoimmune disease: cytotoxic or regulatory mediator? Immunol Today 1998; 19: 556-561.

Kopppenol WH, Traynham JG: Say NO to nitric oxide: Nomenclature for :nitrogen and oxygen containing compounds Methods Enzymol 1996; 268: 3-7.

Knowles RG, Moncada S: Nitric oxide synthase in mammals. Biochem J 1994; 298: 249-258.

Kunz D, Walker G, Pfeilschifter J: Dexamethasone differentially affects interleukin IB- and cyclic AMP-induced nitric oxide synthase mRNA expression in renal mesangial cells Biochem J 1994; 304: 337-340.

Kurose 1, Ebinuma H, Higuchi H, et al: Nitric oxide mediates mitochondrial dysfunction in hepatoma cells induced by nonactivated Kupffer cells: evidence implicating ICAM-l-dependent process. J Gastroenterol Hepatol 1995; 10: S68-71.

Lippe FT, Holzer P: Participation of endothelium-derived nitric oxide but not prostacyclin in the gastric mucosal hyperemia due to acid back-diffusion. Br J Pharmacol 1992; 105: 708-714.

Liu RH, Hotchkiss 1H: Potential genotoxicity of chronically elevated nitric oxide: a review. Mutat Res 1995; 339:73-89.

Malmstrom RE, Weitzberg E: Endothelin and nitric oxide in inflammation: could there be a need for endothelin-blocking anti-inflammatory drugs? J Hypertens 2004; 22: 27-29.

Marshall M, Keeble J, Moore PK: Effect of a nitric oxide releasing derivative of paracetamol in a rat model of endotoxemia Br J Pharmacol 2006; 149: 516-522.

Matthias Endres: Statins: potential new indications in inflammatory conditions. Atherosclerosis supplements 2006; 7: 31-35.

Miller M1S, Clark DA: Nitric oxide synthase inhibition can initiate or prevent gut inflammation: role of enzyme source Agents Actions 1994; 41: C231-232.

Moncada S, Palmer RMJ, Higgs EA: Nitric oxide: physiology, pathophysiology, and pharmacology. Pharmacol Rev 1991; 43: 109-142.

Moncada S, Higgs EA: Nitric oxide and the vascular endothelium. Handb Exp. Pharmacol 2006a; 166 (Ptl): 213-254.

Moncada S, Higgs EA: The discovery of nitric oxide and its role in vascular biology Br J Pharmacol 2006b; 147 (Suppl I): S193-S201.

Muhl H, Kunz, D, Rob P, et al: Cyclosporin derivatives inhibit interleukin IB induction of nitric oxide synthase in renal mesangial cells Eur J Pharmacol 1993; 49: 95-100.

Muscara MN, Wallace 1L: COX-inhibiting nitric oxide donors (CINODs): potential benefits on cardiovascular and renal function. Cardiovasc Hematol Agents Med Chem 2006; 4: 155-164.

Pfeilschifter 1, Eberhardt W, Hummel R, et al: Therapeutics strategies for the inhibition of inducible nitric oxide synthase-potential for a novel class of anti-inflammatory agents. Cell Biol Int 1996; 20: 51-58.

Radomski MW, Palmer RMJ, Moncada S: Glucocorticoids inhibit the expression of an inducible, but not the constitutive, nitric oxide synthase in vascular endothelial cells. Proc Nalt Acad Sci USA 1990; 87: 10043-10047.

Ralston SH, Helfrich M, Grabowski PS, et al: A role for nitric oxide in the regulation of cytokine-induced bone resorption Bone Miner Res 1993; 8: 383.

Reynaert NL, Ckless K, Wouters EF, et al: Nitric oxide and redox signaling in allergic airway inflammation. Antioxid Redox signal 2005; 7: 129-143.

Sato E, Simpson KL, Grisham MB, et al: Reactive nitrogen and oxygen species attenuate interleukin-8-induced neutrophil chemotactic activity in vitro. J Biol Chem 2000; 275: 10826-10830.

Scales WE, Vander AJ, Brown MB, et al: American Journal of Physiology 1988; 65: 1840.

Stichtenoth DO, Fauler J, Zeidler H, et al: Urinary nitrate excretion is increased in patients with rheumatoid arthritis and reduced by prednisolone. Ann Rheum Dis 1995; 54: 820-824.

Stichtenoth DO, Frolich JC: Nitric oxide and inflammatory joint disease. Br J Rheumatol 1998; 37: 246-257.

Subczynski WK, Lomnicka M, Hyde JS: Permeability of nitric oxide through lipid layer membranes. Free Radic Res 1996; 24(5): 343-349.

Sugi K, Musch MW, Field M, et al: Inhibition of Na+, K+ATPase by interferon gamma downregulates intestinal epithelial transport and barrier function. Gastroenterology 2001; 120: 1393-1403.

Suschek CV, Schnorr O, Kolb-Bachofen V: The role of iNOS in chronic inflammatory processes in vivo: is it damage-promoting, protective, or active at all? Curr Mol Med 2004; 4: 763-775.

Tallet D, Soldato PD, Oudart N, et al: NO-Steroids: Potent anti-inflammatory drugs with bronchodilating activity in vitro. Biochemical and biophysical research communications 2002; 290: 125-130.

Ukawa H, Yamakuni H: Effects of cyclooxygenase-2 selective and nitric oxide-releasing nonsteroidal anti-inflammatory drugs on mucosal ulcerogenic and healing responses of the stomach. Dig Dis Sci 1998; 43: 2003-2011.

Van der Vliet A, O'Neill CA, Halliwell B, et al: Aromatic hydroxylation and nitration of phenylalanine and tyrosine by peroxynitrite-evidence for hydroxyl radical production from peroxynitrite. FEBS Lett 1994; 339: 89-92.

Wallace JL: Nitric oxide, aspirin-triggered lipoxinns and NO-aspirin in gastric protection. Inflamm Allergy Drug Targets 2006; 5: 133-137.

Weinberg JB, Granger DL, Pisetsky DS, et al: The role of nitric oxide in the pathogenesis of spontaneous murine autoimmune disease: increased nitric oxide production and nitric oxide synthase expression in MRL-Ipr/Ipr mice, and reduction of spontaneous glomerulonephritis and arthritis by orally administered N^G-monomethyl-L-arginine. J exp Med 1994; 179: 651-660.

Weinberg JB, Misukonis MA, Shami PJ, et al: Human mononuclear phagocyte inducible nitric oxide synthase (iNOS): analysis of iNOS m RNA, iNOS protein, biopterin, and nitric oxide production by blood monocytes and peritoneal macrophages. Blood 1995; 86: 1184-1195.

Weinberger B, Heck BE, Laskin DL, et al: Nitric oxide in the lung: therapeutic and cellular mechanism of action. Pharmacol Therapeut 1999; 84: 401-411.

Chapter 9

The Role of Leukotrienes in the Pathophysiology of Inflammatory Disorders: The prospects of Leukotrienes as Therapeutic Targets

INTRODUCTION

About a decade ago leukotrienes (LTs) had prominence as therapeutic targets in chronic inflammatory diseases but that several lines of evidence suggests there might be a need insights awakened in this field.

LTs are a family of biologically active lipid compounds derived from arachidonic acid (AA) through the 5-lipoxygenase (5-LO) pathway (Henderson, 1994). They play an important role in the pathophysiology of inflammatory diseases such as: asthma, RA and IBD (Sala et al., 1998). The name "leukotriene" is related to their synthesis in leucocytes and their chemical structure with three conjugated double bonds (triene) (Henderson, 1994). LTs can be classified according to their chemical structures and biological activities into two classes: the dihydroxy leukotriene, LTB_4, and the cysteinyl LTs (CysLTs).

LTB_4 has been known as a potent chemoattractant mediator of inflammation. LTB_4, stimulates neutrophils chemotaxis, chemokinesis, and adherence to endothelial cells, and activates neutrophils leading to release of enzymes and mediators, and degranulation (Busse, 1998).

LTC_4, LTD_4 and LTE_4, known as CysLTs, have been shown to be essential mediators in asthma. They mediate features of asthma including bronchoconstriction, bronchial hyperactivity, oedema formation and eosinophilia (Sala et al., 1998). Therefore, anti-LTs represent an important therapeutic advance in the management of inflammatory diseases. Many inhibitors, aimed at LTs biosynthesis, or receptor antagonists are being developed. This paper is intended to review the role of LTs in inflammatory conditions and the use of LTs inhibitors and antagonists in the treatment of these conditions.

BIOSYNTHESIS

The biosynthesis of LTs occurs predominantly in leucocytes. The initial step in the biosynthesis of LTs is the release of AA from cell membrane phospholipids upon cell stimulation (Henderson, 1998; Samuelsson et al., 1987). This reaction is catalyzed by phospholipase A_2. Then, 5-LO catalyzes the insertion of molecular oxygen into AA to form 5-hydroperoxyeicosatetraenoic acid (5-HPETE). 5-HPETE undergoes dehydration enzymatic reactions through the actions of 5-LO to form the unstable epoxide leukotriene A_4, (LTA_4). 5-lipoxygenase activating protein (FLAP), a perinuclear membrane protein, is required before 5-LO can synthesize 5-HPETE. FLAP appears to represent AA to 5-LO. LTA is either hydrolyzed into leukotriene B_4 (LTB_4) by the enzyme LTA_4 hydrolase or conjugated with reduced glutathione to form LTC4, through the enzymatic action of LTC_4 synthase. LTC_4, is actively transported out of the cells and metabolized to LTD_4, and then to LTE_4, LTC_4.), LTD_4 and LTE_4 are known as CysLTs because of their chemical structure (Samuelsson et al., 1987).

METABOLISM

LTs are metabolized to less active compounds in various cells. Chain-shortening via β-oxidation from the w-end has been known as the degradation pathway of LTB_4, and CysLTs. LTB_4 may be hydroxylated, through the action of a microsomal P450 LTB_4, hydroxylase, to form a partially active 20-hydroxy LTB4, (20-OH-LTB4) and the unstable intermediate, 20-aldehyde LTB_4. A 20-aldehyde dehydrogenase then converts 20-aldehyde LTB_4, to inactive 20-carboxyl LTB_4 (20-COOH LTB_4).

LTC_4 is metabolized through the action of gammaglutamyl transpeptidase to the active product, LTD_4.LTD_4 is further metabolized to LTE_4, by various dipeptidases. LTE_4 is excreted in the urine directly or after N-acetylation. It may also undergo (ω-hydroxylation and β-oxidation to yield smaller, more polar molecules (Morelli et al., 1990).

RECEPTORS

LTB_4 receptor

LTB_4 acts as a potent chemoattractant mediator of inflammation. The main targets of LTB_4 are leucocytes where it induces chemotaxis, immigration and activation. Hence, LTB_4 is an important chemical mediator involved in inflammatory diseases such as RA, asthma and IBD (Wang et al., 2000). It appears to signal leucocytes through a seven transmembrane-spaning G protein-coupled receptors (Huang et al., 1998). Two classes of LTB_4, receptors have been identified: LTB_4 receptor-1 (LTB4-R1) and LTB_4 receptor-2 (LTB_4, R-2) (Wang et al., 2000). The two receptors differ in their affinity and specificity for LTB_4, LTB_4, R-1 is the high affinity receptor; on the other hand, LTB_4, R-2 is the low affinity receptor. These receptors have different tissue distribution, and the exact roles of each receptor remain elusive

(Yokomizo et al., 2001). Studies showed that LTB$_4$ causes intracellular calcium mobilization and inhibition of forskolin stimulated cAMP production.

CysLT receptor

CysLTs, previously known as "slow-reacting substances of anaphylaxis (SRS-A)", play an important role in inflammatory disorders, particularly in asthma. They are recognized as the most potent bronchoconstrictors known. They also play an important role in the pathophysiology of other inflammatory disorders such as RA, IBD and psoriasis (Sarau et al., 1999; Figueroa et al., 2003). Binding and functional studies showed that the biological effects of the CysLTs are mediated via G protein-coupled receptors, and that they induce calcium mobilization (Sarau et al., 1999). CysLTs receptors are classified into two types CysLT receptor-1 (CysLT R-1) and CysLT receptor-2 (CysLT R-2). The human CysLT R-1 is expressed on lung macrophages and smooth muscle cells and in peripheral blood eosinophils and subsets of basophiles, monocytes, B lymphocytes and CD34+ stem cells. The human CysLT R-2 has been identified on heart Purkinje conducting fibre cells, adrenal chromaffin cells, in the brain and in subsets of peripheral blood leucocytes, including eosinophils.

A study was done on nasal lavage samples obtained from patients during their active seasonal allergic rhinitis to examine the expression of CysLT R-1 and CysLT R-2 in inflammatory cells. The study showed that both CysLT R-1 and CysLT R-2 mRNA and proteins were identified on 70-90% of nasal lavage eosinophils, 50% of mononuclear cells, and 30% of mast cells. 40% of neutrophils expressed only CysLT R-1 mRNA and its protein, but not CysLT R-2 mRNA and its protein (Figueroa et al., 2003).

ROLE OF LEUKOTRIENES IN INFLAMMATION

The pathophysiologic effects of LTB4,

LTB$_4$ is one of the most potent chemoattractant metabolites of AA. LTB$_4$ enhances neutrophil chemotaxis. Intratracheal instillation of LTB$_4$, in humans induces a selective neutrophil recruitment into the lungs (Busse, 1998). In in-vivo studies, injected LTB$_4$, in the rat peritoneal cavity results in substantial accumulation of macrophages and polymorphonuclear leucocytes. LTB$_4$ causes adherence of neutrophils to endothelium cells. It is able to enhance the adhesion of neutrophils to nylon wool, Sephadex G-25 and endothelial cells. It activates neutrophils leading to degranulation and the release of mediators, enzymes and superoxides. LTB$_4$ is also involved in inflammatory pain by reducing the nociceptive threshold via neutrophil dependent processes. Intracellularly, LTB$_4$, acts as a ligand for the peroxisome proliferator-activated receptor alpha (PPAR-α), a transcription factor that plays an important role in oxidative degradation of fatty acids and its derivatives, including LTB$_4$, itself (Henderson and Klebanoff, 1983).

The pathophysiologic effects of CysLTs

The CysLTs are pro-inflammatory mediators that play an important role in the pathophysiology of asthma. CysLTs are potent bronchoconstrictors and are at least 100-1000 times more potent than histamine (Bisgaard, 2001). They also produce vasoconstriction and increase vascular permeability allowing the exudation of plasma macromolecules, leading to the airway edema that characterizes asthma. In addition, CysLTs stimulate mucus secretion and inhibit mucociliary clearance. There is evidence that LTD, and LTE, are potent and specific chemoattractants for eosinophils, which appear to be important in asthma pathophysiology (Bisgaard, 2001).

LEUKOTRIENE'S ROLE IN INFLAMMATORY DISEASES

Asthma

Asthma is a chronic inflammatory condition of the airways. Many cells are involved in the pathophysiology of asthma, in particular mast cells, eosinophils and T lymphocytes. The mast cell activation is believed to be important in the initiation of the inflammatory response. Once binding of allergen to cell-hound IgE occurs, mast cells release mediators which in turn induce the inflammatory response. The mediators include histamine, chemotactic factors, platelet activating factor (PAF) and AA metabolites (notably prostaglandins, thromboxane, LTs, and the HETEs (Dipiro et al., 2001). CysLTs play an important role in the pathophysiology of asthma. They act as potent bronchoconstrictors. In addition, they cause vasoconstriction, increased microvascular permeability, exudation of macromolecules and oedema. The CysLTs also have potent chemoattractant properties on eosinophils. They cause eosinophils to influx into the airway mucosa. In addition, CysLTs increase mucus secretion and reduce ciliary motility.

There is evidence that synthesis of CysLTs is increased during naturally occurring asthma and acute asthma attacks as well as allergen and exercise challenge (Bisgaard, 2001). Zaitsu et al. (2003) have shown that the synthesis of LTB_4, and LTC_4, the mRNA expression of 5-LO, LTA_4, hydrolase, and LTC_4, synthase were enhanced in asthmatic children compared to controls. In this study, the synthesis of LTs was determined using specific radioimmunoassay. On the other hand, the mRNA expression of LT-synthesizing enzymes was determined using reverse transcriptase polymerase chain reaction in peripheral polymorphonuclear leucocytes, which were obtained from controls and asthmatic patients (Zaitsu et al., 2003). The use of leukotriene receptor antagonist (LTRA) also has been used to determine the role of LTs in the pathophysiology of asthma. The LTRAs montelukast, zafirlukast, and pranlukast inhibit bronchoconstriction caused by allergen, exercise, cold air, and aspirin in asthmatic patients (Bisgaard, 2001).

Rheumatoid arthritis

RA is a chronic and usually progressive inflammatory disorder of joints. The LTA hydrolase inhibitor, SA6541 has been used to investigate the role LTB_4, in murine arthritis models. In vivo, SA6541 inhibited the severity of collagen-induced arthritis and muramyl dipeptide (MDP)-induced hyper-proliferation of synovial cells. In vitro, SA6541 inhibited LTA,-induced hyper-proliferation of synovial stromal cells. Thus, LTB_4 may play an important role in arthritis models (Tsuji et al., 1999). A study on 25 children with RA and 15 normal subjects showed significantly higher levels of LTB_4, in the active stage of the disease compared with the values obtained from patients during the inactive stage of the disease and from healthy children (Gursel et al., 1997). LTB_4, R2 showed higher expression than LTB_4, R-1 in the synovial tissue from patients with the active disease (Hashimoto et al., 2003). Furthermore, the blockade of LTB_4, synthesis inhibition by MK 886 prevents articular incapacitation in rat zymosan-induced arthritis (da Rosa et al., 2004). It has been also proposed that some agents, such as inhibitors 5-lipoxygenase-omega-3 fatty acid and zileuton –may be most useful in treatment of milder RA manifestations such as moderate synovitis (Schiff, 1997; Weinblatt et al., 1992). In addition, Raisford and his coworkers (Rainsford et al., 1996) have demonstrated that certain 5-lipoxygenase inhibitors regulate the formation of those interleukins involved in joint cartilage destruction as well as those seen in joint inflammatory diseases.

Inflammatory bowel diseases

The colonic mucosa of patients with IBD is infiltrated with lymphocytes, plasma cells, mast cells, macrophages and neutrophils and contains higher levels of LTB_4 compared with similar tissue from normal persons. LTB_4 plays an important role as a neutrophil chemoattractant and enhances their adherence to vascular endothelium. Also the synthesis of LTB_4 from exogenous arachidonate in the mucosa from patients with IBD is higher than that of normal subjects (Sharon and Stenson, 1984). LTB_4 levels are elevated in rectal dialysates and tissues of IBD patients. These findings led to the consideration of leukotriene inhibitor strategies for managing IBD. Rask-Madsen (1998) indicated that established therapies, such as glucocorticoids and 5-aminosalicylic acid, inhibit the production at high concentrations of soluble mediators (LTB_4, PAF, PMNs) in IBD.

USE OF LEUKOTRIENE INHIBITORS AND ANTAGONISTS IN INFLAMMATORY DISEASES

LTs play important roles in the pathogenesis of inflammatory diseases, most commonly asthma, RA and IBD. Therefore, LTs have become therapeutic targets. Many LTs modifier agents aimed either to inhibit LTs biosynthesis or to block LTs receptors. LTs modifiers are classified into two classes: LTs inhibitors, which inhibit the formation of both LTB4, and the CysLTs, and LT antagonists, which selectively block the action of CysLTs at one of their receptors. Inhibition of LT biosynthesis can be achieved by inhibition of phospholipases releasing the precursor AA, direct inhibition of 5-LO and inhibition of FLAP (Werz, 2002). The rationale for LTRAs use in inflammatory disorders, particularly asthma, is to inhibit the bronchconstriction and inflammatory effects caused by LTs. LTRAs competitively blocks LTs receptors on bronchial smooth muscle.

Leukotriene inhibitors

Glucocorticosteroids inhibit the actions of phospholipase and assumed to inhibit the biosynthesis of all eicosanoids; however, the effect on LTs biosynthesis is not significant. The 5-LO catalyzes the first steps in the generation of LTs [5]. 5-LO is considered as a key target in developing drugs which inhibit LTs biosynthesis and thus inhibit their pathophysiological effects. Several compounds were identified as potent 5-LO inhibitors; however, such compounds lack selectivity for 5-LO and cause serious side effects (Rask-Madsen et al., 1992). Compounds, containing hydroxamic acids or N-hydroxyurea groups that chelate the iron in the active site of the enzyme, have been found to be potent and more selective inhibitors of 5- LO (Bell et al., 1992). Boswellic acid, the biologically active agent of the gum resin of Boswellia serrata has been shown to be specific inhibitor of 5-lipoxygenase, which has been used to treat IBD, RA, and asthma successfully (Gupta et al., 1997; Ammon, 2002).

Zileuton

The benzothiophene hydroxyurea, Zileuton, is a selective and reversible inhibitor of 5-LO. It is available in the US for the management of asthma (Werz, 2002; Rask-Madsen, 1992). Zileuton is administered orally, which is a significant advantage over inhalation in the pediatric population. Zileuton cannot inhibit the release of AA. Also, it does not inhibit cycloxygenase or phospholipase A,. It acts via the inhibition of calcium stimulated biosynthesis of LTs by neutrophils (McGill and Bussse, 1992).

These investigators also reported that zileuton is rapidly absorbed upon oral administration with a peak plasma concentration after 1-3 hours after administration. The mean elimination half life of zileuton is about 2.3 hours. Zileuton undergoes rapid first-pass metabolism via hepatic biotransformation. It is metabolized by stereosclective glucuronidation into two enantiomers, the R and S forms. Studies showed that zileuton is well tolerated by patients with renal impairment including those with severe renal impairment or those receiving hemodialysis. Therefore, dose adjustment is not required for patients with various degrees of renal impairment and patients on hemodialysis (Awni et al., 1997).

Zileuton improves lung function, relieves symptoms of asthmatic patients, and is also well tolerated by patients. A 12-month, parallel-group, open-label study was done to assess zileuton efficacy and evaluate liver function in patients treated with this drug. 2,947 patients at 233 centers in the United States were randomly assigned in a 5:1 ratio to treatment with zileuton in addition of usual asthma management or usual asthma management alone. Efficacy parameters included exacerbations of asthma; need for alternative treatment, steroid rescue, emergency management, and hospital admissions; forced expiratory volume in 1 second (FEVI); and asthma symptoms scores. For the safety evaluation, alanine aminotransferase levels were measured. Patients receiving zileuton had significantly fewer corticosteroid rescues (P<0.001), required less emergency managements (P<0.05), had fewer admissions, and had greater increases in FEV1 (P=0.048). Also, asthma symptoms improved significantly. Alanine aminotransferase levels elevated three times or more the upper limit in 4.6% in patients receiving zileuton and 1.1% of those receiving usual asthma care alone treatment (P<0.001); most elevations occurred in the first two to three months. Alanine aminotransferase levels reduced to less than two times the upper limit of normal or to baseline levels zileuton therapy or after zileuton withdrawal. No patient developed jaundice or chronic liver disease during the therapy. This study showed that the addition of zileuton to asthma treatment regimens improved asthma control and decreased utilization of healthcare resources (Lazarus et al., 1998).

Zileuton has also been evaluated in patients with exercise-induced asthma. Twenty-four asthmatic patients, with at least a 20% decrease in FEV1 following an exercise challenge received either zileuton (2.4 g/d) or placebo for 2 days before exercise. Zileuton did not alter baseline pulmonary function in these patients. It inhibited exercise-induced bronchospasm by an average of 41% as compared with placebo. Furthermore, 5 min after exercise, the zileuton-treated group had a mean FEV1 value that was 86% of their baseline value, as compared with a 74% value in the placebo group (p < 0.01) (Horwitz et al., 1998). A trial of zileuton versus mesalazine or placebo in maintenance of remission of ulcerative colitis (UC) was conducted in 1997 by the European zileuton study group for UC (Hawkey et al., 1997). This study showed that zileuton (6000 mg qid) was not significantly better than placebo in the maintenance of remission of UC, thus, may have limited use in the treatment of UC. Zarif et al. (1996) stated that zileuton treatment was successful in significantly decreasing the frequency of severe colitis in rat model, but decrease in PMN count was not significant suggesting that another mechanism may be there in its anti-inflammatory effect.

The LT biosynthesis inhibitor, MK-591, caused highly significant inhibition of LT biosynthesis in UC patients, but did not differ significantly from placebo in clinical efficacy (Roberts et al., 1997). This study raises the question of the involvement of LT in the genesis of UC inflammatory disease. However, it has been suggested that topical administration of LT synthesis inhibitor (FPL 64170XX) may be clinically useful in the treatment of active, distally located UC (Kjeldsen et al. 1995).

The other main class of leukotriene inhibitors are FLAP inhibitors, which inhibit the actions of 5-LO indirectly. These compounds are either synthesized from indole or quinolines structure. Of these the indole, MK886, inhibits FLAP (Datta et al. 1999). It inhibits the 5-LO metabolites production potently in the leucocytes. However, it is less effective in the blood and failed to inhibit the actions of purified 5-LO and 5-LO activity biosynthesis in broken cell preparations. M K886 inhibited LTB_4 biosynthesis partially in vivo in whole blood, reduced LTs levels in exudates and inhibited antigen induced bronchconstriction (Werz, 2002).

Leukotriene antagonists

LTs are important mediators of the pathophysiology of asthma and other inflammatory disorders. In asthmatic patients CysLTs cause bronchoconstriction, airway inflammation, edema, and mucus hypersecretion. LTRAs inhibit these potent effects by selectively blocking the CysLT R-1 receptor. Corticosteroid therapy does not inhibit CysLTs synthesis, which suggests that LTRAs may provide additional benefits with corticosteroid therapy. The use of

LTRAs with corticosteroid therapy improved asthma control significantly in clinical trials. Montelukast and zafirlukast are LTRAs that have been shown to improve symptoms in asthmatic patients (Bisgaard, 2001). The efficacy of fish oil 3-omega-fatty-acid, an inhibitor of LT synthesis, in the treatment of UC was conducted in an open trial by Salomon et al. (1990). They found seven patients out of nine showed moderate to marked improvement. This might suggest that there could be other mediators responsible for the cause of UC. The effect of the LTB_4 receptor antagonist, SC-41930, on colonic inflammation in rats, guinea pig and rabbit had provided the evidence in preventing effectively acute colonic inflammation when given orally (Fretland et al., 1990). No clinical data are available on this compound so far. Also, second-generation of LTB_4 receptor antagonists (S41930, SC-53228 and A-69412) have been developed with the view that they could be beneficial in treating psoriasis and UL (Penning et al., 1995; Fretland et al., 1995; Bell et al., 1993).

Montelukast

This is a selective antagonist of LTD_4 receptor (Cys1:1' R 1). It is used as a once daily oral dose for adults and children. A dose of 10-mg/day was found to be effective in studies using different dosages of montelukast on exercise-induced bronchoconstriction. 5-mg/day of the drug has also proved efficacy in children (Markham and Faulds, 1198). Clinical trials proved the efficacy of montelukast in preventing asthma in 2 to 14 years old children. Compared to inhaled sodium cromoglycate and inhaled beclomethasone, montelukast was more convenient and received greater compliance by patients (6-11 years old) in a 6-month randomized non-blind trial (Muijsers and Noble, 2002). Recently, it has been reported that montelukast does not affect the release of histamine from basophils but mildly inhibits the cysLT release in patients with asthma after four weeks of treatment (Sade et al. 2005). The suppression of inflammation is incomplete in some patients with stable asthma treated with inhaled corticosteroids, however, adding a leukotriene receptor antagonist (montelukast) can provide a complementary effect of controlling inflammation, with a significant improvement in quality of life (Biernacki et al., 2005).

In a double-blind, crossover placebo-controlled study, male volunteers received single 20 to 800 mg doses of montelukast. The drug was well tolerated. 11 of 18 of the volunteers experienced adverse reactions which may be related to the treatment. These included headache, diarrhea, abdominal cramps and discomfort, facial flushes, and tenderness in the right chondrium. All side effects were not serious and none required treatment. Montelukast 10-mg/day was also evaluated for tolerability data in 1,955 patients, participated in placebo-controlled clinical trials. The most common side effect was headache. Other side effects included cough, abdominal pain and influenza. Similar tolerability profile was seen in children (n=320) 6 to 14 years old. (Markham and Faulds, 1998).

Zafirlukast

Zafirlukast is an oral selective antagonist of LTs receptors. It competitively inhibits the actions of CysLTs C_4, D_4, and E_4. It is used for preventing and managing chronic asthma. Zafirlukast is used as one 20-mg oral dose twice daily for patients above 12 years old. In US, a dose of 10-mg twice daily is recommended for children aged 7 to 11 years old. On the other hand, it is contraindicated in UK in children less than 12 years old. In UK, the drug is also contraindicated in patients with hepatic impairment, cirrhosis, and moderately or severely abnormal renal function. US guidelines state that dosage adjustments are not required in patients with impaired renal function (Dunn and Goa, 2001).

NOVEL DEVELOPMENT OF LEUKOTRIENE ANTAGONISTS AS FUTURE THERAPY FOR INFLAMMATORY DISEASES

LTB_4 receptors play an important role in the genesis of inflammatory process in rheumatoid arthritis. LTB_4 receptor-2 was found to mediate the proinflammatory effects of LTB_4, in the synovial tissue of patients with rheumatoid arthritis. This suggests the possibility of using new drugs that act by blocking LTB_4 receptors (Hashimoto et al., 2003). BIIL 284 is a new orally active LTB_4 receptor antagonist that is able to inhibit LTB_4-induced Mac-1 expression in leucocytes of rheumatoid arthritic patients. In addition, it was observed that BBL 284 25 mg and 150 mg inhibited Mac-1 expression on neutrophils effectively in 26 patients suffering from rheumatoid arthritis. The study was a double-blind, randomized, parallel group design. In this study, these patients received BIIL 284 25 mg, 150 mg and/or placebo once daily for two weeks. It is concluded that longer treatment with BIIL 284 may result in clinical improvement of patients with RA (Schmolke et al., 2004).

REFERENCES

Alten R, Gromnica-Ihle E, Pohl C, et al: Inhibition of leukotriene B_4-induced CD11B/ CDI8 (Mac-I) expression by BIIL 284, a new long acting LTB_4 receptor antagonist, in patients with rheumatoid arthritis. Ann Rheum Dis 2004; 63 (2): 170-176.

Ammon HPT: Boswelliasauren (Inhaltsstoffe des Werauchs) als wirksame Prinzipien zur behandlung chronich entzundlicher Erkrankungen. Wien Med Wschr 2002; 152: 373-378.

Awni WM, Wong S, Chu SY, et al: Pharmacokinetics of zileuton and its metabolites in patients with renal impairment. J Clin Pharmacol 1997; 37: 395-404.

Bell RL, Young PR, Albert D, et al: The discovery and development of zileuton: an orally active 5-lipoxygenase inhibitor Int J Immunopharmacol 1992; 14: 505-510.

Bell R L, Bouska J, Young PR, et al: The properties of A-69412: a small hydrophilic 5-lipoxygenase inhibitors. Agents Actions 1993; 38: 178-187.

Biernacki WA, Kharitonov SA, Biernacka HM, et al: Effect of montelukast on exhaled leukotrienes and quality of life in asthmatic patients. Chest 2005; 128: 1958-1963.

Bisgaard H: Pathophysiology of cysteinylleukotrienes and effects of leukotriene receptor antagonists in asthma. Allergy 2001; 56: 7-11.

Busse WW: Leukotrienes and Inflammation. Am J Respir Crit Care Med 1998; 165: S210-S213.

Datta K, Biswal SS, Kehrer JP: The 5-lipoxygenaseactinvating protein (FLAP) inhibitor, MK886, induces apoptosis independently of FLAP. Biochem J 1999; 340: 371-375.

De Rosa FA, Teixeira MM, Rocha JC, et al: Blockade of leukotriene B_4 prevents articular incapacitation in rat zymosan-induced arthritis. Eur J Pharmacol 2004; 497: 81-86.

Dunn CJ, Goa KL: Zafirlukast: an update of its pharmacology and therapeutic efficacy in asthma. Drugs 2001; 61 (2): 285-315.

Dipiro JT, Talbert RL, Yee GC, et al: Pharmacotherapy: A Physiologic Approach. 5th edition. McGraw Hill 2002; P: 475.

Figueroa DJ, Borish L, Baramki D, et al: Expression of cysteinylleukotriene synthetic and signaling proteins in inflammatory cells in active seasonal allergic rhinitis. Clin Exp Allergy 2003; 33: 1380-1388.

Fretland DJ, Widomski D, Tsai B, et al: Effect of the leukotriene B_4 receptor antagonist SC-41930 on colonic inflammation in rat, guinea pig and rabbit. J Pharmacol Exp Ther 1990; 255: 572-576.

Fretland DJ, Anglin CP, Bremer M, et al: Antiinflammatory effects of second-generation leukotriene B_4 receptor antagonists, SC-53228: impact upon leukotriene B_4- and 12(R)-HETE-mediated events. Inflammation 1995; 19: 193-205.

Gupta 1, Parihar A, Malhotra P, et al: Effects of Boswellia serrata gum resin in patients with ulcerative colitis. Eur J Med Res 1997; 2: 37-43.

Gursel T, Firat S, Ercan ZS: Increased serum leukotriene B_4 level in the active stage of rheumatoid arthritis in children. Prosta Leukotri Essential Fatty Acids 1997; 56: 205-257.

Hashimoto A, Endo H, Hayashi 1, et al: Differential expression of leukotriene B_4 receptor subtypes (BLT_1 and BLT_2) in human synovial tissues and synovial fluid leucocytes of patients with rheumatoid arthritis. J Rheumatol 2003; 30: 1712-1718.

Hawkey CJ, Dube LM, Rountree LV, et al: A trial of zileuton versus mesalazine or placebo in the maintenance of remission of ulcerative colitis. The European Zileuton study Group For Ulcerative Colitis. Gastroenterology 1997; 112: 718-724.

Henderson WR: The role of leukotrienes in inflammation. AnnIntern Med 1994; 121: 684-697.

Henderson WR, Klebanoff SJ: Leukotriene production and inactivation by normal, chronic granulomatous disease myeloperoxidase-deficient neutrophils. J Biol Chem 1983; 258: 13522-13527.

Horwitz RJ, McGill KA, Busse WW: The role of leukotriene modifiers in the treatment of asthma. Am J Respir Criti Care Med 1998; 157 (5): 1363-1371.

Huang WW, Garcia-Zepeda EA, Sauty A, et al: Molecular and biological characterization of the murine leukotriene B_4 receptor expressed on eosinophils. J Exp Med 1998; 1063-1074.

Kjeldsen J, Laursen LS, Hillingso J, et al: Selective blockade of leukotriene production by a single dose of the FPL 64170XX 0.5% enema in active ulcerative colitis. Pharmacol Toxicol 1995; 77: 371-376.

Lazarus SC, Lee T, Kemp JP, et al: Safety and clinical efficacy of zileuton in patients with chronic asthma. Am J Managed Care 1998; 4: 841-848.

Markham A, Faulds D: Montelukast Drugs 1998; 56: 251-256.

McGill KA, Busse WW: Zileuton. Lancet 1996; 348: 519-524.

Morelli JG, Norris DA, Lyons MB, et al: Metabolism of exogenous leukotrienes by cultured human keratinocytes. J Investi Dermatol 1990; 94: 681-684.

Muijsers RB, Noble S: Montelukast: a review of its therapeutic potential in asthma in children 2 to 14 years of age. Paediatric Drugs 2002; 4: 123-139.

Penning TD, Djuric SW, Miyashiro JM, et al: Second - generation of leukotriene B$_4$ receptor antagonists related to SC41930: hetercyclic replacement of the methyle ketone pharmacophore. J Med Chem 1995; 38: 858-868.

Rainsford KD, Ying C, Smith F: Effects of 5-lipoxygenase inhibitors in interleukin production by human synovial tissue in organ culture:comparison with interleukin-I-synthesis inhibitors. J Pharma Pharmacol 1996; 48: 46-52.

Rask-Madsen J: Soluble mediators and the interaction of drugs in IBD. Drugs Today 1998; 34: 45-63.

Rask-Madsen J, Bukhave K, Laursen LS, et al: 5-Lipoxygenase inhibitors for the treatment of inflammatory bowel disease. Agents Actions 1992; Spec No: C37-46 Roberts WG, Simon TJ, Berlin RG, et al: Leukotrienes in ulcerative colitis. Results of a multicenter trial of a leukotriene biosynthesis inhibitor, MK-591. Gastroenterology 1997; 112: 725-732.

Sade K, Kivity S, Fireman E, et al: Effect of montelukast on basophil releasability in patients with asthma. Isr Med Assoc J 2005; 7:792-795.

Sala A, Zarini S, Bolla M: Leukotrienes: lipid bio-effectors of inflammatory reactions. Biochemistry 1998; 63: 84-92.

Salomon P, Kornbluth AA, Janowitz HD: Treatment of ulcerative colitis with fish oil n-3-omega-fatty acid: an open trial J Clin Gastroenterol 1990; 12: 157-161.

SamuelssonB, Dahlen SE, Lindgren JA, et al: Leukotrienes and lipoxins: structures, biosynthesis, and biological effects. Science 1987; 237: 1171-1176.

Sarau HM, Ames RS, Chambers J, et al: Identification, molecular cloning, expression, and characterization of a cysteinyl leukotriene receptor. Mol Pharmacol 1999; 56: 657-663.

Schiff M: Emerging treatments for rheumatoid arthritis. Am J Med 1997; 102: 11S-15S.

Sharon P, Stenson WF: Enhanced synthesis of leukotriene B$_4$ by colonic mucosa in inflammatory bowel disease. Gastroenterology 1984; 86: 453-460.

Tsuji F, Oki K, Fujisawa K, et al: Involvement of leukotriene B$_4$ in arthritis models. Life Sci 1999; 64: PL51-56.

Wang S, Gustafson E, Pang L, et al: A novel hepatointestinal leukotriene B$_4$ receptor. J Biol Chem 2000; 275: 40686-40694.

Weinblatt ME, Kremer JM. Coblyn JS, et al: Zileuton, a 5-lipoxygenase inhibitor in rheumatoid arthritis. J Rheumatol 1992; 19: 1537-1541.

Werz O: 5-Lipoxygenase: Cellular Biology and Molecular Pharmacology. Current Drug Targets - Inflammation & Allergy 2002; 1: 23-44.

Chapter 10

Therapeutic Prospects of Bradykinin Receptor Agonists in the Treatment of Cardiovascular Diseases

INTRODUCTION

Kinins are potent vasorelaxant polypeptides located in both the vascular smooth muscle and the heart. A number of observations obtained from clinical and experimental models of hypertension, cardiac failure, ischemia, myocardial infarction and left ventricular hypertrophy (LVH) have suggested that the kallikrein-kinin system (KKS) may be involved in the induction of cardiovascular-related diseases (Sharma JN and Sharma J, 2002). A role for the KKS in the central regulation of blood pressure has been demonstrated in hypertensive rats (Sharma et al., 1996). Reduction of peripheral and cardiac KKS components may cause high blood pressure in both humans and animals (Sharma et al., 1996).

Locally administered kinins exert beneficial cardiac effects (Sharma JN and Sharma J, 2002). In both in vitro and in vivo studies in isolated rat hearts, bradykinins (BKs) reduced the duration and incidence of ischemia In Studies undertaken in rats, dogs and humans have revealed that kinins are released under conditions of ischemia and myocardial infarction (Linz et al. 1996; Emanueli C. and Madeddu P. 2001), while BK antagonists worsen ischemia-induced effects (Sharma JN and Sharma J. 2002; Emanueli C. and Madeddu P. 2001; Sharma JN 2003). BKs can contribute to the cardioprotective effects of preconditioning (Sharma JN and Sharma J. 2002), a protective adaptive mechanism produced by short periods of ischemic stress that involves reduction in ischemic cellular damage and life-threatening ventricular arrhythmias (Linz et al., 1996). The beneficial reduction in cardiac infarct size by BK after preconditioning in rabbits was prevented by administration of the BK antagonist icatibant (I, Jerini AG/Sanofi-Aventis; Figure 10.1) (Sharma JN, 2003). In addition, BKs play a role in protection of the heart against the development of LVH through release of nitric oxide (NO) ((Sharma JN and Sharma J, 2002; Sharma JN, 2003).

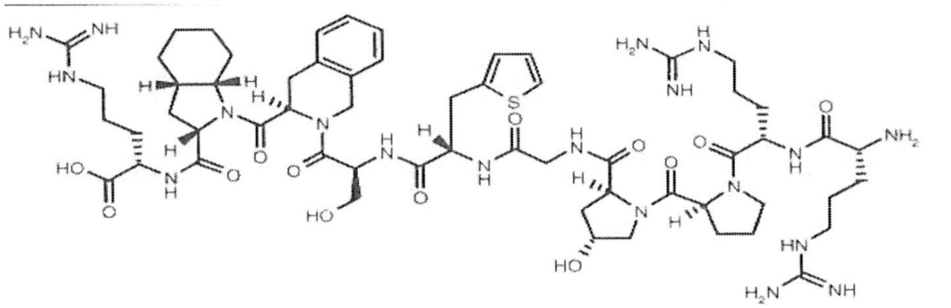

Figure 10.1. The structure of icatibant.

Stimulation of the BK B_2 receptor by kinins is associated with pathophysiological as well as pronounced beneficial effects (Heitsch H. 2003). Consequently, interference with B_2 receptors by either antagonism or agonism offers promise for the development of therapeutic approaches for the treatment of various human diseases (Heitsch H. 2003). B_2 receptor agonists have the potential to become valuable therapeutic agents in the treatment of cardiovascular diseases, and have already demonstrated efficacy in various animal models of human disease (Heitsch H. 2003). However, none of the potent and selective peptide and non-peptide agonists of the B_2 receptor that have been investigated, such as labradamil (2: RMP-7), LF-943 (3; JMV-1116), FR-190997 (4) and FR-191413 (Figure 10.2) have progressed to clinical assessment in cardiovascular indications (Heitsch H. 2003). The aim of this review is to discuss the current knowledge on the role of kinin agonists in the treatment of cardiovascular diseases.

THE KALLIKREIN-KININ SYSTEM

The most important members of the kinin family are BK (Arg-Pro-Pro-Gly-Phe-Ser-Pro-Phe-Arg), kallidin (Lys-Arg-Pro-Pro-Gly-Phe-Ser-Pro-Phe-Arg) and methionyl-lysyl-BK (Met-Lys-Arg-Pro-Pro-Gly-Phe-Arg) (Sharma JN and Sharma J. 2002; Sharma JN. 2003; Campbell DJ 2001). These are pharmacologically active polypeptides derived from circulating precursors (kininogens) by the action of serine proteases, called kallikreins. Once released into the circulation kinins are rapidly (< 15 s) inactivated by enzymes called kininases (Sharma JN and Sharma J. 2002; Sharma JN. 2003; Campbell DJ 2001). Kininogens are typical secretory multifunctional proteins derived from α2-globulin in the liver, which circulate in the plasma and other body fluids (Sharma JN and Sharma J. 2002; Sharma JN. 2003). Two forms of kininogens are present in the mammalian circulation: high-molecular-weight kininogen (HMWK) and low-molecular-weight kininogen (LMWK) (Sharma JN and Sharma J. 2002; Sharma JN. 2003; Campbell DJ 2001) which have completely different biochemical immunological and functional characteristics (Sharma JN and Sharma J. 2002; Sharma et al. 1996). In addition, T-kininogen is found in the rat myocardium and is considered to be an acute-phase reactant of inflammation (Yayama et al. 2000). In rats, T-kininogen releases T-kinin by the enzymatic action of T-kallikrein (Yayama et al. 2000).

Tissue kallikreins are more widely distributed in the tissues (organs), such as the kidneys (urine), pancreas, salivary glands, intestine, prostate gland and synovial tissue (Sharma JN and Sharma J. 2002; Sharma JN. 2003; Campbell DJ 2001). These kallikreins are single-chain acidic glycoproteins that differ from one another in molecular weight, biological function, and physicochemical and immunological properties (Sharma JN and Sharma J. 2002; Sharma JN. 2003; Campbell DJ 2001). In tissues, the inactive enzyme is converted into the active form by the cleavage of an amino-terminal peptide. Active tissue kallikrein liberates kallidin from LMWK (Sharma JN and Sharma J. 2002; Sharma JN. 2003; Heitsch H. 2003; Campbell DJ 2001).

Plasma kallikrein circulates in an inactive state and is also known as prekallikrein or Fletcher factor. Prekallikrein can be activated to form kallikrein by activated Hageman factor or Factor XIIa, and subsequently liberates BK from HMWK (Sharma JN and Sharma J. 2002; Sharma JN. 2003; Heitsch H. 2003; Campbell DJ 2001). In addition, prekallikrein is able to convert inactive Factor XII to XIIa through a positive feedback reaction (Sharma JN and Sharma J. 2002). Two plasma prekallikreins and one HMWK form a complex (Sharma JN and Sharma J. 2002; Sharma JN. 2003), which circulates with Factor XIIa and Factor XI (Sharma JN and Sharma J. 2002; Sharma JN. 2003; Heitsch H. 2003; Campbell DJ 2001). Inactive Factor XI is converted to active Factor XIa through HMWK to participate in the intrinsic coagulation pathway (Sharma JN and Sharma J. 2002; Sharma JN. 2003; Heitsch H. 2003; Campbell DJ 2001).

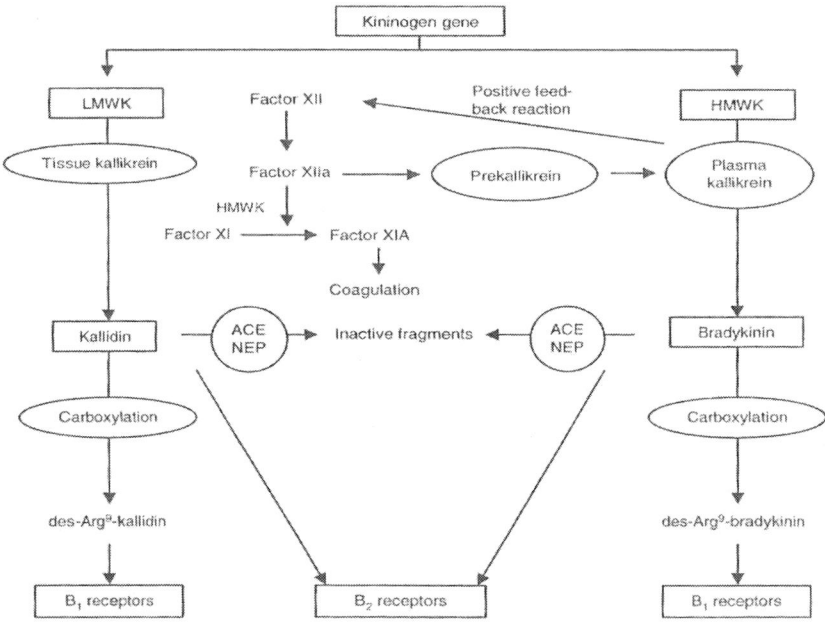

ACE angiotensin-converting enzyme, HMWK high molecular-weight kininogen, LMWK low-molecular-weight kininogen, NEP neutral endopeptidase.

Figure 10.3. The formation and metabolism of kinins.

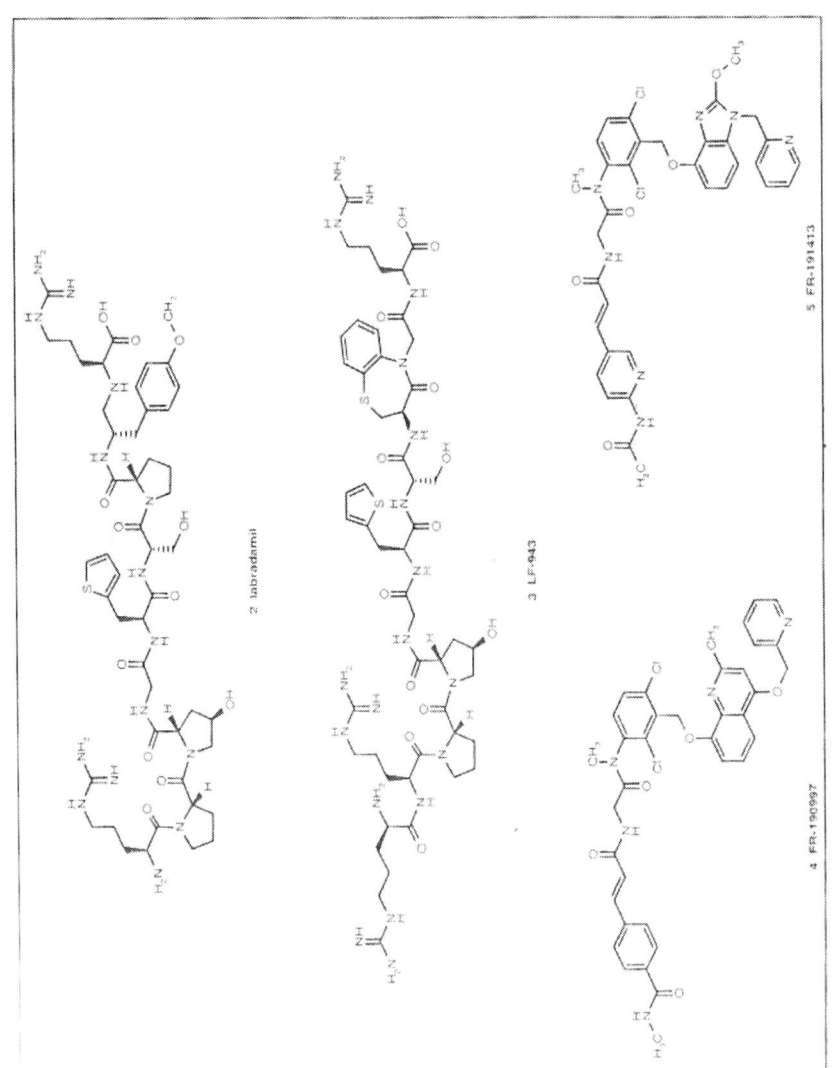

Figure 10.2. The structure of selected bradykinin B_2 receptor agonists.

Kininases (kinin-inactivating enzymes) are present in the plasma, urine, tissue, endothelial cells and body fluids (Sharma JN and Sharma J. 2002; Sharma JN. 2003). Their prime function is to monitor the concentration of BK in the body to enable it to perform the necessary physiological activities (Sharma JN and Sharma J. 2002; Sharma JN. 2003; Heitsch H. 2003; Campbell DJ 2001). Carboxypeptidases or kininases I cleave the C-terminal Arg residue from BK and kallidin to produce their corresponding des-Arg derivatives (Heitsch, 2003). Two metalloproteases, neutral endopeptidase (NEP) and angiotensin-converting enzyme (ACE; also called kininase II) degrade BK and kallidin into inactive fragments .ACE is regarded as the most important kinin degrading enzyme in the cardiovascular system and kidneys (Sharma JN. 2003; Heitsch H. 2003; Campbell DJ 2001) and has a higher affinity for BK than for angiotensin I (Ang I), resulting in more favorable kinetics for BK than for angiotensin degradation (Heitsch H. 2003). Hence, ACE links the KKS with the renin-angiotensin system (RAS). Inhibitors of ACE and NEP increase BK peptide levels In although the effect on kinin peptide levels vary in the blood, urine and tissues. This may account for the differential contribution of ACE and NEP to kinin-peptide metabolism in the multiple compartments in which kinin-peptide generation occurs (Campbell DJ, 2000). The steps involved in kinin formation are outlined in Figure 10.3

Kinin peptides are implicated in many physiological and pathological processes. Several of the major physiological roles of kinins have been described in parallel with their discovery (Campbell DJ 2001). Data suggest that kinins act as mediators of endogenous cardioprotective mechanisms (Sharma JN and Sharma J. 2002; Sharma et al. 1996; Linz et al 1996; Campbell DJ 2001); kinins stimulate smooth muscle, produce hypotension and protect against ischemia, as will be discussed later. However, kinins also participate in the cardinal features of inflammation, producing swelling (edema), redness, heat (vasodilation) and pain (Campbell DJ. 2001). The discovery of this inflammatory role of kinins stimulated a large number of studies of their role in inflammation, tissue damage, antigen-antibody interactions and shock (Campbell DJ. 2001). In addition, BK-like activity was detected in the spinal fluid of individuals with degenerative diseases of the central nervous system, migraine and chronic schizophrenia, and a bronchoconstricting action of intravenous BK has been documented.

There is therefore a need to understand how the generation of kinin peptides is regulated, which will allow exploitation of the beneficial actions of these peptides and avoidance of their adverse effects. At the molecular level, these contributions are mediated through activation of B_1 andor B_2 receptors, and downstream activation of various second messenger systems, such as NO, cGMP, cAMP, arachidonic acid and inositol phosphate (IP3,), which leads to increased intracellular Ca2 levels (Sharma JN and Sharma J. 2002; Heitsch H. 2003).

KININ RECEPTOR CLASSIFICATION

Kinins exert a variety of biological actions by acting through specific receptors that are widespread and belong to two major categories B_1 and B_2 which have been defined pharmacologically using a variety of peptidergic agonists and antagonists (Regoli et al. 2001). More recent pharmacological findings from various studies suggest the existence of new receptor types: B_3, B_4, and B_5; (Regoli et al. 2001). These receptors mediate the contractile and relaxant responses of the opossum esophagus to BK (Regoli et al. 2001). However, B_3,

B_4, and B_5 receptors have not been sufficiently characterized with either agonists or antagonists to be evaluated for their therapeutic potential (Regoli et al. 2001).

B_1 and B_2 bradykinin receptors

B_2 receptors normally predominate, whereas B_1 receptors are induced by tissue injury (Campbell DJ. 2001). Furthermore, and in contrast to B_2 receptors, B_1 receptors occur only in certain species (Sharma JN and Sharma J. 2002; Sharma JN 2003). B_2 receptors have been cloned and belong to the family of seven transmembrane-spanning domain receptors that are coupled via G proteins to a number of biochemical pathways through a system of second messengers (Sharma JN and Sharma J. 2002; Sharma JN 2003; Campbell DJ 2001). The B_1 receptor displays high affinity and is preferentially activated by kinin metabolites lacking the C-terminal Arg residue, ie, des-Arg^9-BK and des-Arg^9-kallidin (Sharma JN and Sharma J. 2002; Sharma JN 2003; Campbell DJ 2001). The B_1 receptor is rarely expressed in certain vascular tissues, but can be expressed in response to inflammation and tissue injury (Sharma JN and Sharma J. 2002; Sharma JN 2003; Heitsch H. 2003). B_1 receptor activation may induce stimulation of smooth muscle, increased cell proliferation and collagen synthesis (Sharma JN and Sharma J. 2002; Sharma JN 2003).

Agata et al evaluated the effect of the KKS on the proliferation and migration of primary cultured vascular smooth muscle cells (VSMCs) in vitro, and neointima formation in balloon-injured rat carotid arteries in vivo (Agata et al. 2000). Data obtained indicate that the B_1 receptor contributes to reduction of neointima formation via the promotion of reendothelialization. B_1 receptors were originally defined in terms of agonist rank order of potencies, with des-Arg^9-BK being the most potent relative to BK. This, along with an appreciable affinity for the antagonist des-Arg^9-[Leu^8]-BK, was taken to demonstrate the presence of B_1 receptors in various cells and tissues (Sharma JN and Sharma J. 2002; Sharma JN 2003).

The majority of the prominent physiological actions of BK appear to be mediated by stimulation of the constitutive B_2 receptor (Sharma JN and Sharma J. 2002; Sharma JN 2003; Heitsch H.2003), which exhibits a higher affinity for BK and kallidin (Sharma JN 2003). BK activates sensory nerve terminals, induces the release of pro-inflammatory and hyperalgesic mediators (eg, neuropeptidase, leukotrienes and cytokines), increases vascular permeability and induces vasodilation via stimulation of B_2 receptors (Heitsch H. 2003). These pharmacological effects are the underlying cause of the strong pro-inflammatory and nociceptive properties of BK (Heitsch H. 2003). B_2 receptors may therefore participate in pathological conditions such as septic shock pancreatitis, edema, asthma, rhinitis, colitis, arthritis and pain (Heitsch H. 2003) and hence there is potential for the development of B_2 receptor antagonists as therapeutic agents.

Kinin acts on B_2 receptors to release NO and prostaglandins (PGI_2, and PGE_2), which are the underlying cause of its vasodilatory, antihypertensive and anti-atherosclerotic action (Sharma JN and Sharma J. 2002; Sharma JN 2003; Heitsch H.2003). Stimulation of B_2 receptors may therefore have potential for the treatment and prevention of cardiovascular diseases such as hypertension, cardiac failure, ischemia, and myocardial hypertrophy (Sharma JN and Sharma J. 2002; Sharma JN 2003; Heitsch H.2003).

Antagonist affinity has been pursued for more than two decades (Sharma JN and Sharma J. 2002; Sharma JN 2003; Heitsch H.2003). Des-Arg9- [Leu^8]-BK was the first synthetic antagonist prepared, which acts at B1 receptors (Sharma JN and Sharma J. 2002; Sharma JN 2003; Regoli et al. 2001; Heitsch H.2002). The second generation of antagonists came with the introduction of icatibant, which shows high affinity in all preparations tested, has no residual agonistic activities and is a highly selective B_2 receptor antagonist (Sharma JN and Sharma J. 2002; Heitsch H.2002). The third category of antagonists, exemplified by FR-167344 (6; Figure 4), FR-173657 (7; Fujisawa Pharmaceutical Co Ltd; Figure 10.4) and a series of bradyzides (Novartis AG), are extremely potent, selective and orally active non-peptide B_2 receptor antagonists (Sharma JN and Sharma J. 2002; Sharma JN 2003; Heitsch H.2002). These BK receptor antagonists will allow rapid progress in analyzing the pathological states that relate to hyperactivity of kinins (Sharma JN and Sharma J. 2002; Sharma JN 2003; Heitsch H.2002). The functions and the antagonists of the BK receptors are outlined in Table10. 1.

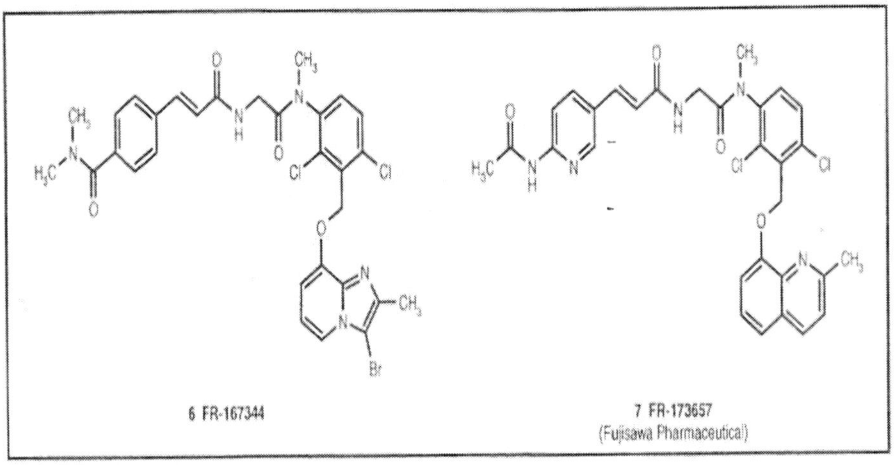

Figure 10.4. The structure of FR-167344 and FR-173657.

Bradykinin B_2 receptor agonists

By stimulating B_2 receptors, kinins exert a wide variety of diverse biological actions (Heitsch H. 2003). In various studies in both humans and animals, stimulation of B_2 receptors has been implicated in cardioprotective mechanisms (Heitsch H. 2003; Heitsch H. 2002). The best characterized peptide B_2 receptor agonists are labradamil and LF-943 (Amblard M. 1999). The key feature of these two potent and selective agonists is their improved resistance to enzymatic degradation by kininases, which makes them valuablepharmacological tools for studying the effects of B_2 receptor stimulation without the accompanying rapid metabolism of BK (Heitsch H. 2003). In vitro, LF-943 exhibited a high affinity toward the human cloned B_2 receptor in a radioligand-binding assay (Amblard M. 1999). Moreover, LF-943 behaved as a full B_2 receptor agonist on human umbilical vein and rat uterus preparations, with the same efficacy as BK (Amblard M. 1999).

Table 10.1. Pharmacological Properties of Bradykinin Receptors

BK receptor	Functions	Antagonist
B_1	Stimulation of vascular smooth muscle, contraction of venous and arterial smooth muscle, and increased collagen synthesis and cell proliferation.	des-Arg^9-[Leu^5]-BK
B_2	Stimulation of rat uterus and guinea pig ileum. Mediation of pain, vasodilation and hypotension. Also induces release of NO, PGI_2 and PGE_2.	Icatibant Novartis bradyzide antagonists FR-167344 FR-173657

BK bradykinin, **NO** nitric oxide, **PG** prostaglandin.

Preliminary clinical trials in oncology indications confirmed that labradamil permeabilized the blood-brain-tumor barrier to increase the delivery of agents such as carboplatin to tumors (Shimuta et al. 1999). Moreover, labradamil enhanced drug delivery to solid peripheral tumors (Shimuta et al. 1999; Emerich DF. 2002). The first potent, selective non-peptide B_2 receptor agonists, FR-190997 and FR-191413, were discovered in 1997 (Heitsch H. 2003; Heitsch H. 2002; Rizzi et al. 1999). The structures of FR-190997 (a 4-(2-pyridyl-methoxy)-quinolone derivative) and FR-191413 (a 3-(2-pyridylmethyl)-benzimidazole derivative) (Heitsch H. 2003; Heitsch H. 2002) are closely related to those of non-peptide B2 antagonists, such as the quinolone FR-173657 and the benzimidazole FR-167344 [12]. The key difference between these B2 receptor antagonists and previously studied agonists is the substitution at position 4 of the quinolone moiety (FR-190997 has a 2-pyridylmethoxy substituent) and the substitution at position 3 of the benzimidazole moiety (FR-191413 has a 2-pyridylmethyl substituent) (Heitsch H. 2003; Heitsch H. 2002).

FR-190997 is a highly potent non-peptide B_2 receptor agonist (Heitsch H. 2003; Heitsch H. 2002) that stimulates IP3 hydrolysis in Chinese hamster ovarian (CHO) cells transfected with the human B_2 receptor, and increases PGE_2 production in human fibroblasts (Heitsch H. 2003; Heitsch H. 2002). However, detailed in vitro evaluation on human, rabbit and pig vascular B_2 receptors have revealed that this agonist shows different intrinsic activity depending on the tissue preparation (Rizzi et al. 1999). FR-190997 acts as a partial agonist in the human umbilical vein and the rabbit jugular vein, but as a pure antagonist in the pig coronary artery (Rizzi et al. 1999). This study suggested that the addition of a 2-pyriclylmethoxy group to the basic structure of the antagonist FR-173657 may not be sufficient to change the pharmacological spectrum of a pure antagonist to that of a full agonist (Rizzi et al. 1999). In a second study, FR-190997 induced a hypotensive response in anesthetized spontaneously hypertensive rats after continuous infusion into the abdominal aorta (Ueno et al. 1999). Furthermore, FR-190997 induced natriuresis and diuresis without any influence on urinary potassium excretion in anesthetized rabbits (Majima et al. 2000).

FR-191413 belongs to a promising second series of non-peptide B, receptor agonists, although the pharmacological properties of FR-191413 have been less intensively evaluated than those of FR-190997 (Heitsch H. 2003). The potency of FR-191413 was similar to that of FR-190997 on membranes of CHO cells transfected with human B_2 receptor (Heitsch H. 2002).

FR-191413, FR-190997 and other potent non-peptide B_2 agonists have been discovered, but the oral efficacy of these agonists is limited due to inadequate pharmacokinetic properties, and this excludes their development as potential therapeutic agents for the treatment of all cardiovascular conditions (Heitsch H. 2003).

THE KININ SYSTEM IN CARDIOVASCULAR DISORDERS

Hypertension

Hypertension is a major risk factor for the development of cardiovascular diseases, for example, coronary heart disease, congestive heart failure, and peripheral vascular and renal diseases (Sharma JN and Sharma J. 2002; Sharma et al. 1996; Sharma JN 2003;). Deficiency of the KKS may participate in the genesis of hypertension (Sharma et al. 1996). Kinins have potent diuretic and natriuretic effects that regulate sodium excretion from the kidney (Heitsch H. 2003). Moreover, kinins have a vasodilatory action on peripheral blood vessels (Sharma JN and Sharma J. 2002; Sharma et al. 1996; Sharma JN 2003; Heitsch H. 2003). The involvement of kinins in blood pressure regulation has been confirmed in transgenic mice that overexpress the human B_2 receptor (Wang et al. 2000), which develop sustained lifetime hypotension. Administration of aprotinin, a tissue kallikrein inhibitor, or icatibant to the transgenic mice restored their blood pressure to normal levels (Wang et al. 2000). The suppression of the hypotensive response of ACE inhibitors by aprotinin in spontaneously hypertensive rats has been documented Sharma et al. 1995).

Studies of systemic changes in the KKS has provided further insight regarding various hypertensive conditions (Sharma JN and Sharma J. 2002; Sharma JN 2003). In essential and malignant hypertension, kininogen levels and kinin-potentiating factor are reduced (Sharma JN and Sharma J. 2002; Sharma et al. 1996; Sharma JN 2003). In individuals who develop hypertension after mild exercise, the deficiency in plasma HMWK may be due to decreases in liver synthesis (Sharma JN and Sharma J. 2002; Sharma et al. 1996). In addition, deficient kallikreinkininogens-kinin formation may be a significant factor in the pathophysiology of hypertension. The renal KKS may cause excretion of excessive sodium in the urine (Sharma JN and Sharma J. 2002; Sharma et al. 1996; Sharma JN 2003; Heitsch H. 2003). Studies of the role of the renal KKS, using congenitally kininogen-deficient Brown-Norway Katholiek rats and B_2 receptor knockout mice, revealed that this system induces natriuresis and diuresis in the presence of high concentrations of sodium ions, which may be caused by excess sodium intake or excessive aldosterone release (Katori M. and Majima M. 2003). Thus, it can be hypothesized that the renal KKS functions as a safety valve for sodium accumulation (Katori M. and Majima M. 2003). A compound that has renal kallikrein-like activity may help the body to excrete excess amounts of sodium (Sharma JN and Sharma J. 2002; Sharma JN. 2003).

Tissue kallikrein gene delivery into various hypertensive models has been reported to be protective, for example, reducing high blood pressure, attenuating cardiac hypertrophy, inhibiting renal damage and fibrosis, and enhancing capillary growth in spontaneously hypertensive rats (Bledsoe et al. 2003). These findings indicate the potential of kallikrein gene therapy for cardiovascular and renal pathology (Sharma JN and Sharma J. 2002; Sharma JN. 2003).

ACE inhibitors such as captopril and enalapril are currently used in the treatment of hypertension (Sharma JN and Sharma J. 2002; Sharma et al. 1996; Sharma JN. 2003), as they lower blood pressure by blocking the conversion of Ang I to Ang II, and increase levels of BK (Sharma et al. 1996). In patients with essential hypertension, abnormality in the urinary kallikrein excretion has been corrected with administration of nifedipine, a calcium channel blocker (Sharma JN and Sharma J. 2002; Sharma et al 1996). The BK-induced blood pressure lowering effect is mediated by the B_2 receptor, but the B_1 receptor may also be involved under certain circumstances (Sharma JN and Sharma J. 2002). The B_2 receptor antagonist FR-173657 significantly attenuated the hypotensive action of captopril (Sharma et al. 1996). Hence, it would be reasonable to suggest that the hypotensive response of ACE inhibitors is mainly mediated via B_2 receptor activation (Sharma JN and Sharma J. 2002; Sharma et al. 1996). The accumulation of BK after administration of ACE inhibitors, with subsequent release of the endothelium-derived relaxants NO, PGE_2 and PGI_2, could also be involved in the antihypertensive effects of captopril-like drugs (Sharma JN and Sharma J. 2002; Sharma et al. 1996; Sharma JN. 2003). However, BK antagonists can abolish the efficacy of antihypertensive drugs, and therefore these drugs are contraindicated in patients with hypertension (Sharma JN and Sharma J. 2002; Sharma JN. 2003).

CARDIAC FAILURE AND ISCHEMIA

Cardiac failure and ischemia are the leading causes of death in both developing and developed countries (Sharma JN and Sharma J. 2002; Emanueli C. and Madeddu P. 2001, Sharma JN. 2003). They are characterized by narrowed or blocked arteries, which impair the supply of blood and starve tissues of necessary nutrients and oxygen (Emanueli C. and Madeddu P. 2001). Kinins increase coronary perfusion, and reduce preload, afterload and oxidative stress via stimulation of the release of NO and PGs, mainly from the coronary cardiac endothelium, which protects the heart from acute ischemic damage (Sharma JN and Sharma J. 2002; Sharma JN 2003; Heitsch H. 2003). However, the potentially beneficial effects of kinins in the heart were neglected for a long time (Sharma JN and Sharma J. 2002; Emanueli C. and Madeddu P. 2001; Sharma JN 2003). ACE not only acts as a kinin-degrading enzyme, but also contributes to Ang II generation (Emanueli C. and Madeddu P. 2001). Preventing the formation of Ang II could limit ventricular dilation, delay the progression of clinical symptoms and improve mortality rate (Sharma JN and Sharma J. 2002; Sharma JN 2003). The ability of ACE inhibitors to prevent kinin-degradation represents a relevant mechanism contributing to cardioprotection (Sharma JN and Sharma J. 2002; Emanueli C. and Madeddu P. 2001; Sharma JN 2003). This concept has initiated many studies, which have provided evidence demonstrating the presence of a local KKS in the heart ((Sharma JN and Sharma J. 2002; Emanueli C. and Madeddu P. 2001).

Kinins released from the vascular endothelium activate B1, and B2 receptors on endothelial cells and VSMCs (Emanueli C. and Madeddu P. 2001; Sharma JN 2003) and, as already mentioned, studies have revealed that kinins are released under conditions of ischemia and myocardial infarction (Linz et al. 1996). Binding to B1 and B2 receptors conjointly promotes the formation of PGs and NO, which increase intracellular concentrations of cAMP and cGMP (Emanueli C. and Madeddu P. 2001), thus exerting vasodilator, anti-ischemic and antiproliferative effects, and preserving myocardial stores of energy-rich phosphate and glycogen (Emanueli C. and Madeddu P. 2001; Sharma JN 2003). Circumstantial evidence also suggests that a dysfunctional KKS may contribute to the pathogenesis of heart failure (Sharma JN and Sharma J. 2002; Emanueli C. and Madeddu P. 2001; Sharma JN 2003). Indeed, reduced kinin outflow from the heart and blunted NO formation have been reported in microvessels of the failing human heart (Sharma JN and Sharma J. 2002; Sharma JN 2003). Icatibant has been used as a tool to evaluate the role of kinins in cardiac ischemia. In isolated rat hearts, perfusion with icatibant reversed the beneficial cardioprotective effects of BK and facilitated the development of cardiac failure (Ito et al. 2003). Kinins act as a cardioprotective agent in perfusion and participate in the process of ischemic preconditioning. BK infused into the coronary artery of anesthetized dogs significantly reduced the severity of ischemia-induced arrhythmia (Linz et al. 1996; Sharma JN 2003).

Increased plasma levels of kallikrein, kininogen and BK were found following myocardial infarction, and the increase in plasma kallikrein levels was positively correlated with the early survival rate for post-myocardial infarction patients (Tschope et al. 2000; Tschope 2000). Kinins are released directly from the myocardium during myocardial infarction and contribute to the impact of ischemic damage (Tschope et al. 2000; Tschope et al. 2000). Moreover, the influence of the B_2 receptor on infarct size in rats with permanently ligated coronary arteries has been confirmed using a non-peptide B_2 receptor antagonist and agonist, respectively. In this model, the infarct size was reduced by a continuous infusion of FR-190997, whereas it was increased upon oral administration of FR-173657 (Ito et al. 2003). The effect of locally administered BK on the limitation of infarct size has been investigated in anesthetized dogs in which the left descending coronary artery was ligated for 6 h. One group of dogs received saline into the main stern of the left coronary artery, while the second group received a sub-hypotensive dose of BK (1 ng/kg/min). The intracoronary route and the low dose of BK were chosen to obtain a local cardiac effect with little or no effect on systemic hemodynamics. Within 6 h of coronary occlusion, infusion of BK had no significant effect on systemic bloodpressure; however, BK limited infarct size, providing evidence for the involvement of kinins in ischemic events (Linz et al. 1996). Kinins may therefore act as mediators of endogenous cardioprotective agents.

The cardioprotective profiles of kinins resemble those of ACE inhibitors. However, more investigations of the molecular biology and gene mapping of KKS in the heart during health and cardiovascular disorders are required, which may provide answers to the many questions regarding the role of KKS in cardiovascular pathophysiology (Sharma JN and Sharma J. 2002; Sharma JN 2003).

MYOCARDIAL HYPERTROPHY

LVH is an independent predictor for increased morbidity and mortality from cardiac diseases Sharma JN and Sharma J. 2002; Sharma JN 2003; Heitsch H. 2003). The antihypertrophic efficacy of BK is due to B2 receptor-mediated release of the endothelial cardioprotectants NO and the PGs (Sharma JN 2003; Heitsch H. 2003). However, B2 receptor antagonists and NO synthetase inhibitors can counteract this effect (Sharma JN and Sharma J. 2002; Sharma JN 2003). Indeed, the lack of cardiac kinin-forming components in the development of LVH has been documented in hypertensive and diabetic rats (Sharma et al. 1998). Reduced cardiac tissue kallikrein and cardiac kininogen may therefore be responsible for reduced BK generation in the heart that can lead to LVH (Sharma JN and Sharma J. 2002; Sharma JN 2003). In a more recent study, the importance of elevation of cardiomyocyte cGMP as an antihypertrophic mechanism caused by BK was demonstrated in adult rat isolated cardiomyocytes, and BK was demonstrated to exert a direct inhibitory action against the acute hypertrophic response to Ang II in Langendorff-perfused rat hearts (Rosenkranz et al. 2002). In a further study in hypertensive rats, blood pressure reduction and regression of LVH with captopril treatment was considered to be potentially caused by enhanced renal tissue kallikrein activity (Sharma JN and Kesavarao U. 2002). This may further support the view that tissue kallikrein can act as a cardioprotective agent (Sharma JN and Sharma J. 2002; Sharma JN 2003).

The most conclusive evidence to date that B_2 receptor agonists may have potential for the treatment of cardiovascular disorders comes from a study by Ebrahim et al, which suggests that B_2 receptor activation limits the infarct size and lowers the threshold for myocardial preconditioning of ACE inhibitor treatment in the isolated rat heart. In addition, BK is able to induce mitochondrial reactive oxygen, cGMP, protein kinase G and mitochondrial ATP-sensitive K channel opening, which is cardioprotective in rabbit cardiornyocytes (Oldenburg et al. 2004).

Interestingly, BK inhibits development of myocardial infarction through B_2 receptor signaling by an increment of regional blood flow around the ischemic lesion in rats (Ito et al. 2003). Furthermore, administration of BK during reperfusion reduces infarction in rabbit hearts through PI3K, extracellular-regulated kinase and NO (Yang et al. 2004). The mechanical load caused by pressure overload may downregulate B2 receptor expression during the initial stage of LVH (Yayama et al. 2003).

These findings highlight the significance of BK in the protection of the heart in various disorders. The discovery of the first non-peptide full agonist for the human B_2 receptor (Figure10.5), currently being investigated by Fujisawa Pharmaceutical Co Ltd (Sawada et al. 2004), may provide greater prospects for the application of B_2 agonists in cardiology treatment.

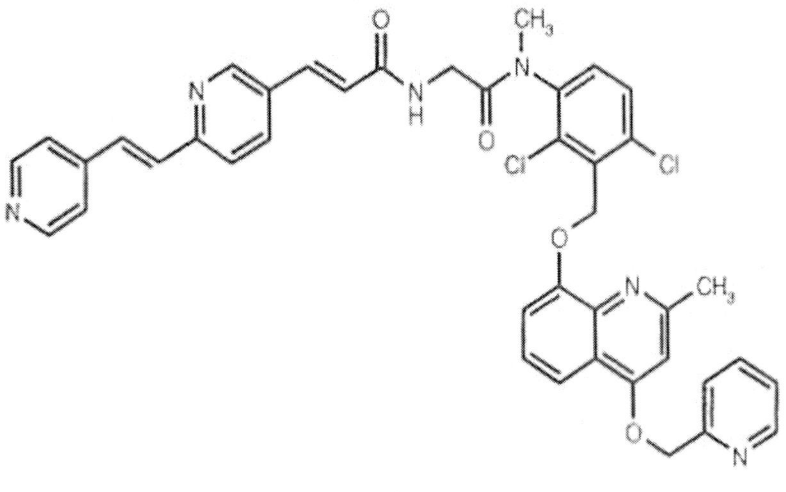

Figure 10.5. The structure of a non-peptide B2 receptor full agonist.

UNDESIRABLE SIDE EFFECTS OF KININ AGONISTS

Zxxir

Kinin agonists displayed pronounced and long-lasting pro-inflammatory properties in vivo (Heitsch H. 2003, Heitsch H. 2002), kinin vascular permeability increased upon intradermal injection into the dorsal skin of rats in a dose-dependent and sustained manner; paw swelling was markedly induced upon subcutaneous injection into the hind paws of mice; the frequency of writhing reactions was enhanced in mice upon intraperitoneal injection; and angiogenesis and granulation increased upon topical application in mice sponge implants (Ueno et al. 1999). B_2 receptor-mediated activation of cyclooxygenase (COX)-1 or COX-2 and synergism with PGI_2 are suggested as underlying mechanisms of these adverse events (Heitsch H. 2003). Interestingly, FR-190997 proved to be a significantly less active bronchoconstrictor than BK (Ueno et al. 1999).

These observations indicate that pain induction or edemaformations are probably peripheral side effects of stable kinin receptor agonists (Heitsch H. 2003, Heitsch H. 2002). Further studies are therefore required to demonstrate that there is a sufficient therapeutic window between the pathophysiological and beneficial kinin receptor-mediated effects. This therapeutic window would have to allow the treatment of inflammatory disorders and chronic pain with B_2 receptor antagonists without diminution of the beneficial systemic and cardiovascular effects of endogenous kinins. On the other hand, the treatment of cardiovascular and metabolic diseases with B_2 receptor agonists would have to occur without concomitant pro-inflammatory side effects, especially upon chronic administration (Heitsch H. 2003, Heitsch H. 2002).

REFERENCES

- Bradykinin B_2 receptors are involved in cardio protection, as demonstrated by the use of B_2 receptor antagonists and agonists.
- Kallikrein-kinin abnormality could contribute to the genesis of hypertension.
- Reduced cardiac bradykinin generation might lead to cardiac hypertrophy.
- Captopril may lower blood pressure via kallikrein activation.
- Decreased kallikrein-kinin formation in the heart may result in the production of left ventriculer hypertrophy in hypertensive and diabetic rats.
- Kallikrein gene delivery reduces cardiac hypertrophy.

Agata J, Miao R, Yayama K, et al: Bradykinin B_1 receptor mediates inhibition of neointima formation in rat artery after balloon angioplasty. Hypertension 2000; 36(3): 364-370.

Amblard M, Daffix I, Bedos P, et al: Design and synthesis of potent bradykinin agonists containing a benzothiazepine moiety. J Med Chem 1999; 42(20): 4185-4192.

Bledsoe G, Chao L, Chao J: Kallikrein gene delivery attenuates cardiac remodeling and promotes neovascularization in spontaneously hypertensive rats. Am J Physiol Heart Circ Physiol 2003; 285(4): H1479-H1488.

Campbell DJ: The kallikrein-kinin system in humans. Clin Exp Pharmacol Physiol 2001; 28 (12): 1060-1065.

Campbell DJ: Towards understanding the kallikrein-kinin system:

Ebrahim Z, Baxter GE, Yellon DM: Omapatrilat limits infarct size and lowers the threshold for induction of myocardial preconditioning through a bradykinin receptor-mediated mechanism. Cardiovasc Drugs Ther 2004; 18(2): 127-134.

Emanueli C, Madeddu P: Targeting kinin receptors for the treatment of tissue ischaemia. Trends Pharmacol Sci 2001; 22 (9): 478-484.

Emerich DF: Use of bradykinin agonist, Cereport, as a pharmacological means of increasing drug delivery to the brain.Curr Med Chem Immunol Endocrine Metabol Agents 2002; 2(2): 109123.

-Evidence suggests that bradykinin B_2 receptor agonists might be useful therapeutic agents in treating cardiac diseases.

Heitsch H: Non-peptide antagonists and agonists of the bradykinin B_2 receptor. Curr Med Chem 2002; 9(9): 913-928.

Heitsch H: The therapeutic potential of bradykinin B_2 receptor agonists in the treatment of cardiovascular disease. Expert Opin Investig Drugs 2003; 12 (5): 759-770.

Insights from measurement of kinin peptides. Braz J Med Bioi Res 2000; 33(6): 665-677.

Ito H, Hayashi I, Izumi T, et al: Bradykinin inhibits development of myocardial infarction through B_2 receptor signaling by increment of regional blood flow around the ischemic lesions in rats. Br J Pharmacol 2003; 138(1): 225-233.

Ito H, Hayashi I, Izumi T, et al: Bradykinin inhibits development of myocardial infarction through B_2 receptor signaling by increment of regional blood flow around the ischaemic lesions in rats. Br J Pharmacol 2003; 138(1): 225-233.

Katori M, Majima M: The renal kallikrein-kinin system: Its role as a safety valve for excess sodium intake, and its attenuation as a possible etiologic factor in salt-sensitive hypertension. Crit Rev Clin Lab Sci 2003; 40(1): 43-115.

Linz W, Wiemer G, Scholkens BA: Role of kinins in the pathophysiology of myocardial ischemia. In vitro and In vivo studies. Diabetes 1996; 45(1): 551-558.

Majima M, Hayashi I, Inamura N, et al: A non peptide mimic of bradykinin blunts the development of hypertension in young spontaneously hypertensive rats. Hypertension 2000; 35(1 pt 2): 437-442.

Oldenburg O, Qin Q, Krieg T, et al.: Bradykinin induces mitochondrial ROS generation via NO, cGMP, PKG, and mitoKATP channel opening and leads to cardioprotection. Am J Physiol Heart Circ Physiol 2004; 286(1): H468-H476.

Regoli D, Rizzi A, Perron 5, et al: Classification of kinin receptors. Biol Chem 2001; 382(1): 31-35.

Rizzi A, Rizzi C, Amadesi 5, et al: Pharmacological characterization of the first non-pepetide bradykinin B_2 receptor agonist FR-190997: An In vitro study on human, rabbit and pig vascular B_2 receptors. Naunyn Schmiedebergs Arch Pharmacol 1999; 360(4): 361-367.

Rosenkranz AG, Hood SG, Woods RL, et al: Acute anti hypertrophic actions of bradykinin in the rat heart: Importance of cyclic GMP. Hypertension 2002; 40(4): 498-503.

Sawada Y, Kayakiri H, Abe Y, et al: Discovery of the first non-peptide full agonists for human bradykinin B_2 receptor incorporating 4-(2picolyloxy) quinolin and 1-(2-picolyl) benzimidazole frameworks. J Med Chem 2004; 47(11): 2853-2863.

Sharma IN, Amrah SS, Noor AR: Suppression of hypotensive responses of captopril and enalapril by kallikrein inhibitor aprotinin in spontaneously hypertensive rats. Pharmacology 1995; 50(6): 363-369.

Sharma IN, Kesavarao U: Effect of captopril on urinary kallikrein, blood pressure and myocardial hypertrophy in diabetic spontaneously hypertensive rats. Pharmacology 2002; 64(4): 196-200.

Sharma IN, Sharma J: Cardiovascular properties of the kallikreinkinin system. Curr Med Res Opin 2002; 18 (1): 10-17.

Sharma IN: Does the kinin system mediate in cardiovascular abnormalities? An overview. J Ciin Pharmacol 2003; 43 (11): 1187-1195.

Sharma JN, Uma K, Noor AR, et al: Blood pressure regulation by the kallikrein-kinin system. Gen Pharmacol 1996; 27 (1): 55-63.

Sharma JN, Uma K, Yusof A: Left ventricular hypertrophy and its relation to the cardiac kinin-forming system in hypertensive and diabetic rats. Int J Cardiol 1998; 63(3): 229-235.

Shimuta 5, Barbosa A, Borges A, et al: Pharmacological characterization of RMP-7, a novel bradykinin agonist in smooth muscle. Immunopharmacology 1999; 45(1-3): 63-67.

-Synthesis of novel bradykinin receptor agonlsts, Including LF-943.

Tschope C, Heringer-Walther S, et al: Regulation of the kinin receptors after induction of myocardial infarction: A mini-review.Braz J Med Bioi Res 2000; 33(6): 701-708.

Tschope C, Heringer-Walther S, Koch M, et al: Myocardial bradykinin B_2-receptor expression at different time points after induction of myocardial infarction. J Hypertens 2000; 18(2): 223-228.

Ueno A, Naraba H, Kojima F, et al: FR-190997, a novel bradykinin B_2 agonist, expresses longer action than bradykinin in paw edema formation and hypotensive response.Immunopharmacology 1999; 45(1-3): 89-93.

Wang D, Yoshida H, Song Q, et al: Enhanced renal function in bradykinin B_2 receptor transgenic mice. Am J Physiol Renal Physiol 2000; 278(3): F484-F491.

Yang XM, Krieg T, Cui L, et al: NECA and bradykinin at reperfusion reduce infarction in rabbit hearts by signaling through PI3K, ERK and NO. J Mol Cell Cardiol 2004; 36(3): 411-421.

Yayama K, Matsuoka S, Nagaoka M, et al: Down-regulation of bradykinin B_2-receptor mRNA in the heart in pressure-overloaded cardiac hypertrophy in the rat. Blochem Pharmacal 2003; 65(6): 1017-1025.

Yayama K, Nagaoka M, Takano M, et al: Expression of kininogen, kallikrein and kinin receptor genes by rat cardiomyocytes. Biochim Biophys Acta 2000; 1495(1): 69-77.

Chapter 11

Therapeutic Prospects Of Bradykinin Receptor Antagonists

Abstract

1. Bradykinin and related kinins may act on four types of receptors designated as B_1, B_2, B_3, and B_4. It seems that the B_2 receptors are most commonly found in various vascular and non-vascular smooth muscles, whereas B_1 receptors are formed in vitro during trauma, and injury, and are found in bone tissues.
2. These BK receptors are involved in the regulation of various physiological and pathological processes.
3. The mode of kinin actions are based upon the interactions between the kinin and their specific receptors, which can lead to activation of several second-messenger systems.
4. Recently, numerous BK receptor antagonists have been synthesized with prime aim to treat diseases caused by excessive kinin production.
5. These diseases are RA, inflammatory diseases of the bowel, asthma, rhinitis and sore throat, allergic reactions, pain, inflammatory skin disorders, endotoxic and anaphylactic shock and coronary heart diseases.
6. On the other hand, BK receptor antagonists could be contraindicated in hypertension, since these drugs may antagonize the antihypertensive therapy and/or may trigger the hypertensive crisis.
7. It is worth suggesting that the BK receptor agonists might be useful antihypertensive drugs.

Introduction

Bradykinin (BK), a nonapeptide (Arg-Pro-Pro-GlyPhe-Ser-Pro-Phe-Arg), which belongs to a family of kinins that also includes kallidin or lysyl-BK (Lys-Arg-Pro-Pro-Gly-Phe-Ser-Pro-Phe-Arg) and methionyl-lysyl-BK (Met-Lys-Arg-Pro-Pro-GlyPhe-Set-Pro-Pbe-Arg). These kinins are released from plasma precursors (kininogens) by the action of plasma and tissue kallikreins to regulate the essential physiological functions (Sharma, 1988a, 1990,

1991a). Figure 11.1 shows the complex mode of kinin forming, activating and inhibitory factors. BK is normally present in very low concentrations (<50 pg/ml) in the body fluids (Shimamoto et al.., 1982) mainly due to its rapid destruction either by removal of Arg via the action of kininase-I (carboxypeptidase N) or by removal of Phe-Arg through the action of kininase-II (angiotensin converting enzyme) from its C-terminal (Erdos, 1990).

Abnormally raised BK release in response to noxious agents, tissue injury and/or lack of circulating kininases can induce several pathological conditions ranging from rheumatoid arthritis (RA) to asthma (Sharma, 1991a, b, 1992; Abe et al., 1967). In contrast, reduced BK-forming activities have been implicated in the genesis of hypertension (Sharma, 1984, 1988a, 1990; Sharma et al., 1992). Recently, important advances have been achieved by Vavrek and Stewart (1985) in developing a novel sequence of competitive BK antagonist. At present numerous BK antagonists are being synthesized to improve the potency. These BK antagonists are intended to block the biological function of BK receptors in diseases caused by excessive BK release. The intention of this article is not to exhaustively review this area of research, but to impress upon the reader that understanding of the role of BK-forming components with respect to disease aetiology and potential for the BK receptor antagonists as new and more versatile therapeutic agents.

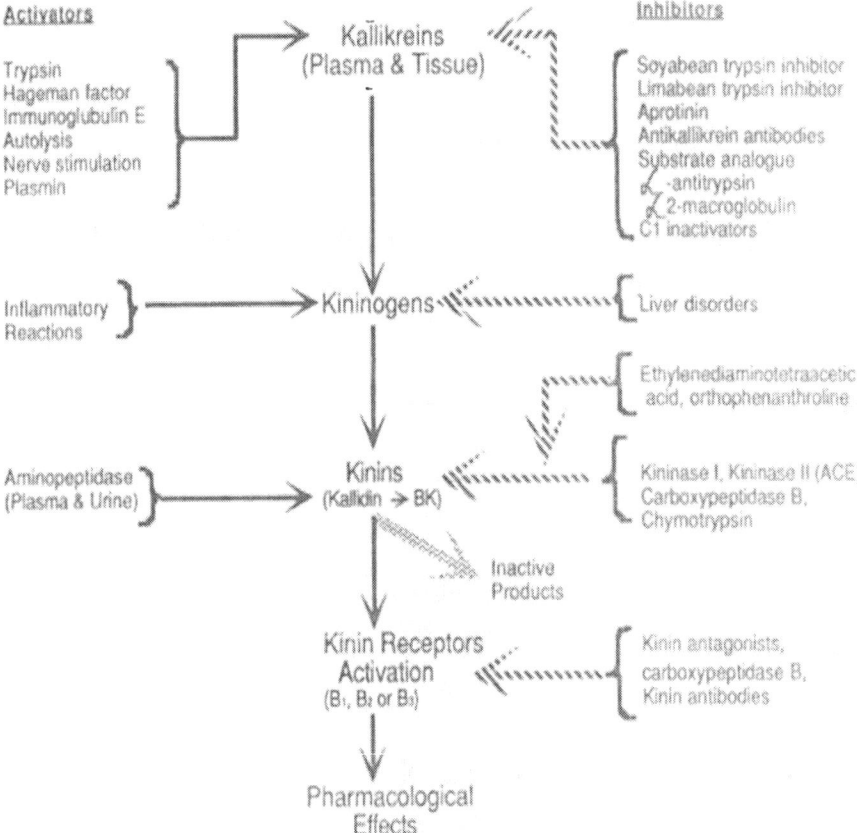

Figure 11.1. The Mode of kinin formation.

BRADYKININ RECEPTORS

The BK receptors have been classified as B_1 and B_2 on the basis of the relative potencies of agonists (kinins) and antagonists (kinin analogues) on various pharmacological preparations (Regoli and Barabe, 1980; Vavrek and Stewart, 1985). B_1 receptors are generated de novo during incubation and antigen-induced arthritis in the vascular smooth muscle (Bouthillier et al., 1987; Farmer et al., 1991a). However it is known that B_1 receptor induction develops in non-vascular tissues and de novo formation of B_1 receptors may result from tissue injury and from inflammatory reactions (Marceau et al., 1980; Couture et al., 1982). Kinin metabolites without the C-terminal arginine residue, such as des-Arg^9-BK and des-Arg^{10}-kallidin are generated during the action of plasma kininase I (Erdos et al., 1965; Proud et al., 1987). Under physiological conditions, these kinin metabolites are devoid of biological actions. However, des-Arg^9-BK and des-Arg^{10}-kallidin show significant biological activities (des-Arg10 kallidin > des-Arg9-BK > kallidin > BK) via activating B_1 receptor in various vascular and non-vascular smooth muscles (Marceau et al., 1980; Regoli et al., 1981). The pharmacological classification of the B_1 receptor was further strengthened by the substitution of Phe^8 with leucine (des-Arg^9-[Leu^8]-BK) gives rise to a potent B_1 antagonist (Regoli and Barabe, 1980). B_1 receptor activation may produce stimulation of smooth muscle cells, increased cell proliferation and high collagen synthesis (Regoli, 1984). Stimulation of B_1 receptor causes release of endothelium-derived relaxing factor (EDRF) and prostacyclin (PGI$_2$) from bovine aortic endothelial cells grown in culture (D'Orleans-Juste et al., 1989). Kinins stimulate tumor necrosis factor (TNF) and interleukin (IL-1) formation from macrophages via B_1 receptors (Tiffany and Burch, 1989). In addition, B_1 receptor agonist (des-Arg^9-BK) induces release of 45Ca, PGE$_2$, and PGI$_2$ and subsequent bone resorption from neonatal mouse calvarial bones (Ljunggren and Lerner, 1990). Hence, B_1 receptors could mediate the inflammation-induced bone resorption in areas of chronic inflammatory processes seen in rheumatoid arthritis (RA), periodontitis and osteomyelitis.

Numerous studies have shown that the predominant pathological responses, such as pain (Whalley et al, 1987a), inflammation (Burch and De Haas, 1990), bronchoconstriction (fin a al., 1989) and hypotension (Sharma et al, 1992) caused by BK involves B_2 receptor participation, however, it is becoming increasingly clear that B_2 receptor subtypes do exist (Llona et al., 1987; Plevin and Owen, 1988; Farmer et al., 1989). The B_2 receptor is thought to mediate contraction of the rat uterus, cat, guinea-pig ileum (Barabe et al., 1977; Farmer et al., 1991b) and guinea-pig tracheal strips (Farmer et al., 1991b). Subsequently, it has been demonstrated that B_2 receptors can cause increased vascular permeability after application of kinins in rabbit skin (Schachter et al., 1987; Whalley et al., 1987b). Kinins act on B_2 receptors to release conjointly EDRF and PGI$_2$, from bovine aortic endothelial cells in vitro (D'Orleans-Juste et al., 1989). B_2 receptors exhibit much higher affinity for kallidin or BK than for des-Arg^{10}–kallidin or des-Arg^9-BK ([Tyr(Me)8-BK = kallidin > BK > des-Arg^{10}kallidin > des-Arg^9-BK) in rabbit jugular vein preparation (Regoli et al., 1989).

Table 11.1. Pharmacological Properties of Bradykinin Receptors

Bradykinin Receptors	Functions	Antagonists
B_1 (formed by de novo synthesis in isolated aortic vascular smooth muscle and by pathological states in vivo)	Stimulation of smooth muscle, increased cell proliferation, increased collagen synthesis, contraction of venous and arterial preparation hi vitro and relaxation of peripheral resistance vessels in vivo, EDRF and PGI, release from aortic endothelial cells	Des-Arg^9-[Leu^8]-BK
B_2	Stimulation of rat uterus, cat and guinea-pig ileum mediation of pain and vasodilation, increased vascular permeability, hypot-ension, release of histamine and PGs. Relaxation of arteries and contraction of vein, bronchoconstriction, EDRF and PGI, release from aortic endothelial cells	D-Arg^8-[Hyp^3-$Thi^{5,8}$, D-Phe^7]-BK [$Thi^{5,8}$, D-Phe^7]-BK D-Arg; [Hyp^3, Thi^5-D-Tic, Oic^8]-BK
B_3	Contraction of airways, opossum oesophageal longitudinal with rapid desensitization (action involves PGs)	D-Arg[Hyp^3-Thi^5-D-Tic^7-Tic^8-]-BK
B_4	Contraction of opossum oesophageal longitudinal muscle with no tachphylaxis (action does not involve PGs)	

Recent findings by Farmer et al. (1989) suggest that pulmonary tissues, particularly in the large airways, contain a novel B_3 receptor, which might be involved in BK-induced bronchoconstriction. These investigators noted that several B2 antagonists (D-Arg[Hyp^3, D-Phe^7-BK and D-Arg[Hyp^3, $Thi^{5,8}$ D-Phe^7-BK) as well as B_1 antagonist (desArg^9[Leu^8-BK) did not inhibit BK-induced guinea-pig tracheal contraction. The presence of B_3 receptor has been proposed in the opossum oesophageal longitudinal smooth muscle (Saha et al., 1990). This receptor has been characterized by rapid desensitization, causes contraction of longitudinal smooth muscle via PG release, and is activated by Phes-D-Phe^7-BK and D-Phe^7–Hyp8-BK (B_2 receptor antagonists). Saha et al. (1990) have suggested also the presence of B_4 receptors in the opossum oesophageal longitudinal smooth muscle. The B_4 receptor shows no tachyphylaxis; its action does not involve PGs, and it is activated by B_2 receptor antagonists, [$Thi^{5,8}$-D-Phe^7]-BK and B6572. The pharmacological properties of BK receptors and their possible biological functions are presented in Table 11.1.

MODE OF KININ ACTION

Interaction between the kinins and their specific receptors can lead to activation of several second-messenger systems. The BK receptor stimulation in intact cells or tissues appeared to initiate the second-messenger systems, such as biologically active arachidonic acid products and activation of calcium-sensitive system (Burch, 1990; Freay et al., 1989). Elevation of cellular inositol phosphates by BK involves G-protein coupled activation of phospholipase A_1 and C that are used in the synthesis of eicosanoid (Burch and Axelrod, 1987; Burch, 1989). Indomethacin, a cyclooxygenase inhibitor, caused potentiation of the BK-induced contraction of the isolated oestrous rat uterus preparations (Sharma and Zeitlin, 1977). The finding may suggest that there could be non-eicosanoid pathways for the cellular and molecular pharmacological actions of kinins. Furthermore, inositol phosphates and BK cause calcium release from intracellular stores in cultured bovine endothelial cells (Freay et at, 1989). In this regard, it has been demonstrated that BK significantly stimulates phosphoinositide hydrolysis in guinea-pig ileum longitudinal muscle that may result in the elevation of cytosolic calcium ion levels to induce contractile actions (Ransom et at, 1992).

Schini et al. (1990) have indicated that the B_2 receptor stimulation causes production of cyclic GMP, but not of cyclic AMP, in cultured porcine aortic endothelial cells. The production of cyclic GMP may be an important step for the biological responses as well as release of EDRF evoked by BK in endothelial cells.

BRADYKININ RECEPTOR ANTAGONISTS AND THEIR THERAPEUTIC PROPSECTS

Since the amino acid sequence of BK was determined in 1960, a number of BK analogues have been synthesized in an effort to define structure-activity relationships and in the search for competitive receptor antagonists. Vavrek and Stewart (1985) made a significant advancement in synthesizing the first sequence of analogue as competitive BK receptor antagonist. In recent years, many additional antagonist sequences have been synthesized in an attempt to improve potency (see Table11.2). These antagonists have been evaluated on several pharmacological experiments involving both in vitro and in vivo investigations.

Table 11.2. Structure-activity Relationships of Some Important Bradykinin Receptor Antagonists

Structure	Receptors	References
D-Arg-Mrp^3, Thi^5, D-Tic^7, Oic^8]-BK	B_2	Hock et al. (1991)
D-Arg-Hyp^2, Thi^{5,8},-D-Phe^7]-BK	B_2	Vavrek and Stewart (1985)
Des-Arg^9-[Leu^8]-BK	B_1	Regoli and Barabe (1980)
D-Arg-[Hyp^3-D-Phe^7]-BK	B_2	Steranka et al. (1985)
D-Artg[Hyp^3-Thi^5-D-Tic^{7}Tic^8]-BK		Farmer et al. (1991) Repoli et al. (1991)
D-Arg[Hyp^3-D-Phe^7-Leu^8]-BK		Regoli et al. (1991)
D-Arg[Hyp^3-Gly^6-D-Phe^7-Leu^8-BK		Stewart and Vavrek (1987)
[Hyp^3-Thi^{5,8}-D-Phe^7-BK		Stewart and Vavrek (1987)
Lys-Lys[Hyp^{2,3}-Thi^{5,8}-D-Phe^7]-BK		Lammek et al. (1990)
[D-Arg-Arg-Pro-Hyp-Gly-Thi-Ser-DPhe-Thi-Arg.TFA		Sharma et al. (1993)

1. Isolated preparations

The ileum of several species has been used extensively to investigate functional activities of BK receptors (Burch et at, 1990; Ranson et al., 1992). Kinin-induced contraction in the guinea-pig ileum preparations' are antagonized by B2 receptor antagonists, such as D-Arg-[Hyp^3-Thi^5-D-Tic^7-Oic^8]-BK (pA$_2$ = 6.18). In cultured bovine endothelial cells, D-Arg-[Hyp3-Thi5-D-Tic7-Oicsl-BK abolished the BK-induced PGI, and EDRF release, whereas D-Arg[Hyp^2-Thi^{5,8}-D-Phe^7]-BK showed a weaker antagonistic activity (Hock et al., 1991). Regoli et al. (1991) demonstrated that BK-induced contractions of rabbit jugular vein are competitively antagonized by a novel B$_2$ receptor antagonist (D-Arg-Hyp^{3}D-Phe^7-Lue^8]-BK). Moreover, B$_1$ receptor antagonist, [Leu^8-des-Arg^9-BK] is found to be inactive on this preparation. These findings further indicate that rabbit jugular vein provides a sensitive bioassay in which the potency and specificity of B$_2$ receptor antagonists can be adequately evaluated. The rabbit aortic isolated preparation possesses the B$_1$ type receptors for kinins, which implies that des-Arg^{9}BK is more potent than BK and both peptides are antagonized by B$_1$ receptor antagonist, [Leu^8]desArg^9-BK (Regoli and Barabe, 1980).

2. Blood pressure

Blood pressure (BP)-lowering effects of BK can be antagonized by B$_2$ receptor antagonists (Lys-Lys^3-Hyp^{5,8}-Thi^7-D-Phe-BK and D-Arg-Arg-Pro-HypGly-Thi-Ser-Dhe-Thi-Arg. TFA in SpragueDawley normotensive rats (Griesbacher et al., 1989) and in spontaneously hypertensive rats (Sharma et al., 1992). In addition, it has been observed that the B$_2$ receptor antagonist, such as D-Arg-[Hye-Thi^5- D-Tic^7-Oic^8]-BK abolishes the antihypertrophic effect of an angiotensin converting enzyme inhibitor, ramipril, in rats (Linz and Scholkens, 1992). These findings suggest that the BK receptor antagonists have unwanted effects in hypertension, and they should be contraindicated in patients with high BP. In a rat model of endotoxic shock, the fall in arterial BP in response to an i.v. injection of lipopolysaccharide from E. coli is significantly attenuated after the administration of B2 receptor blocker (Lys-LysHyp^2-Thi^{5,8}-D-Phe-BK) (Weipert et al., 1988). This finding has been contradicted by Berg et al. (1989) who reported that B$_2$ receptor antagonists do not protect against the hypotensive response to endotoxin, anaphylaxis or acute pancreatitis in experimental rat models. Lammek et al. (1990) have indicated that the acylatation of the N-terminus of [D-Arg^0-Hyp^3-Thi^{5,8}-D-Phe^7-BK with 1-adamantane-acetic acid can result in one of the most potent antagonists known to date. This B$_2$ receptor antagonist does not increase the plasma catecholamines at doses sufficient to inhibit by more than 90% the vasodepressor response to 250 ng of exogenously given BK in normotensive rats. In fact, BK antagonists synthesized at early stages showed partial agonistic activities and were found to be potent histamine releasers (see Regoli et al., 1989).

3. Pain

Kinins have been implicated in the physiopathological processes of inflammatory reactions, such as pain, oedema, redness and loss of function (Sharma, 1991a, b, 1992; Sharma and Mohsin, 1990). A study using the human blister base technique of Armstrong et al. (1951) has revealed that the analgesic action of BK is significantly reduced by the B_2 receptor antagonist (D-Arg-Arg-Pro-Hyp-Gly-Thi-Ser-D-Phe-Thi-Arg-TFA), but not by the B_1 receptor antagonist (des-Are-Leu^8-BK) (Whalley et al, 1987a). These findings support the view that B2 receptor antagonists could be useful analgesic agents. Kinins are probably the most painful endogenous chemical mediators. Juan and Lembeck (1974) have shown that the stimulation of nociceptors by intraarterial injection of BK and acetylcholine into the circulation of rabbit ear (separated from the head but remaining in contact with the body only by the auricular nerve) can cause a reflex fall in systemic BP, which has been quantified to study the degree of nociceptor stimulation. In these experiments, B_2, receptor antagonist, Lys-Lys[Hyp^{2,3}-Thi^{5,8}-D-Phe^7]-BK, abolishes the analgesic effect of BK, but it did not inhibit the pain-inducing effect of acetylcholine (Griesbacher and Lembeck, 1987; Lembeck and Griesbacher, 1990). Furthermore, the duration of action of B_2 receptor antagonist has been found to be shorter. This may limit its use in clinical situations. Hence, long-acting blockers of B_2 receptor are needed to establish the therapeutic application in the management of various pain disorders.

4. Inflammatory disorders

Kinins have long been proposed as prominent inflammatory mediators in the pathogenesis of RA and inflammatory bowel diseases (Sharma 1988b, 1991a, b, c; Sharma and Buchanan, 1979; Sharma and Mohsin, 1990), because they can induce all the cardinal signs of inflammatory reactions due to their endogenously raised concentrations.

The role of the kinin system in rheumatology has been substantiated by the fact that BK mediates osteoblast formation and subsequent enhancement of bone resorption in vitro from cultured mouse calvarian bones (Ljunggren and Lerner, 1990). The bone resorption property is due to the activation of B_1 receptor present in the osteoblasts. Also, in porcine cultured articular chondrocytes, BK causes inositol phosphate generation, intra-cellular free calcium ions and PG release via activating B_2 receptor (Benton et al., 1989). The functions of BK receptors in the pathophysiology of joint inflammatory disease are presented in Table11.3. None the less, the involvement of the B_1 and B_2 receptors in inflammatory intestinal diseases has yet to be investigated. However, it would be reasonable to suggest that the main therapeutic goals should be directed to blocking either enhanced formation or inadequate destruction of kinins by the application of specific BK receptor antagonists in the inflammatory diseases of joints and the gut.

Bradykinin antagonists have been indicated as being useful anti-inflammatory compounds. It is reported that specific B_2 kinin antagonist, D-Arg-[Hyp^3-D-Phe^7]-BK, infusion (100 nmol/hr) via ileac artery for 2 hr can inhibit carrageenan-induced inflammation in the rat paw (Burch and De-Haas, 1990). We evaluated the anti-inflammatory action of D-Arg-[Hyp^3-Thi^5-D-Tic^7-Oic^8]-BK (a B_2 receptor antagonist) on mycobacterial-induced chronic inflammatory disease, and observed that the i.p. (1.5 mg/kg) administration of the antagonist for 9 days reduces the swelling significantly in the rat (Sharma et al., unpublished observations). However, vigorous experimental studies are required to achieve the therapeutic potential of BK receptor antagonists as anti-inflammatory and antirheumatic agents (see Figure11.2). Proud and Kaplan (1988) provided a large body of evidence indicating that kinins might be involved in the pathogenesis of several types of rhinitis. Kinins have the ability to induce rhinitis and a sore throat, and it has also been demonstrated that they are generated in human nasal secretions during symptomatic rhinovirus infections and during allergic rhinitis (Proud et al., 1988). These findings provide strong support that BK might be an important mediator of inflammatory processes of the upper respiratory tract. Thus B_2 receptor antagonist, D-Arg-[Hyp^3-D-Phe^7]-BK, has been synthesized to conduct clinical trials for the treatment of rhinitis symptoms (Steranka et al, 1989).

Table 11.3. Actions of Bradykinin Receptors in Joint Inflammatory Disease

Receptors	Actions
B_1 receptors	Calcium release from bones
	Bone resorption
	PGE_2 and PGI_2 release from osteoblasts
	Interleukin-1 and tumor necrosis factor release
B_2 receptors	Pain
	Increased vascular permeability
	Vasodilatation
	Inflammation
	Bone resorption

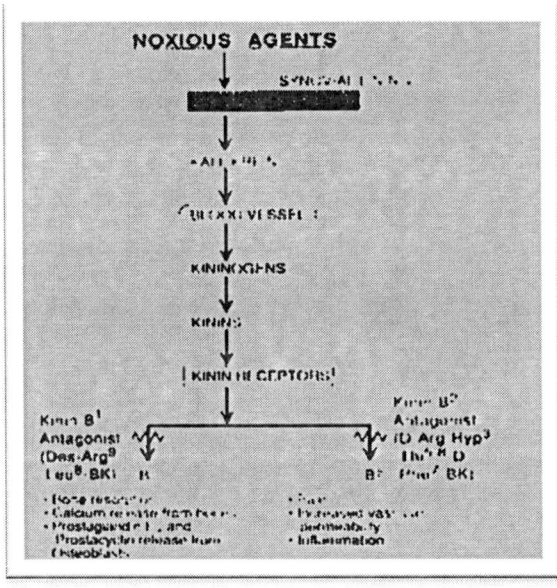

Figure11.2. The mechanism of abnormal kinin formation in inflamed rheumatoid joints, and the role of B_1 and B_2 receptors in the physiopathology of rheumatoid disease. Kinin receptor antagonists might represent novel therapeutic agents for the treatment of rheumatoid arthritis.

5. Vascular permeability

Increases in vascular permeability after intradermal injection of BK have been demonstrated in guinea-pig, man, rabbit and rat (Holdstock et al., 1957; Herxheimer and Schachter, 1959; Carr and Wilhelm, 1964). The kinin receptor mediating an increase in vascular permeability has been evaluated in a variety of experimental animals. It appears that B_2 receptors are involved in rabbit, since B_2 receptor antagonist, D-Arg-[Hyp^{3}Thi^{5,8}-DPhe^7-BK] markedly reduces the increased vascular permeability produced by intradermal administration of BK (Whalley et al., 1987b; Schachter et al., 1987). The B_1 antagonist [Leu^8]des-Arg^9-BK was, however, ineffective. However, a kinin receptor causing an increase in skin vascular permeability is unlikely to be of the B_2 type (Whalley et al., 1987b). Thus, B_2 receptor antagonists may be useful in controlling the skin lesions associated with a local increase in vascular permeability.

6. Asthma

The tendency of kinins to raise pulmonary arterial pressure may contribute to the symptom of bronchial asthma. Plasma kinin levels in asthmatic patients are found to be 10 times higher than in normal subjects (Abe et at, 1967). Bradykinin, whether administered as an aerosol (Hencheimer and Stresemann, 1963) or by i.v. infusion (Bishop et al., 1965) provokes bronchospasm in patients with asthma or chronic bronchitis more readily than in healthy subjects. In addition, BK has been implicated in the genesis of asthma, in that bronchoalveolar kinin levels are raised following allergen challenge in allergic asthmatics (Christiansen et al., 1987). Bradykinin is a potent bronchoconstrictor in vivo and causes contractions of guinea-pig epithelium denuded trachea preparations (Farmer et al., 1989). These researchers indicated also that the B_2 receptor antagonists, D-Arg[Hyp^3-D-Phe^7]-BK and D-Arg-[Hyp^3-Thi^{5,8}-D-Phe^7-BK] are found to be weak inhibitors of BK-induced bronchoconstrictor in vivo, and they were virtually inactive as antagonists of BK-induced airway smooth muscle contraction in guinea-pigs. These results led to the proposal that a novel receptor, designated B_3, mediates BK-induced tracheal contraction (Farmer et al., 1989). Its existence has been confirmed by the discovery of B_3 receptor antagonist, D-Arg[Hyp^3-Thi^5-D-Tic^{7}Tic^8]-BK, (Farmer et al., 1991b). This antagonist potently inhibits BK-induced contractile responses in guinea-pigs. Furthermore, B_1 receptors in the guinea-pig trachea are blocked by D-Arg[Hyp^3-Thi^5- D-Tic^7-Oic^8-BK, a B_2 receptor antagonist (Field et al., 1992). Nevertheless, Jin et al. (1989) noted that BK-induced bronchoconstriction in the guinea-pig could be antagonized by a synthetic B_2 receptor antagonist (D-Arg-[Hyp^3-Thi^{5,8}-D-Phe^7-BK]. It is therefore suggested that the combinations of B_2 and B_3 receptor antagonists might be clinically useful drugs in the treatment of bronchoconstriction occurring in asthmatic patients.

7. Coronary heart diseases

The role of the plasma kallikrein-kinin system has been investigated in patients with acute myocardial infarction by several investigators (Sicuteri et al., 1977; Hashimoto et al., 1978; Shimamoto et al., 1989). High concentrations of plasma kinin have been indicated in patients with acute myocardial infarction (Hashimoto et al., 1978; Shimamoto et al, 1989). Cardiac tissue injury or trauma may initiate the activation of kinin-forming components, and pain induction associated with acute myocardial infarction may result, due to excessive kinin release by the cardiac tissue. In this regard, it is known that the plasma prekallikrein and kininogen levels are reduced in patients with myocardial infarction (Torstilo, 1978) in the process of kinin generation. Increased plasma kinin levels in a dog myocardial ischemic model also indicate the pathogenic role of kinins in coronary diseases (Shimamoto et al., 1989). However the significance of BK receptor functions in the coronary heart diseases remains unclear. In these disorders, BK receptor antagonists may help us to investigate the functional states of B_1 and B_2 receptor involvement in pathophysiology and in the development of specific antagonists as potential therapeutic agents.

REFERENCES

Abe K, Watanabe N, Kumagai N, et al: Circulating plasma kinin in patients with bronchial asthma. Experientia 1967; 23: 626-627.

Armstrong D, Dry RML, Keele CA, et al: Method for studing chemical excitants of cutaneous pain in man. J Physiol (Lond) 1951; 120: 326-351.

Barabe J, Droulin JN, Regoli D, et al: Receptors for bradykinin in intestine and uterine smooth muscle. Can J Physiol Pharmac 1977; 96: 920-926.

Benton HP, Jackson TR, Hanley MR: Identification of a novel inflammatory stimulant of chondrocytes. Biochem J 1989; 269: 861-867.

Berg T, Schlichting E, Ishida H, et al: Kinin antagonist does not protect against the hypotensive response to endotoxin, anaphylaxis or acute pancreatitis. J Pharmac exp Ther 1989; 251: 731-734.

Bishop JM, Harris P, Segel N: The circulatory effects of bradykinin in normal subjects and patients with chronic bronchitis. Br J Pharmac Chemother 1965; 25: 456-460.

Bouthiller J, Deblois D, Marceau F: Studies on the induction of pharmacological responses to des-Arg9-bradykinin in vitro and vivo. Br J Pharmac 1987; 92: 257-264.

Br J Pharmac 1989; 96: 531-538.

Burch RM, Axelrod J: Dissociation of bradykinin-stimulated arachidonic acid release from inositol phosphate formation in Swiss 3T3 fibroblasts. Evidence for a G protein-coupled phospholipase A_2. Proc natn Acad Sci USA 1987; 84: 6374-6378.

Burch RM, DeHaas C: A bradykinin antagonist inhibits carrageenan edema in rats. Naunyn-Sehmiedeberg's Arch Pharmac 1990; 342: 189-193.

Burch RM, Farmer SS, Steranka LR: Bradykinin receptor antagonists. Med Res Rev 1990; 10: 237-269.

Burch RM: Diacylglycerol in the synergy of bradykinin and thrombin stimulation of prostaglandin synthesis. Eur J Pharmac 1989; 168: 39-42.

Burch RM: Kinin signal transduction: role of phosphoinositides and eicosanoids. J Cardiovasc Pharmac 1990; 15 (Suppl. 6): S44-S45.

Carr J, Wilhelm DL: The evaluation of increased vascular permeability in the skin of guinea-pig. Aust J exp Biol med Sci 1964; 42: 511-517.

Christiansen SC, Proud D, Cochrane CG: Detection of tissue kallikrein in the bronchoalveolar lavage fluid of asthmatic subjects. J clin Invest 1987; 79: 188-197.

Couture R, Mizrahi J, Regoli R, et al: Peptides and the human colon: an in vitro pharmacological study. Can J Physiol Pharmac 1982; 59: 957-970.

D'Orleans-Juste P, de Nucci G, Vane JR: Kinins act on Bt or B2 receptors to release conjointly endothelium-derived relaxing factor and prostacyclin from bovine aortic endothelial cells. Br J Pharmac 1989; 96: 920-926.

Erdos EG, Wohler IM, Levine MI: Carboxy-peptidase in blood and other fluids.

Erdos EG: Some old and some new ideas on kinin metabolism. J cardiovasc Pharmac 1990; 15 (Suppl. 6): S20-S24.

Farmer SG, Burch RM, Meeker SA, et al: Evidence for a pulmonary B_3 bradykinin receptor. Molec Pharmac 1989; 36: 1-8.

Farmer SG, McMillan BA, Meeker SN, et al: Induction of vascular smooth muscle bradykinin B_1 receptors in vitro during antigen arthritis. Agents Actions 1991a; 34: 191-193.

Farmer SS, Burch RM, Kyle DJ, et al: D-Arg[Hyp^3-Thi^5D- Tic^7- Tic^8]-bradykinin, a potent antagonist of smooth muscle BK_2 receptors and BK_3 receptors. Br J Pharmac 1991b; 102: 785-787.

Field JL, Hall JM, Morton IKM: Bradykinin receptors in the guinea-pig taemia caeci are similar to proposed BK_3 receptors in the guinea-pig trachea, and are blocked by HOE 140. Br J Pharmac 1992; 105: 293-296.

Freay A, Johns A, Adams DJ, et al: Bradykinin and inositoll,4,5-triphosphate-stimulated calcium release from intracellular stores in cultured bovine endothelial cells. Pflugers Arch 1989; 414: 377-384.

Griesbacher T, Lembeck F, Saria A: Effect of bradykinin antagonist B4310 on smooth muscles and blood pressure in rats, and its enzymatic degradation.

Griesbacher T, Lembeck F: Effect of bradykinin antagonists on bradykinin-induced plasma extravasation, venoconstriction, prostaglandin E_2 release, nociceptor stimulation and contraction of the iris sphincter muscle in the rabbit. Br J Pharmac 1987; 92: 333-340.

Hashimoto K, Hamamoto H, Honda Y, et al: Changes in components of kinin system and hemodynamics in acute myocardial infarction. Am Heart J 1978; 95: 619-626.

Herxheimer A, Stresemann E: Bradykinin and ethanol in bronchial asthma. Archs int Pharmacodyn Ther 1963; 144: 315-321.

Hock FJ, Wirth K, Aebus D, et al: Hoe 140 a new potent and long acting bradykinin-antagonist: in vitro studies. Br J Pharmac 1991; 102: 769-773.

Holdstock DJ, Mathias AP, Schachter M: A comparative study of kinin, kallidin and bradykinin. Br J Pharmac Chemother 1957; 12: 149-154.

Jin LS, Seeds E, Page CP, et al: Inhibition of bradykinin-induced bronchoconstriction in the guinea-pig by a synthetic B_2 receptor antagonist. Br J Pharmac 1989; 97: 598-602.

Juan H, Lembeck F: Action of peptides and other algesic agents on paravascular pain receptors of isolated perfused rabbit ear. Naunyn Schniedeberg's Arch Pharmac 1974; 283: 151-164.

Lammek B, Wang YS, Gavras 1, et al: A new highly potent antagonist of bradykinin. Peptides 1990; 11: 1041-1043.

Lembeck F, Griesbacher T: Functional analysis of kinin antagonists. J Cardiovasc Pharmac 1990; 15 (Suppl 6): S75-S77.

Linz W, Scholkens A: A specific B_2-bradykinin receptor antagonist HOE 140 abolishes the antihypertensive effect of ramipriL Br J Pharmac 1992; 105: 771-772.

Ljunggren O, Lerner DH: Evidence for BK_1 bradykinin receptor-mediated prostaglandin formation in osteoblasts and subsequent enhancement of bone resorption. Br J Pharmac 1990; 101: 382-386.

Llona 1, Vavrek R, Stewart J, et al: Identification of pre- and postsynaptic bradykinin receptor sites in the vas deference: evidence for structural prerequisites. J Pharmac exp Ther 1987; 241: 608--614.

Values in human blood in normal and pathological conditions. Clin Chim Acta 1965; 11: 39-43.

Index

A

absorption, 97, 99, 101, 102
acetic acid, 58, 62, 136, 174
acetylcholine, 175
acid, 4, 5, 6, 10, 27, 28, 38, 43, 44, 45, 48, 58, 59, 60, 62, 63, 64, 65, 66, 67, 68, 70, 72, 95, 97, 98, 101, 103, 108, 114, 119, 127, 128, 130, 133, 135, 137, 141, 142, 145, 146, 148, 151, 157, 172, 173, 174, 178
acute asthma, 144
acute respiratory distress syndrome, 134
adamantane, 174
adaptation, 38
adenine, 126, 127
adenosine, 101
adhesion, 128, 129, 132, 136, 143
adjustment, 146
adult respiratory distress syndrome, 54, 66
adverse event, 165
aetiology, 2, 28, 170
afferent nerve, 68
aggregation, 35, 42, 45, 46, 49, 71, 135, 136
agonist, 158, 159, 160, 163, 164, 165, 166, 167, 171
AIDS, 130
airway inflammation, 138, 147
airways, 11, 12, 114, 136, 144, 172
alanine, 146
alanine aminotransferase, 146
aldosterone, 27, 28, 30, 35, 37, 87, 161
aldosteronism, 31, 37
alkalosis, 28, 34
allele, 81
allergen challenge, 177
allergic asthma, 177
allergic inflammation, 52, 74, 107, 109
allergic reaction, 94, 105, 169
allergic rhinitis, 19, 143, 150, 176
allergy, 52
alveolar macrophage, 62, 107
amines, 50, 74, 84
amino acids, 27, 54, 57, 94
amyotrophic lateral sclerosis, 130
analgesic, 2, 102, 175
analgesic agent, 175
anaphylactic reactions, 54
anaphylactic shock, 44, 108, 169
anaphylaxis, 120, 143, 174, 178
angiogenesis, 1, 133, 165
angioplasty, 136, 166
angiotensin converting enzyme, 6, 20, 33, 36, 40, 41, 87, 89, 121, 170, 174
angiotensin II, 27, 28, 29, 32, 33, 38, 41, 42, 77, 78, 81, 82, 83, 86, 87, 89, 128
anhydrase, 98
ankylosing spondylitis, 131
antagonism, 59, 63, 136, 154
antibody, 50, 53, 157
antidiuretic hormone, 27, 29
antigen, 10, 16, 39, 50, 52, 53, 70, 98, 106, 147, 157, 171, 179
antihypertensive agents, 79, 88
antihypertensive drugs, 82, 162, 169
anti-inflammatory agents, 54, 73, 138
anti-inflammatory drugs, 2, 17, 43, 47, 62, 63, 72, 73, 79, 98, 102, 131, 134, 135, 136, 138, 139
antioxidant, 131, 133
aorta, 39, 101, 119, 160
apoptosis, 123, 125, 128, 132, 149
ARDS, 134
arginine, 6, 10, 15, 28, 38, 41, 42, 78, 91, 112, 113, 125, 126, 127, 128, 134, 135, 136, 137, 139, 171

arrhythmia, 117, 122, 163
arterial hypertension, 35
arteries, 12, 158, 162, 163, 172
artery, 29, 31, 35, 94, 96, 115, 117, 118, 137, 160, 163, 166, 175
arthritis, 1, 2, 10, 13, 15, 16, 17, 19, 20, 42, 49, 50, 51, 52, 53, 58, 59, 60, 62, 63, 64, 65, 67, 69, 70, 71, 72, 73, 75, 98, 102, 105, 106, 108, 109, 125, 131, 135, 138, 139, 145, 149, 150, 151, 158, 170, 171, 176, 179
Asia, 120
asthma, 108, 134, 141, 142, 143, 144, 145, 146, 147, 148, 149, 150, 151, 158, 169, 170, 177, 178, 179
asthma attacks, 144
asthmatic children, 144
atherosclerotic plaque, 131
ATP, 164
authors, 50, 51, 52, 53, 58, 106
autoimmune disease, 130, 137, 139
autonomic nervous system, 40, 71

B

bacteria, 53, 61, 129, 130
bacterial infection, 128, 130
balloon angioplasty, 136, 166
basement membrane, 60, 64
basophils, 53, 59, 105, 148
beneficial effect, 154, 162
beta blocker, 79
bile, 92, 94, 133
bile acids, 92, 94
binding, 53, 57, 116, 127, 128, 144, 159
bioavailability, 125, 131
biochemistry, 62
biodegradation, 27, 32, 77, 81, 116
biological activity, 49, 51, 109
biological processes, 126, 133
biological responses, 173
biologically active compounds, 47, 73, 99
biosynthesis, 16, 26, 42, 47, 65, 66, 95, 97, 99, 103, 125, 134, 141, 142, 145, 146, 147, 151
bladder, 28, 35, 36
blocks, 83, 146
blood flow, 8, 23, 27, 28, 29, 38, 47, 58, 67, 70, 78, 82, 86, 96, 99, 101, 103, 115, 116, 119, 133, 164, 166
blood monocytes, 16, 139
blood plasma, 41, 62, 94
blood pressure, 2, 23, 36, 37, 38, 39, 40, 41, 42, 55, 60, 69, 77, 85, 86, 87, 88, 89, 92, 111, 120, 121, 153, 161, 162, 163, 164, 166, 167, 179
blood pressure reduction, 164
blood stream, 23, 131
blood supply, 91
blood vessels, 29, 65, 161
body fluid, 5, 6, 78, 111, 112, 154, 157, 170
body weight, 47, 96
bonds, 141
bone, 1, 2, 8, 9, 10, 12, 13, 17, 18, 51, 52, 106, 132, 138, 169, 171, 175, 180
bone resorption, 2, 8, 9, 12, 17, 18, 132, 138, 171, 175, 180
bones, 8, 18, 171, 175, 176
bowel, 44, 47, 49, 55, 58, 62, 70, 72, 95, 102, 125, 132, 145, 151, 169, 175
bradykinin, 1, 3, 7, 13, 14, 15, 16, 17, 18, 19, 20, 23, 34, 35, 36, 37, 38, 39, 41, 42, 54, 61, 62, 64, 65, 66, 67, 70, 71, 73, 74, 85, 87, 88, 89, 99, 100, 101, 118, 119, 120, 121, 122, 156, 158, 160, 166, 167, 168, 178, 179, 180
brain, 130, 143, 160, 166
Brazil, 3
breakdown, 116, 132
bronchial asthma, 177, 178, 179
bronchial epithelium, 131
bronchiectasis, 134
bronchitis, 177, 178
bronchoconstriction, 11, 12, 17, 62, 64, 71, 108, 114, 119, 144, 147, 148, 171, 172, 177, 179
bronchoconstrictors, 143, 144
bronchospasm, 147, 177

C

calcium, 4, 13, 17, 33, 47, 52, 53, 60, 79, 107, 114, 115, 116, 127, 128, 132, 143, 146, 162, 172, 175, 179
calcium channel blocker, 162
calvaria, 2, 17
CAP, 85
capillary, 70, 162
cardiac arrhythmia, 114
cardiovascular disease, 32, 115, 117, 154, 158, 161, 166
cardiovascular system, 108, 111, 120, 121, 125, 128, 157
carotid arteries, 158
carrier, 135
cartilage, 1, 9, 16, 51, 52, 62, 70, 106, 132, 145
catecholamines, 174
cDNA, 15, 19
cell, 1, 7, 8, 9, 10, 12, 15, 44, 47, 50, 52, 53, 60, 61, 63, 66, 67, 73, 81, 86, 95, 96, 97, 98, 102, 112, 113, 126, 128, 129, 130, 133, 134, 137, 142, 144, 147, 158, 160, 171, 172
cell death, 128
cell line, 8, 137

cell membranes, 126
central nervous system, 126, 130, 157
channel blocker, 33, 116, 162
chemical structures, 141
chemokines, 130
chemotaxis, 43, 52, 57, 61, 66, 68, 106, 129, 132, 141, 142, 143
children, 62, 144, 145, 148, 150
CHO cells, 161
chondrocyte, 70, 132
chromosome, 5
chronic granulomatous disease, 61, 74, 150
cimetidine, 50, 75
circulation, 4, 6, 7, 8, 24, 26, 28, 29, 39, 40, 53, 54, 55, 71, 81, 91, 94, 99, 103, 112, 115, 154, 175
cirrhosis, 149
classes, 141, 142, 145
classification, 10, 157, 171
cleavage, 69, 101, 112, 120, 155
cleavages, 39
clinical assessment, 154
clinical symptoms, 49, 116, 162
clinical trials, 98, 148, 160, 176
cloning, 4, 15, 19, 136, 151
coagulation, 1, 4, 6, 8, 24, 37, 51, 55, 57, 68, 69, 72, 92, 112, 122, 155
colitis, 47, 49, 50, 62, 64, 68, 70, 75, 94, 96, 99, 101, 131, 132, 147, 150, 151, 158
collagen, 9, 10, 12, 92, 113, 145, 158, 160, 171, 172
colon, 15, 58, 72, 92, 94, 95, 99, 102, 103, 131, 179
color, iv
complement, 43, 44, 49, 53, 54, 57, 61, 63, 65, 66, 68, 69, 71, 72, 74
complementary DNA, 4, 6
compliance, 148
complications, 66
components, 7, 8, 25, 44, 47, 52, 53, 58, 60, 63, 77, 94, 106, 111, 117, 153, 164, 170, 178, 179
compounds, 47, 52, 68, 73, 82, 99, 107, 117, 125, 135, 137, 141, 142, 146, 147, 175
concentration, 6, 28, 29, 31, 37, 42, 52, 102, 105, 128, 130, 131, 146, 157
confusion, 97
congestive heart failure, 115, 117, 161
connective tissue, 7, 51
constitutive enzyme, 135
consumption, 96, 101
control, 27, 28, 36, 38, 40, 41, 69, 74, 83, 84, 89, 96, 103, 147, 148
control group, 84
conversion, 26, 27, 30, 48, 53, 55, 65, 77, 81, 125, 127, 162
coronary arteries, 163

coronary heart disease, 115, 161, 169, 178
correlation, 27, 29, 31, 47
cortex, 27, 34, 57
corticosteroid therapy, 147
corticosteroids, 49, 148
corticotropin, 27
critical analysis, 84
culture, 11, 42, 72, 151, 171
cyclooxygenase, 9, 44, 47, 49, 95, 96, 103, 114, 139, 165, 173
cytochrome, 44, 95, 126, 127
cytokines, 9, 128, 130, 131, 134, 158
cytotoxicity, 63, 132

D

death, 116, 128, 130, 162
defense, 132, 133, 134
deficiency, ix, 4, 24, 29, 32, 35, 37, 41, 54, 57, 64, 65, 68, 69, 74, 92, 99, 100, 115, 119, 122, 161
deficit, 118, 119
degradation, 6, 33, 51, 62, 87, 142, 143, 157, 159, 162, 179
delivery, 115, 123, 160, 162, 166
dementia, 130
deposition, 36, 71
derivatives, 69, 107, 129, 135, 138, 143, 157
dermatoses, 60
desensitization, 11, 12, 101, 114, 172
destruction, 7, 13, 44, 51, 64, 129, 130, 145, 170, 175
detachment, 60, 61, 67
detection, 39, 70
developed countries, 162
developing countries, 116
diabetes, 37, 117, 121
diastolic blood pressure, 85
diastolic pressure, 117
diffusion, 126, 137
digestion, 20, 37, 67, 100
discomfort, 148
disease activity, 20, 40, 75, 135
disease progression, 132
diseases, ix, 1, 7, 17, 32, 43, 44, 47, 49, 50, 51, 52, 54, 58, 59, 60, 64, 66, 67, 71, 87, 94, 100, 105, 107, 115, 117, 118, 125, 126, 130, 131, 132, 133, 134, 135, 136, 141, 142, 144, 145, 153, 154, 157, 158, 161, 164, 165, 166, 169, 170, 175, 178
disorder, 36, 145
disseminated intravascular coagulation, 51
distribution, 4, 5, 15, 24, 54, 142
diuretic, 28, 77, 161
diversity, 128
DNA, 4, 6, 15, 19, 130, 132

DNA damage, 132
dogs, 2, 27, 38, 39, 59, 64, 67, 70, 82, 87, 89, 101, 117, 122, 153, 163
dominant allele, 81
double bonds, 141
drug delivery, 160, 166
drug therapy, 121
drugs, ix, 2, 17, 33, 42, 43, 49, 52, 54, 62, 65, 67, 71, 73, 77, 79, 83, 84, 98, 102, 107, 116, 128, 130, 134, 135, 138, 139, 146, 149, 151, 162, 169, 177
dumping, 103
duodenal ulcer, 98, 103
duration, 28, 41, 85, 117, 153, 175

E

edema, 15, 58, 64, 71, 144, 147, 157, 158, 165, 167, 178
electrolyte, 29, 91, 96, 99, 101, 133
emergency management, 146
enantiomers, 146
encephalopathy, 66
endocrine glands, 78
endothelial cells, 1, 6, 8, 10, 11, 12, 15, 16, 17, 19, 52, 65, 66, 72, 78, 88, 91, 105, 112, 113, 115, 119, 121, 125, 126, 129, 131, 132, 135, 138, 141, 143, 157, 163, 171, 172, 173, 174, 179
endothelium, 10, 16, 64, 78, 88, 119, 126, 127, 128, 129, 135, 137, 138, 143, 145, 162, 163, 171, 179
endotoxemia, 53, 138
endotoxins, 130
energy, 116, 123, 163
environment, 100
enzyme inhibitors, 77, 87, 89, 119, 121
enzymes, 4, 5, 6, 17, 24, 26, 37, 54, 55, 57, 67, 78, 91, 100, 112, 126, 127, 128, 129, 130, 132, 135, 141, 143, 144, 154, 157
eosinophilia, 141
eosinophils, 105, 143, 144, 150
epidemic, 116
epithelial cells, 134
epithelial transport, 138
epithelium, 118, 131, 177
equilibrium, 68
erosion, 10, 51, 52
erythrocytes, 105, 108
esophagus, 157
ester, 73, 135, 136
ethanol, 97, 179
etiology, 74, 134
excretion, 23, 26, 27, 29, 31, 32, 33, 34, 35, 36, 37, 38, 39, 55, 61, 69, 81, 82, 88, 94, 101, 115, 118, 120, 122, 131, 132, 137, 138, 160, 161, 162
exercise, 32, 37, 115, 119, 144, 147, 148, 161

exploitation, 157
extravasation, 52, 60, 66, 107, 179
exudate, 74, 96, 109

F

FAD, 127
failure, 66, 83, 98, 116, 117, 130, 153, 158, 162, 163
family, 2, 3, 4, 5, 18, 24, 44, 53, 57, 92, 95, 111, 112, 113, 120, 134, 141, 154, 158, 169
fatty acids, 143
feedback, 4, 26, 29, 55, 95, 112, 130, 155
fever, 45, 46, 47, 51
fibers, 60
fibrin, 65, 108
fibrinolysis, 18, 24, 37, 40, 57, 65, 69, 74, 92, 122
fibroblasts, 15, 37, 51, 59, 70, 131, 160, 178
fibrosis, 137, 162
fish, 148, 151
fish oil, 148, 151
fluid, 1, 2, 7, 8, 9, 10, 15, 16, 17, 18, 20, 24, 26, 35, 47, 49, 52, 55, 58, 59, 60, 63, 64, 67, 71, 72, 73, 75, 92, 94, 106, 118, 129, 130, 131, 133, 136, 150, 157, 179
Ford, 49, 63, 65
fragments, 53, 112, 157
free radicals, 65, 130, 132
fructose, 73
functional changes, 129

G

gastric mucosa, 98, 99, 102, 136, 137
gastric ulcer, 100
gastrointestinal tract, 54, 94, 100, 102, 103
gel, 98
gene, 4, 5, 6, 15, 16, 17, 18, 19, 86, 112, 115, 117, 118, 120, 123, 135, 162, 163, 166
gene expression, 15
gene mapping, 117, 163
gene therapy, 116, 118, 162
generation, 13, 16, 23, 24, 29, 35, 37, 40, 51, 56, 57, 58, 61, 69, 74, 114, 115, 117, 122, 133, 146, 148, 150, 151, 157, 159, 162, 164, 166, 167, 175, 178
genes, 4, 6, 16, 19, 112, 168
genetic defect, 26, 31, 55
Germany, 3, 17
gland, 4, 15, 26, 35, 39, 40, 55, 62, 63, 70, 71, 87, 92, 94, 99, 100, 103, 155
glutathione, 142
glycerol, 51, 108
glycogen, 116, 163
glycoproteins, 6, 155
goals, 13, 175

goblet cells, 92, 94
gout, 8, 49, 71
gouty arthritis, 58
Greeks, 43
groups, 24, 31, 52, 54, 82, 91, 107, 125, 126, 146
growth, 16, 116, 162
gut, 1, 2, 58, 91, 94, 95, 96, 98, 125, 126, 132, 138, 175

H

HE, 57, 120
headache, 148
healing, 136, 139
health, 5, 61, 66, 69, 117, 163
heart disease, 115, 136, 161, 169, 178
heart failure, 115, 117, 161, 163
heart rate, 83, 84
heat, 43, 97, 157
heme, 125, 127, 133
hemodialysis, 146
hepatic encephalopathy, 66
hepatic failure, 66
hepatoma, 137
high blood pressure, 153, 162
histamine, 1, 10, 12, 43, 44, 47, 50, 51, 53, 58, 60, 61, 62, 63, 64, 65, 66, 67, 71, 72, 74, 144, 148, 172, 174
histidine, 50
homeostasis, 26, 28, 30, 35, 54, 55, 63, 68, 117
homologous genes, 5
Honda, 179
hormone, 27, 28, 29, 78
host, 130, 133, 134
human genome, 6
human neutrophils, 107
hydrocortisone, 132
hydrogen, 61, 66, 126, 129
hydrogen peroxide, 61, 66, 129
hydrolysis, 60, 115, 160, 173
hydroxyl, 136, 139
hyperactivity, 114, 141, 159
hyperaldosteronism, 28
hyperemia, 47, 67, 137
hyperplasia, 28, 128
hypersensitivity, 59, 72, 74
hypertension, 19, 23, 26, 27, 28, 29, 31, 32, 33, 34, 35, 36, 37, 38, 39, 40, 41, 55, 67, 69, 77, 81, 82, 83, 84, 86, 87, 88, 89, 92, 101, 102, 111, 114, 115, 117, 118, 119, 120, 121, 122, 136, 153, 158, 161, 162, 166, 169, 170, 174
hypertrophy, 111, 116, 117, 119, 121, 153, 158, 162, 166, 167, 168
hypokalemia, 28
hypotension, 11, 12, 23, 78, 82, 83, 84, 85, 105, 122, 130, 137, 157, 160, 161, 171, 172
hypotensive, 2, 20, 28, 32, 41, 77, 82, 83, 84, 85, 88, 89, 115, 121, 122, 160, 161, 162, 163, 167, 174, 178
hypothesis, 32, 60, 83, 117
hypoxia, 117

I

IBD, 141, 142, 143, 145, 146, 151
ibuprofen, 72, 109
ICAM, 137
identification, 68, 108, 122
IFN, 1, 9, 13
ileum, 2, 3, 11, 12, 95, 101, 114, 115, 120, 160, 171, 172, 173, 174
immigration, 142
immune reaction, 59
immune response, 125
immune system, 51, 128
immunity, 51, 61, 64
immunoglobulin, 50
immunomodulatory, 131
immunoreactivity, 64
immunosuppressive agent, 137
in vitro, 3, 7, 8, 11, 12, 13, 15, 16, 17, 20, 27, 44, 45, 51, 52, 60, 64, 74, 100, 106, 114, 118, 122, 138, 139, 153, 158, 160, 169, 171, 173, 175, 178, 179
in vivo, 6, 12, 20, 44, 45, 51, 53, 60, 62, 64, 68, 73, 100, 132, 138, 147, 153, 158, 165, 172, 173, 177
inbreeding, 31
incidence, 153
incubation time, 24, 55, 92
indication, 84
indices, 133
indigenous, 72, 109
inducer, 128
induction, 10, 15, 47, 53, 60, 117, 130, 133, 136, 137, 138, 153, 165, 166, 167, 171, 178
induration, 49, 96
infarction, 117, 123, 153, 163, 164, 166, 167, 178, 179
infection, 64, 128, 130, 134
infectious disease, 134
inflammation, 1, 7, 8, 10, 11, 14, 15, 17, 18, 20, 40, 43, 44, 47, 49, 50, 51, 52, 53, 54, 57, 58, 59, 61, 62, 64, 65, 66, 67, 68, 70, 71, 72, 73, 74, 75, 88, 89, 94, 96, 100, 102, 105, 107, 108, 109, 112, 113, 121, 125, 126, 129, 130, 133, 135, 136, 137, 138, 141, 142, 148, 150, 154, 157, 158, 171, 175
inflammatory bowel disease, 47, 58, 62, 70, 72, 102, 132, 151, 175
inflammatory cell migration, 1, 9

inflammatory cells, 10, 15, 52, 69, 105, 107, 131, 143, 150
inflammatory disease, 1, 2, 7, 13, 14, 20, 43, 44, 47, 49, 52, 53, 54, 59, 60, 72, 94, 103, 107, 125, 132, 134, 135, 141, 142, 144, 145, 147, 169, 175
inflammatory mediators, 1, 2, 7, 8, 10, 43, 47, 48, 52, 66, 70, 101, 107, 130, 144, 175
inflammatory responses, 51, 52, 73, 108, 131
ingestion, 37
inhibition, 6, 7, 13, 15, 17, 27, 28, 30, 31, 32, 36, 41, 47, 48, 70, 77, 78, 83, 87, 88, 89, 93, 96, 97, 102, 103, 112, 116, 122, 128, 130, 131, 132, 134, 135, 138, 143, 145, 146, 147, 166
inhibitor, 7, 28, 29, 32, 36, 40, 41, 57, 61, 83, 87, 89, 92, 95, 114, 115, 117, 121, 145, 146, 147, 148, 149, 151, 161, 164, 167, 173, 174
initiation, 2, 24, 51, 54, 57, 144
injections, 58, 70, 83
injury, 1, 8, 10, 59, 60, 61, 67, 68, 72, 74, 88, 113, 128, 132, 133, 158, 169, 170, 171, 178
inositol, 13, 114, 157, 172, 175, 178
insertion, 142
insight, 115, 161
institutions, ix
integrin, 136
interaction, 28, 30, 51, 59, 79, 81, 97, 129, 136, 137, 151
interactions, 2, 27, 28, 43, 50, 59, 63, 95, 107, 136, 157, 169
interference, 99, 154
interferon, 9, 18, 138
interferon gamma, 138
interleukin-8, 138
interleukins, 44, 145
intervention, 135
intestinal tract, 91, 95
intestine, 4, 15, 19, 26, 55, 73, 89, 91, 92, 95, 96, 98, 99, 100, 101, 118, 122, 133, 155, 178
ions, 13, 53, 161, 175
iris, 179
iron, 125, 127, 132, 146
ischemia, 111, 116, 117, 123, 136, 153, 157, 158, 162, 163, 166
isolation, 51, 66, 99
isozymes, 136
issues, 6, 169

J

Japan, 81, 100
jaundice, 147
joint damage, 132
joints, 1, 2, 7, 8, 9, 10, 11, 13, 14, 49, 58, 106, 131, 145, 175, 176

K

K^+, 138
keratinocytes, 150
kidney, 4, 15, 18, 26, 27, 28, 29, 31, 35, 36, 38, 39, 40, 55, 57, 61, 74, 88, 91, 92, 94, 95, 101, 112, 115, 120, 131, 161
kidneys, 4, 38, 155, 157

L

laparotomy, 58
lateral sclerosis, 130
laxatives, 96
leakage, 50, 61
lesions, 10, 62, 97, 102, 103, 166, 177
leucine, 10, 171
leukotriene modifier, 150
leukotrienes, 11, 44, 49, 65, 66, 73, 74, 95, 102, 106, 107, 141, 149, 150, 158
lifetime, 126, 161
ligand, 128, 143
lipids, 129
lipooxygenase, 44, 49, 61, 66, 95, 98
liquid phase, 35, 71, 99
liver, 4, 5, 32, 38, 63, 78, 79, 86, 88, 94, 108, 112, 115, 136, 146, 154, 161
liver disease, 147
localization, 5, 15, 91
locus, 16, 112
lower esophageal sphincter, 120
LTA, 142, 145
LTB4, 8, 9, 10, 45, 47, 49, 52, 73, 96, 98, 107, 141, 142, 143, 144, 145, 147, 148, 149
LTD, 144
lung disease, 134
lung function, 146
lymph, 62, 78, 91
lymphocytes, 10, 47, 51, 60, 70, 132, 143, 144, 145
lymphoid, 50
lysis, 53, 61
lysosome, 129

M

macromolecules, 52, 60, 94, 107, 129, 144
macrophages, 1, 8, 10, 11, 20, 47, 51, 52, 60, 62, 66, 67, 105, 107, 113, 122, 125, 128, 129, 130, 131, 132, 134, 136, 139, 143, 145, 171
maintenance, 52, 117, 147, 150
majority, 31, 132, 158
malignant hypertension, 115, 161
mammalian tissues, 19, 78
management, 125, 141, 146, 175

mapping, 117, 163
mast cells, 47, 50, 53, 60, 105, 134, 143, 144, 145
measurement, 38, 50, 83, 131, 166
membranes, 55, 57, 95, 126, 129, 138, 161
mesangial cells, 137, 138
messenger RNA, 6, 17
messengers, 129, 158
metabolism, 13, 16, 19, 20, 48, 49, 54, 62, 65, 66, 70, 100, 116, 119, 134, 146, 155, 157, 159, 179
metabolites, 6, 10, 43, 44, 45, 47, 50, 51, 62, 65, 67, 68, 96, 101, 113, 130, 136, 137, 143, 144, 147, 149, 158, 171
metabolizing, 6
metalloproteinase, 122
mice, 98, 102, 115, 118, 119, 122, 137, 139, 161, 165, 167
microcirculation, 54, 60, 61, 64
microspheres, 47
migration, 1, 9, 52, 53, 60, 61, 78, 107, 108, 158
mineralocorticoid, 31
model, 1, 17, 31, 36, 47, 49, 50, 52, 59, 70, 79, 96, 101, 106, 117, 122, 138, 147, 163, 174, 178
models, 1, 54, 61, 82, 114, 116, 118, 145, 151, 153, 154, 162, 174
mole, 6
molecular biology, 117, 163
molecular mass, 6
molecular oxygen, 142
molecular structure, 5, 78
molecular weight, 2, 4, 6, 9, 14, 18, 20, 24, 37, 54, 55, 57, 65, 68, 69, 70, 72, 78, 91, 92, 99, 100, 101, 102, 103, 112, 119, 120, 122, 155
molecules, ix, 6, 50, 53, 126, 129, 132, 136, 142
monolayer, 66
montelukast, 144, 148, 149, 151
morbidity, 164
mortality, 116, 135, 162, 164
mortality rate, 116, 162
mRNA, 137, 143, 144, 168
mucosa, 47, 60, 70, 72, 91, 94, 95, 96, 97, 98, 99, 100, 120, 131, 132, 133, 136, 144, 145, 151
mucus, 98, 100, 133, 144, 147
mucus hypersecretion, 147
multiple sclerosis, 130, 131
muscles, 10, 78, 114, 115, 169, 171, 179
mutagenesis, 132
myocardial infarction, 117, 123, 153, 163, 164, 166, 167, 178, 179
myocardial ischemia, 118, 123, 136, 166
myocardium, 154, 163
myoglobin, 126

N

Na^+, 138
naphthalene, 136
necrosis, 9, 16, 18, 20, 51, 64, 113, 122, 171, 176
neovascularization, 166
nephrectomy, 58
nephron, 26, 38, 40, 55, 72
nerve, 55, 67, 99, 158, 175
nervous system, 26, 40, 54, 55, 71, 126, 128, 130, 157
neurodegeneration, 130
neuronal cells, 134
neurons, 70, 126
neuroprotection, 130
neurotransmission, 126, 133
neurotransmitter, 125, 130
neutrophils, 47, 71, 105, 107, 108, 129, 132, 134, 141, 143, 145, 146, 149, 150
nicotinamide, 126
nitric oxide, 113, 123, 126, 128, 131, 134, 136, 137, 138, 139, 153, 160
nitric oxide synthase, 126, 136, 137, 138, 139
nitrogen, 125, 127, 134, 136, 137, 138
nitrogen dioxide, 134
nitrogen oxides, 136
NO synthases, 135
non-steroidal anti-inflammatory drugs, 47, 63, 72, 97, 102, 131, 135, 136
Norway, 112, 161
NSAIDs, 47, 49, 51, 97, 131
nucleotides, 52, 107
nutrients, 162

O

observations, 14, 26, 28, 29, 60, 81, 111, 115, 153, 165, 176
occlusion, 118, 163
oedema, 1, 7, 10, 12, 13, 47, 52, 62, 65, 106, 121, 141, 144, 175
oil, 58, 108, 148, 151
omega-3, 145
opportunities, 118
order, 158
organ, 4, 5, 72, 78, 130, 151
organism, 130
osteoarthritis, 131
osteomyelitis, 1, 171
overload, 164
overproduction, 130, 134, 135
ox, 16
oxidation, 127, 142

oxidative damage, 131
oxidative stress, 132, 133, 134, 162
oxides, 136
oxygen, 61, 65, 101, 125, 127, 129, 136, 137, 138, 142, 162, 164
oxygen consumption, 101

P

Pacific, 120
pacing, 117
pain, 1, 7, 8, 11, 12, 21, 43, 45, 46, 47, 50, 57, 58, 59, 64, 68, 74, 78, 79, 90, 94, 114, 122, 137, 143, 148, 157, 158, 160, 165, 169, 171, 172, 175, 178, 180
pancreas, 2, 4, 16, 18, 26, 36, 55, 69, 92, 100, 155
pancreatitis, 158, 174, 178
pannus formation, 1, 9
paradigm, 137
parallel, 112, 131, 146, 149, 157
parameters, 63, 109, 146
parasympathetic nervous system, 26, 55
parenchyma, 29
parenchymal cell, 5
partial thromboplastin time, 24, 55
passive, 108
pathogenesis, 9, 20, 32, 43, 49, 52, 55, 58, 60, 66, 69, 82, 84, 105, 106, 109, 115, 117, 125, 130, 139, 145, 163, 175, 176
pathogens, 132
pathology, 9, 34, 62, 98, 116, 162
pathophysiology, 7, 51, 54, 81, 95, 115, 117, 138, 141, 143, 144, 147, 161, 163, 166, 175, 178
pathways, 1, 35, 44, 48, 53, 54, 60, 64, 65, 78, 86, 95, 112, 114, 115, 117, 158, 173
penicillin, 54
peptidase, 179
peptides, 4, 5, 18, 23, 26, 54, 57, 65, 74, 89, 157, 166, 174, 180
perfusion, 117, 123, 130, 136, 162, 163
periodontitis, 1, 171
peripheral blood, 16, 58, 143, 161
peritoneal cavity, 143
permeability, 7, 8, 11, 12, 28, 35, 36, 40, 43, 45, 46, 47, 49, 50, 52, 53, 54, 57, 58, 59, 60, 61, 63, 66, 67, 69, 70, 72, 74, 79, 94, 106, 108, 133, 144, 158, 165, 171, 172, 176, 177, 179
peroxide, 61, 66, 129
peroxynitrite, 139
perseverance, 106
PGE, 8, 27, 28, 51, 57, 59, 88, 98
pH, 60
phagocyte, 78, 129, 133, 134, 139
phagocytosis, 53, 129

pharmacogenetics, 98
pharmacology, ix, 19, 64, 97, 99, 100, 102, 119, 138, 150
phenylalanine, 6, 139
phosphates, 114, 116, 123, 172
phosphoinositides, 15, 118, 179
phospholipids, 44, 47, 52, 70, 73, 95, 107, 109, 142
physicochemical properties, 55
physiology, ix, 32, 62, 98, 138
physiopathology, 20, 26, 32, 92, 97, 121, 176
pigs, 64, 108, 177
placebo, 58, 147, 148, 149, 150
plasma cells, 50, 145
plasma levels, 58, 163
plasma membrane, 129
plasma proteins, 53, 75, 94
plasminogen, 37, 51, 64, 69
platelet activating factor, 10, 11, 15, 20, 62, 68, 69, 73, 98, 105, 107, 108, 109, 144
platelet aggregation, 135, 136
platelets, 47, 49, 51, 52, 54, 61, 66, 71, 92, 105, 108, 109
pleurisy, 58, 63, 66, 67, 73, 106, 109
PM, 15, 20, 40, 42, 63, 66, 68, 75, 88, 89
polymerase, 144
polymerase chain reaction, 144
polymorphism, 120, 122
polymorphisms, 112
polypeptide, 2, 3, 6
population, 81, 146
positive correlation, 47
positive feedback, 4, 95, 112, 130, 155
potassium, 37, 59, 160
pranlukast, 144
pregnancy, 116
pressure, 2, 23, 36, 37, 38, 39, 40, 41, 42, 55, 60, 69, 77, 84, 85, 86, 87, 88, 89, 92, 111, 116, 120, 121, 153, 161, 162, 163, 164, 166, 167, 168, 174, 177, 179
prevention, 103, 158
pro-inflammatory, 2, 43, 50, 52, 60, 125, 128, 130, 131, 132, 134, 135, 144, 158, 165
proliferation, 1, 9, 10, 12, 113, 132, 145, 158, 160, 171, 172
properties, 4, 12, 13, 19, 24, 26, 43, 45, 46, 51, 54, 55, 58, 60, 73, 74, 82, 84, 91, 112, 120, 121, 131, 133, 137, 144, 149, 155, 158, 161, 165, 167, 172
prostaglandins, 19, 27, 36, 38, 39, 41, 43, 59, 62, 64, 66, 67, 68, 73, 78, 88, 89, 91, 97, 100, 101, 102, 103, 106, 107, 120, 122, 136, 144, 158
prostate, 4, 16, 18, 155
prostate gland, 4, 155
prostate specific antigen, 16

proteases, 4, 5, 19, 23, 26, 54, 60, 72, 91, 154
protective mechanisms, 111
protein kinase C, 47
proteinase, 94
proteins, 5, 20, 40, 51, 53, 60, 75, 78, 94, 112, 133, 143, 150, 154, 158
proteinuria, 77, 87
proteoglycans, 7
proteolysis, 74
proteolytic enzyme, 53
psoriasis, 52, 106, 143, 148
publishers, xi
purification, 3, 15, 18, 136
pyrophosphate, 60

Q

quality of life, 148, 149

R

race, 31, 37, 38, 109
radicals, 61, 65, 72, 130, 132
radio, 35
range, 27
reactant, 112, 154
reaction mechanism, 63, 127
reactions, 2, 6, 7, 8, 10, 40, 43, 44, 47, 51, 54, 58, 59, 60, 61, 64, 65, 72, 74, 78, 105, 112, 119, 128, 131, 137, 142, 148, 151, 165, 169, 171, 175
reactive oxygen, 125, 136, 164
reactivity, 32
reason, 98, 125, 126, 134
receptor sites, 18, 180
receptors, 1, 4, 9, 10, 11, 12, 13, 14, 15, 16, 18, 19, 50, 51, 57, 63, 67, 78, 79, 83, 84, 88, 96, 113, 114, 116, 119, 120, 121, 122, 129, 133, 136, 142, 143, 145, 148, 149, 154, 157, 158, 159, 160, 163, 165, 166, 167, 169, 170, 171, 172, 174, 175, 176, 177, 179, 180
recognition, 70
recommendations, iv
recovery, 123
rectum, 68
regression, 36, 40, 89, 118, 164
regulation, 19, 24, 26, 27, 28, 29, 30, 31, 32, 38, 54, 55, 57, 61, 66, 69, 70, 78, 79, 81, 82, 83, 84, 86, 87, 91, 96, 99, 103, 115, 120, 121, 125, 128, 131, 133, 136, 138, 153, 161, 167, 168, 169
regulations, 83
relationship, 20, 32, 38, 39, 40, 41, 64, 75, 89, 98, 100, 103, 120
relaxation, 12, 126, 172
relevance, 2, 10, 20, 43, 66, 68, 88, 136

remission, 147, 150
renal medulla, 28
renin, 27, 28, 29, 30, 32, 34, 35, 37, 38, 40, 41, 77, 79, 81, 83, 87, 88, 157
reparation, 11, 160, 171
replacement, 151
resistance, 12, 23, 29, 35, 81, 115, 136, 159, 172
respiration, 132
respiratory, 54, 60, 66, 133, 134, 176
respiratory distress syndrome, 54, 66, 134
restenosis, 136
restriction fragment length polymorphis, 112
retention, 23, 81
reverse transcriptase, 144
rheumatic diseases, 51, 64, 71, 100, 136
rheumatoid arthritis, 1, 16, 17, 20, 42, 49, 51, 52, 53, 59, 60, 62, 64, 67, 69, 72, 98, 102, 105, 106, 131, 138, 149, 150, 151, 170, 171, 176
rheumatoid factor, 16
rhinitis, 19, 60, 71, 143, 150, 158, 169, 176
rhinovirus infection, 176
risk, 81, 115, 117, 161
RNA, 6, 17, 137, 139
rolling, 129

S

safety, 146, 161, 166
salicylates, 135
salivary glands, 4, 55, 155
salt, 26, 27, 28, 31, 35, 37, 41, 82, 116, 121, 166
scavengers, 135
schizophrenia, 157
search, 52, 106, 173
second generation, 114, 159
secretion, 2, 16, 26, 39, 40, 55, 70, 72, 91, 92, 95, 97, 98, 99, 101, 103, 133, 135, 144
selectivity, 113, 146
sensitivity, 6, 33, 41, 78, 116
sepsis, 51, 130, 133, 135
septic shock, 130, 158
serine, 4, 5, 19, 23, 26, 40, 54, 72, 94, 154
serotonin, 44, 47, 54, 70, 101
serum, 54, 68, 131, 136, 150
severity, 31, 117, 122, 145, 163
shock, 44, 74, 105, 108, 122, 130, 157, 158, 169, 174
side effects, 146, 148, 165
signal transduction, 15, 47, 117, 118, 179
signs, 43, 47, 71, 96, 175
skin, 11, 47, 49, 52, 54, 59, 62, 63, 65, 66, 67, 70, 71, 73, 74, 79, 106, 107, 108, 165, 169, 171, 177, 179
small intestine, 55, 92, 100

smooth muscle, 2, 6, 10, 11, 12, 15, 16, 19, 32, 53, 60, 78, 81, 87, 91, 95, 96, 113, 114, 118, 120, 128, 134, 143, 146, 153, 157, 158, 160, 167, 169, 171, 172, 177, 178, 179
smooth muscle cells, 10, 134, 143, 158, 171
sodium, 23, 29, 31, 34, 38, 41, 81, 85, 94, 101, 115, 118, 137, 148, 161, 166
species, 4, 6, 26, 54, 55, 98, 102, 105, 112, 125, 134, 136, 138, 158, 174
spectrum, 44, 49, 62, 95, 160
sphincter, 120, 179
spleen, 28, 36, 95, 99
sponge, 165
Spring, 70
stability, 135
stabilization, 131
stable asthma, 148
stem cells, 143
stenosis, 116, 136
stent, 136
steroids, 38, 41
stimulant, 2, 8, 15, 178
stomach, 92, 100, 139
strain, 58, 70, 105
strategies, 138, 145
strategy, 134
stress, 127, 132, 133, 134, 153, 162
stromal cells, 145
students, ix
subcutaneous injection, 58, 165
substitution, 10, 160, 171
substrates, 17, 18, 24, 37, 53, 57, 69, 70, 92
sugar, 94
sulfur, 132
supply, 91, 135, 162
suppression, 115, 134, 148, 161
surveillance, 133
survival, 117, 118, 122, 163
survival rate, 163
susceptibility, 24, 35, 37, 57, 92, 112
swelling, 43, 50, 52, 57, 58, 157, 165, 176
sympathetic nervous system, 26
symptom, 43, 177
symptoms, 2, 49, 116, 146, 148, 162, 176
syndrome, 28, 34, 37, 41, 57, 118
synovial fluid, 1, 2, 7, 8, 9, 10, 16, 17, 18, 20, 47, 49, 52, 58, 64, 67, 71, 72, 73, 74, 106, 131, 136, 150
synovial membrane, 50, 55, 57, 58, 70, 131
synovial tissue, 1, 2, 4, 7, 8, 9, 14, 16, 20, 26, 40, 51, 58, 59, 64, 71, 92, 102, 112, 121, 145, 149, 150, 151, 155
synovitis, 1, 8, 9, 10, 49, 106, 145

synthesis, 8, 10, 12, 13, 15, 28, 29, 31, 32, 36, 37, 41, 44, 51, 52, 58, 72, 73, 86, 92, 94, 95, 101, 107, 113, 114, 115, 118, 122, 126, 130, 134, 135, 136, 137, 141, 144, 145, 147, 151, 158, 160, 161, 166, 171, 172, 173, 179
systemic change, 31, 115, 161

T

T lymphocytes, 70, 144
targets, 97, 135, 141, 142, 145
terminals, 67, 158
testosterone, 101
therapeutic agents, ix, 84, 154, 158, 161, 166, 170, 176, 178
therapeutic approaches, 154
therapeutic benefits, 134
therapeutic goal, 13, 175
therapeutic targets, 141, 145
therapeutics, ix, 117
therapy, 28, 32, 42, 43, 58, 72, 98, 116, 118, 121, 131, 135, 147, 162, 169
threshold, 143, 164, 166
thrombin, 1, 37, 92, 112, 179
thrombosis, 52, 106, 136
thromboxanes, 49
tissue perfusion, 130
TNF, 1, 8, 11, 51, 171
toxic effect, 97
toxic substances, 135
trachea, 177, 179
transcription, 135, 143
transduction, 15, 47, 117, 118, 179
translation, 135
transmission, 101
transplantation, 39
transport, 78, 87, 94, 96, 99, 101, 133, 138
trauma, 1, 169, 178
trial, 87, 147, 148, 150, 151
triggers, 129
trypsin, 3, 70, 88, 101
tryptophan, 54
tumor, 8, 16, 18, 20, 43, 51, 64, 113, 122, 133, 160, 171, 176
tumor necrosis factor, 8, 16, 18, 20, 51, 64, 113, 122, 171, 176
tyrosine, 131, 139

U

UK, 149
ulcer, 103, 136
ulcerative colitis, 47, 64, 68, 94, 96, 99, 131, 132, 147, 150, 151

underlying mechanisms, 29, 165
United Kingdom, 72
United States, 146
upper respiratory tract, 60, 176
urea, 35, 66
urinary bladder, 28, 35
urine, 2, 4, 6, 15, 17, 23, 26, 28, 29, 35, 39, 40, 41, 55, 61, 72, 101, 112, 142, 155, 157, 161
uterus, 11, 12, 114, 121, 159, 160, 171, 172, 173

V

valuation, 40, 72, 146, 160
variations, 96
vas deferens, 18
vasculature, 50, 82
vasoactive intestinal peptide, 74
vasoconstriction, 23, 27, 81, 125, 128, 135, 136, 144
vasodilation, 7, 26, 35, 43, 47, 54, 55, 57, 60, 62, 66, 70, 78, 94, 96, 128, 133, 136, 157, 158, 160, 172
vasodilator, 27, 29, 50, 79, 81, 94, 116, 133, 163
vasomotor, 128

vasopressin, 28, 36, 38, 42
vasopressin level, 36
vasopressor, 32, 78
vasospasm, 136
vein, 11, 137, 159, 160, 171, 172, 174
velocity, 128
ventricular arrhythmias, 153
venules, 129, 132
vessels, 12, 29, 65, 120, 161, 172
viral infection, 134
vitamin B1, 94
vitamin B12, 94
vitamin E, 62, 96, 100

W

water permeability, 28
workers, 78, 92, 98, 118

Y

yeast, 53